# Genetic Engineering

## A Christian Response

# THE CHRISTIAN RESPONSE SERIES
Timothy J. Demy and Gary P. Stewart, editors

*Genetic Engineering: A Christian Response*
*Suicide: A Christian Response*

# Genetic Engineering

## A Christian Response

Crucial Considerations in Shaping Life

**Timothy J. Demy & Gary P. Stewart, editors**

Foreword by Hessel Bouma III

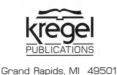

kregel
PUBLICATIONS

Grand Rapids, MI  49501

*Genetic Engineering: A Christian Response*

Copyright © 1999 by Timothy J. Demy and Gary P. Stewart

Published by Kregel Publications, a division of Kregel, Inc., P.O. Box 2607, Grand Rapids, MI 49501. Kregel Publications provides trusted, biblical publications for Christian growth and service. Your comments and suggestions are valued.

Scripture quotations marked NASB are from the *New American Standard Bible.* Copyright © the Lockman Foundation 1960, 1962, 1963, 1968, 1971, 1972, 1973, 1975, 1977.

Scripture quotations marked NIV are from the *Holy Bible, New Internatinoal Version®.* Copyright © 1973, 1978, 1984 by International Bible Society. Used by permission of Zondervan Publishing House. All rights reserved.

Scripture quotations marked NKJV are from *The New King James Version.* Copyright © 1979, 1980, 1982, Thomas Nelson, Inc., Publishers.

Scripture quotations marked RSV are from the *Revised Standard Version.* Copyright © 1946, 1952, 1971, 1973 by the Division of Christian Education of the National Council of the Churches of Christ in the United States of America.

Scripture quotations marked TEV are from *Today's English Version, Good News Bible*—New Testament. Copyright © American Bible Society 1966, 1971, 1976.

For more information about Kregel Publications, visit our web page at http://www.kregel.com.

Cover and book design: Nicholas G. Richardson

All views expressed in this work are solely those of the authors and do not represent or reflect the position or endorsement of any governmental agency or department, military or otherwise.

**Library of Congress Cataloging-in-Publication Data**
Demy, Timothy J.
    Genetic engineering: a Christian response: crucial considerations in shaping life / by Timothy J. Demy and Gary P. Stewart.
        p.    cm.
    Includes bibliographical references and index.
    1. Medical genetics—Religious aspects—Christianity. 2. Medical genetics—Moral and ethical aspects. 3. Genetic engineering—Religious aspects—Christianity. 4. Genetic engineering—Moral and ethical aspects. I. Stewart, Gary (Gary P.) II. Title.
RB155.D425        1998        241'.64957—dc21        98-45988
                                                                         CIP

ISBN 0-8254-2357-0

Printed in the United States of America

1  2  3  /  05  04  03  02  01  00  99

To Christians in
medicine, nursing, health care, and science
who daily wrestle with the issues of life and death
on a very personal level—we express to you
our highest esteem.

Also, to the memory of
Thomas E. Elkins, M.D.

# CONTENTS

## Part 3: Genetic Engineering and the Individual

# CONTRIBUTORS

J. Kerby Anderson, M.S., M.A., is President of Probe Ministries and the author of several books, including *Genetic Engineering, Origin Science*, and *Signs of Warning—Signs of Hope*.

Raymond G. Bohlin, Ph.D., is Director of Communications and Research, Probe Ministries and the coauthor of *The Natural Limits of Biological Change* as well as numerous journal articles.

Douglas Brown, Ph.D., is an assistant professor at the University of Tennessee School of Medicine, Knoxville, Tennessee.

Byron C. Calhoun, M.D., is Assistant Chief, Obstetrical Service, Madigan Army Medical Center, Tacoma, Washington.

J. Daryl Charles, Ph.D., is Affiliate Fellow of the Center for the Study of American Religion, Princeton University, Princeton, New Jersey; and Assistant Professor of Religion and Philosophy, Taylor University, Upland, Indiana.

Francis S. Collins, M.D., Ph.D., is Director, The Human Genome Project.

Melissa Cox is former editor of *Physician* magazine and is now associated with the Medical Institute for Sexual Health in Austin, Texas.

William Cutrer, M.D., M.A., is a board-certified obstetrician-gynecologist and Regional Representative, Christian Medical and Dental Society. He is the coauthor of several books on issues of medicine and the family.

Brock L. Eide, M.D., is Fellow of the MacLean Center for Clinical Medical Ethics, University of Chicago, and a Ph.D. candidate at the Committee on Social Thought, University of Chicago.

Thomas E. Elkins, M.D., F.A.C.O.G., was Professor and Chair of Gynecology, and Director of Pelvic Reconstructive Surgery and Urogynecology at Johns Hopkins Hospital, Baltimore, Maryland.

Sandra Glahn is completing theological studies at Dallas Theological Seminary and is a former board member of RESOLVE, a national organization for couples facing infertility and the professionals who treat them. She is the coauthor of several books and articles dealing with family and infertility issues.

Nathan J. Hoeldtke, M.D., is Chief, Antepartum Diagnostic Center, Tripler Regional Medical Center, Honolulu, Hawaii.

Dennis P. Hollinger, Ph.D., is Dean of College Ministries and Professor of Christian Ethics at Messiah College, Grantham, Pennsylvania.

Edward J. Larson, J.D., Ph.D., is Professor of History and Law at the University of Georgia and the author of the 1998 Pulitzer Prize-winning volume *Summer of the Gods*. He is also the author of several other volumes, including *Sex, Race, and Science: Eugenics in the Deep South*.

Jim Leffel, Ph.D., is Lecturer in Philosophy at Ohio Dominican College, Columbus, Ohio.

Michael McKenzie, Ph.D., is Associate Professor of Philosophy and Theology at Liberty University, Lynchburg, Virginia.

Eugene H. Merrill, Ph.D., is Professor of Old Testament Studies at Dallas Theological Seminary. He is the author of numerous books and articles, including *Kingdom of Priests* and *Deuteronomy* (New American Commentary), and a contributing editor of the multivolume *New International Dictionary of Old Testament Theology and Exegesis*.

Sonya Merrill, Ph.D., received her doctorate in moral philosophy with an emphasis in medical ethics from the University of London. She has taught medical ethics courses at Beeson Divinity School and Harvard Divinity School and is currently completing her medical training at Harvard Medical School.

C. Ben Mitchell, Ph.D., is Visiting Professor of Christian Ethics at Southern Baptist Theological Seminary, Louisville, Kentucky; editor of the journal *Ethics and Medicine;* and consultant on biomedical and life issues for the Christian Life Commission of the Southern Baptist Convention.

Dónal P. O'Mathúna, Ph.D., is Associate Professor of Medical Ethics and Chemistry at Mount Carmel College of Nursing, Columbus, Ohio.

Rebecca D. Pentz, Ph.D., is Clinical Ethicist and Associate Professor of Clinical Ethics, University of Texas at M. D. Anderson Cancer Center, Houston, Texas. She is also a board member of the American Society for Bioethics and Humanity.

Scott B. Rae, Ph.D., is Associate Professor of Biblical Studies and Christian Ethics at Talbot School of Theology, La Mirada, California. He is the author of *An Introduction to Ethics* and *Brave New Families: Biblical Ethics and Reproductive Technologies*.

James S. Reitman, M.D., M.A., is Chief, Internal Medicine Service, 52d Medical Group, USAF Hospital, Bitburg, Germany; and Medical Consultant for Medical Ethics to the USAF Surgeon General.

Frank E. Young, M.D., Ph.D., is former Commissioner, U.S. Food and Drug Administration, and served also as Deputy Assistant Secretary for Health. He currently serves as Executive Director of Reformed Theological Seminary in Washington, D.C., and Director of Adult Education and Ministries at Fourth Presbyterian Church in Bethesda, Maryland.

# FOREWORD

GENETIC ENGINEERING IS PART OF an imposing revolution in our society. It has the potential to affect virtually every aspect of our lives. Through genetic engineering, bacteria now produce human hormones. Several plant varieties bear a bacterial insecticide. Human-mouse hybrid cells make monoclonal antibodies for diagnostic tests and new therapies. Strains of mice express human genetic diseases for research. Viruses transfect bone marrow stem cells for human gene therapy. In the near future, we anticipate reengineering organs from pigs for human transplantation.

Add to this revolution new assisted reproductive technologies that have humans reproducing in heretofore unimaginable ways. We now can asexually reproduce not only embryonic mammals but also adult mammals; the cloning of humans is a distinct possibility. Concurrently, the Human Genome Project has passed the halfway point toward mapping and sequencing the sixty to eighty thousand genes in the human genome. We are about to learn the molecular basis for more than four thousand human genetic conditions. Ready or not, we have the scientific and technical ability to reengineer ourselves and future generations.

Like impatient pioneers, scientists blaze a path with genetic engineering on a frenzied race toward a better medicine, often with scant time used to consult a moral compass. The potential rewards are great. So are the potential harms. Our morality, ethics, and public policies struggle to keep up. To envision what we can do in the future is mind-boggling; to contemplate what we should do (and should not do) is sobering. And for a pluralist society where autonomy and utility are trump, the technological imperative—We can, we should!—has an alluring magnetism that threatens to draw us off course.

Religious traditions in general, and the Christian tradition in particular, have much to contribute toward exploring the future directions of genetic engineering. These traditions ask, Who are we? Why and how do we value ourselves and others? What are the moral boundaries we may not cross? Why?

This revolution presents several challenges and opportunities for the Christian community and society. First, to truly engage the issues, we need to be knowledgeable. To be informed about genetics, theology, and ethics is no small task. It requires every participant to be conversant outside specialty areas, to learn about science, philosophy, ethics, religion, and the making of public policy.

Second, we need to evaluate our moral positions very carefully and thoroughly, in open dialogue within our religious communities and with society. In our pluralist society, we have largely come to accept public policies based on a minimal morality founded on a freedom of scientific inquiry and the autonomy of parental reproductive decisions. But best-case scenarios involving a useful application of genetic engineering ought not to be sufficient moral justification to make the technology available without regulations for any and all uses. Similarly, however, worst-case scenarios, slippery-slope arguments, or admonitions to avoid "playing God" are insufficient moral justifications to prohibit these technologies unless firmly based on deontological principles commonly shared in society. Can we craft regulations on genetic engineering that preserve common deontological principles while maximizing the good and minimizing the harm? When we apply these technologies to children-to-be, should we not insist on asking, "Is this in the best interests of the child-to-be?"

Third, we need to remember and to care about the present and the past, even as we look to the future. Many of the anticipated applications of genetic engineering may benefit—or harm—the young and future generations. Those benefits should not come at the expense of caring for persons with genetic conditions for whom the applications of genetic engineering come too late. History reminds us how we have devalued persons who were not considered "normal." The Christian tradition—in faith, hope, and love—has much to offer society in its rich history of Christlike caring for persons who are incurable and for those perceived to be "the least of these." Christians count them among the first. In situations where we would limit genetic engineering, it is incumbent upon us to develop and to support caring alternatives for those who bear the consequences of such restrictions. In so doing, we will "let justice roll down like waters and righteousness like an ever-flowing stream" (Amos 5:24 NASB); we will be honoring God's command "to do justice, to love kindness, and to walk humbly with your God" (Micah 6:8b NASB).

Fourth, we need to wrestle with how to translate our faith values into public policy in a pluralist democracy. The doctrine of separation of church and state does not preclude the state from regulating religion. Nor should it be sufficient reason for faith values not to be incorporated into public policy regulations. But when and how? The National Bioethics Advisory Committee Report titled "Cloning Human Beings" includes a chapter on religious perspectives, drawn from a report written by Dr. Courtney Campbell. In the final recommendations to the president and Congress, the importance of religious perspectives was largely ignored. Dr. Campbell later mused, "the contributions of religious perspectives were deemed politically important [but] ethically insignificant."[1]

---

1. Courtney S. Campbell, "Prophecy and Policy," Hastings Center Report 27.5 (September–October 1997): 17.

In the aftermath of the Civil War, Americans encountered two revolutions. One involved recognizing the equality of humans regardless of race. The second was an industrial revolution fostered by the rapid development of railroads. American politician William Seward noted, "I know, and all the world knows, that revolutions never go backward." As we face this new and now inevitable revolution in genetic engineering, we do so with the mantle of responsibility to be caretakers and stewards of God's creation. We do so too with confidence knowing that God—Creator, Provider, Sustainer—is in control. The essays in this book are a welcome step toward assuming these responsibilities and opportunities in light of the Christian faith.

Hessel Bouma III, Ph.D.
Professor of Biology, Calvin College
Grand Rapids, Michigan

# ACKNOWLEDGMENTS

THE EDITORS ARE GRATEFUL TO Kregel Publications for the opportunity to present this timely material for dissemination and thought. Publisher Dennis Hillman shared our concern for the topic and enthusiasm for the work. It was a pleasure to work with the staff at Kregel. We are especially grateful to Rachel Warren, Nick Richardson, Steve Barclift, Mike Leming, and Wendy Leep for their efforts behind the scenes. Without them there would be no book. Jan Ortiz has also been an integral part in accurately communicating the message of this volume. We are especially thankful to Virginia A. Coburn, whose daily prayers move mountains unseen by us in the fog of life. As always, Lyn Demy and Kathie Stewart have patiently sacrificed family time for one more project to reach completion. Several chapters were reprinted or expanded from previous journals. We are grateful for permission to use them. Specifically:

Chapter 1: "Joy in the Journey: A Physician Talks About the Importance of Genetic Research," *Physician* (November–December 1996), Copyright 1996, Focus on the Family. All rights reserved. International copyright secured. Used by permission.

Chapter 3: "Genetics and Christianity: An Uneasy but Necessary Partnership," *Christian Research Journal* (fall 1995): 11–17, 41.

Chapter 8: "Engineering Life: Human Rights in a Postmodern Age," *Christian Research Journal* (Sept.–Oct. 1997): 39–44.

Chapter 11: "'The Least That a Parent Can Do': Prenatal Genetic Testing and the Welcome of Our Children," *Ethics & Medicine* 13 (1997): 59–66.

Chapter 13: "Perinatal Hospice: A Response to Early Termination for Severe Congenital Anomalies," *Issues in Law & Medicine* 13, no. 3 (fall 1997): 125–44.

Chapter 14: "The Cost of Choice: A Price Too High in the Triple Screen for Down's Syndrome," *Clinical Obstetrics and Gynecology* 36, no. 3 (September 1993): 532–40.

# INTRODUCTION

FROM A PURELY PHYSICAL PERSPECTIVE, disease can arguably be considered the greatest threat to human survival. Every generation since the fall of humanity (at the time of Adam's and Eve's rebellion) has struggled with the problem of humanity's susceptibility to disease. It is interesting that in the definition of disease, we find the concept of *disorder*—disease is abnormal; it is an intruder, a corrupter of what is good or healthy, something that is not a part of the original design of the Creator. Disorder in the human body can occur because of nutritional deficiency, environmental factors, toxicity, infection, and from developmental or genetic errors.

Disease is a more than able adversary. It is one that will not be thoroughly defeated until after the second coming of Christ when the creation of a new heaven and earth will exist without it (1 Cor. 15:51–58; Rev. 21:4–5; 22:1–5). Until that time, it is an enemy with which we must and should contend. The suffering that accompanies disease is a human experience that provokes compassion in the heart of each of us. The heart of God is also grieved by the suffering of humanity. Jesus regularly played the role of a physician by reaching out to those who suffered from disease, many of whom had genetic abnormalities. His love and mercy for the ill compels us to pursue means that would enable us to free as many people as we can from the debilitating effects of disease. For this reason, Christians should applaud the efforts of the United States government for funding a program to identify the blueprint from which each human being develops.

The Human Genome Project (HGP) has already identified many genetic abnormalities and will no doubt identify many more. New treatments, and better and safer treatments, are likely to follow as a result. For this reason, we believe that the HGP is the single most important scientific project of this century and, probably, the most important of all time. Although it is based on the findings of many researchers over many years, the efforts of the HGP have the potential for creating more good for humanity than any single scientific venture in world history and is, therefore, worthy of our prayers and support.

This compilation of essays is not designed to cast any shadow on the project or on technology itself. Both of the editors and many of our readers are alive today because of medical and scientific research. Because this volume cannot possibly identify or cover every application of genetic engineering or identify all the ethical issues, our desire is to provide Christians (and hopefully others who will consider or are sympathetic with our concerns) with an ethical guide for the use of genetic technology. For every good that a technology can bring to society, there is also a potential for abuse. Ethical guidelines are essential to the success of the HGP. It is such a worthy enterprise that potential misuses must be identified in advance and averted—the enormous good that can come from a greater understanding of the uniqueness of God's handiwork in designing human life cannot be underestimated; therefore, the research of the human genome must never be overshadowed or lost because of the possibility of abuse.

In the pages that follow, contributors write of both the benefits and dangers inherent to understanding the intricate workings of the human body. They extol its benefits for alleviating human misery and critically evaluate its past, present, and potential misuses. The research that is produced by the Human Genome Project should never be used to *improve* what is genetically normal but, rather, to correct what is genetically abnormal. The application of genetic technology should focus on disease management and alleviation, for it is the disease that is the disorder and is the enemy of humanity, not the person who carries the disease.

---

# PART 1

---

# GENETIC ENGINEERING
# AND SOCIETY

*An Overview*

The Human Genome Project is one of the most extensive endeavors in the history of science. The mapping and sequencing of the human genome will provide scientists and physicians with significant information to assist in fighting genetic diseases and disorders as well as information that enhances gene therapy and furthers medical research. In this interview with Dr. Francis S. Collins, director of the Human Genome Project, we are given insight into the scope and purpose of the project as well as glimpses into his personal faith—his religious beliefs have a direct influence on his professional life. In these pages, Dr. Collins provides a balanced perspective on the challenges and the necessary safeguards that accompany the future of genetic research.

Chapter One

# JOY IN THE JOURNEY
## *A Physician Talks About the Importance of Genetic Research*

### Francis S. Collins, M.D. and Melissa Cox

When man becomes capable of instructing his own cells, he must refrain from doing so until he has sufficient wisdom to use the knowledge for the benefit of mankind.

—Marshall W. Nirenberg
Nobel Prize for Medicine, 1968

*PHYSICIAN* RECENTLY SPENT A FEW HOURS interviewing Francis S. Collins, M.D., Ph.D., the director of the Human Genome Project based at the National Institutes of Health in Bethesda, Maryland. Dr. Collins showed great passion for his project—the mapping and sequencing of the human genome. As an enthusiastic Christian, Collins is concerned about how the public, especially physicians, view genetic research. He strongly believes that genetic research can provide seeds of hope for healing and alleviating human suffering. The Human Genome Project is a bold effort to decode the 3 billion base pairs of the human DNA molecule. The project began in 1989, and its goal is to have a completed human sequence by 2005.

Our conversation focused on his involvement in the field of medical genetics, how physicians can understand genetics apart from the media's sensationalized reports, and how we as Christians can possibly affect the future of genetics. When we asked Dr. Collins why he chose medical genetics as a specialty, his answer was simple: "The simplicity and elegance of the DNA molecule immediately appealed to me."

***Why are people so worried about the outcomes of genetic research?***
Genetics has been a natural extension of the medical research agenda for the last several decades. It happens to be a particularly powerful approach because it operates at such a fundamental level. Because it allows you to look at the instruction book rather than looking at outcomes and consequences, it is enormously appealing to scientists.

But in a public forum, I think the perception of the progress of genetics is often distorted. On the one hand, we have the discovery of a specific gene—

a complicated process in itself—being reported, by excited scientists who have been working on it for years, to reporters who aren't particularly knowledgeable about genetic research. Then the media often communicate the message inaccurately because of their lack of understanding. So, instead of reporting that a gene thought to be linked to breast cancer has been found, it's reported that *the* breast cancer gene has been found, and you should be tested for it today.

On the other hand, the public reads, sees, and hears about totally unrealistic scenarios of genetics gone wild. *Jurassic Park* and *The Island of Dr. Moreau* are dramatic examples, and so is Sigmund Brouwer's *Double Helix*. In these examples, people see scientists manipulating embryos to create a superior race, mixing human and animal genes, or recreating something from the past. The problem with these scenarios is they have the ability to make people believe that researchers are doing those kinds of experiments today. The truth is that we are light years away from those sorts of applications.

***But everyone knows fiction is just for fun.*** Yes, but some of the sci-fi scenarios are the ones that people are using to try to convince people that we shouldn't proceed with genetic research.

I'm deeply concerned that we are wasting too much energy wrestling with these science-fiction scenarios when we ought to be spending our energy dealing with the very real dilemmas that are here right now—the ones that are going to affect patients who are going to be walking into physician's offices seeking guidance on specific concerns.

***What sort of concerns will the clinical physician be addressing in the next few months or years?*** I already suspect that many a physician has had somebody walk into the office, waving a recent copy of *Time* or *Newsweek*, wanting to know whether she should be tested for breast cancer susceptibility or whether her child is at risk for having some sort of genetic anomaly.

Because genetics has developed so rapidly, and mostly in research labs, many physicians aren't up on the ethical and social implications of specific tests and may not be prepared to answer their patients' questions.

***How can physicians prepare themselves for these kinds of questions?*** Continuing medical education is the key. Only half of the medical schools in the United States offer any training in genetics. Because of this, we don't have a well-prepared professional group to deal with these issues.

It's fortunate that genetic principles are rather straightforward. This isn't rocket science. Physicians and nurses do, however, need to learn a set of basic principles and gain experience applying them in clinical settings. For starters, we need a crash program to get educational materials into the hands of physicians and nurses. Currently, the Genome Project is working with the American Medical Association and the American Nursing Association to develop such a program.

*Until the material reaches the hands of a physician in Smalltown, USA, what are some basic guidelines physicians can use?* The bottom line of whether a patient should proceed with genetic testing comes down to benefits and risks. It's imperative for patients to know this information before they proceed with the testing. This kind of information must be presented in a nondirective fashion. Physicians unfamiliar or uncomfortable with these issues should identify their closest source of genetic expertise (most major medical centers will have a genetics clinic) and make appropriate referrals.

There are potentially some very significant reasons for someone to be tested for breast or colon cancer. A person at risk may be able to take some preventive steps in delaying the onset of the disease or eliminating the risks altogether. Albeit, if a person is found to have the likelihood of developing a disease (such as Alzheimer's) where nothing can be done, most patient's will decide they'd rather not know.

There are also significant risks to receiving this sort of information. The results may not only have lasting medical ramifications but psychological and economic ones as well. A particularly troubling issue is that under our current health-care system, if an individual is found to be at risk for future illness on the basis of genetic test results, he may be charged outrageous premiums for his health insurance, making it impossible for him to take advantage of preventive measures just when they would have the greatest benefit.

*What is a realistic example of how a patient might benefit from the research that is happening today?* When many people think about applications of genetic research, there is a tendency to assume that this means prenatal diagnosis. This is an arena with which I think most Christian physicians are uncomfortable, and I share those feelings. But the major growth area of genetics in clinical medicine in the near future will be in the area of presymptomatic identification of future risks for illness. This means that the person whose health is being predicted is already an adult and is receiving information—while she is still healthy—about her risk of developing a specific disease.

The concept is rather new. We have had in the past some imperfect abilities to do this kind of prediction based on family history. But the notion that you can test for specific genes offers a more precise set of predictable factors. This doesn't mean that the tests will tell you that you'll definitely get colon cancer, but the information will help generate a statistical analysis of your risks. And we are all at risk for something—there are no perfect specimens at the DNA level.

*How will this information be applied?* It will be applied through individualized preventive medicine. Instead of telling the entire population to undergo colonoscopic screening to avoid colon cancer and have them largely ignore the advice, we can individualize treatment programs so they are focused on those who most need the screening.

This is definitely an intermediate technology, however. Genetics will not truly deliver its full promise until we get beyond the diagnostic era into the therapeutic era. At that point, the physician cannot only make a prediction about risk but offer an effective treatment or even a cure before the illness ever strikes.

***What will the therapeutic stage look like?*** In some instances the solution will be to replace the abnormal genes by using gene therapy. But for many diseases, the notion that you can go in and precisely fix the genetic defect is naïve. For instance, in a disease like Alzheimer's, it's daunting to imagine trying to go into the brain to repair the responsible genes within a trillion cells that can't even divide. Even the most optimistic person would think that's unlikely.

Albeit, if we could use the information about the genes involved in Alzheimer's disease—four are known already—to learn what is wrong at the most basic molecular level, there would be good reason to believe the research would lead to a designer drug that could arrest or even prevent the process altogether.

Ironically, I believe that for the next couple of decades many of the therapeutic advances that will come out of gene discovery are likely to be drugs and not gene therapy.

***It seems as though God has placed you in your position as director of the Human Genome Project for a specific reason. If genetics is so wrong, as some claim, why did God put a committed Christian at the helm?*** I've been trying to figure that out too! In many ways I feel that this is a calling. Looking back, it seems to me that God prepared me for this role in ways I wasn't aware of through other experiences I've had in research and in clinical medicine.

I was actually quite reluctant to take this on. I basically turned the job down the first time it was offered. After several months of struggling with the decision and spending time on my knees, I came to the realization that this was something I was called to do at this stage in my life.

***What is it like to be involved in a project of this magnitude?*** It's enormously exciting and energizing to see the Human Genome Project take shape. Progress often happens in small increments but they add up to big things. Currently we're running one to two years ahead of schedule, and the budget is substantially less than predicted—quite a surprise for a federally funded project.

The Human Genome Project ranks right up there at the top of the scale of scientific advances. The opportunity to read our own instruction manual is historic and astounding. What else in science could compete with that? I could be accused of overstating it, but in my view, this is the most important organized scientific endeavor that humankind has ever mounted. This dwarfs going to the moon or splitting the atom.

***Why are you so committed to the work of the Human Genome Project?*** I strongly believe in the message of Matthew 9:35: "Jesus went through all the towns and villages, teaching in their synagogues, preaching the good news of the kingdom and healing every disease and sickness."

If Jesus spent so much of his brief time with us healing the sick, it was something we were meant to notice. The research being conducted through the Human Genome Project is a natural extension of the Christian mandate to heal the sick. To say that genetic research should be stopped because it might be misused is to deny that mandate.

*Some people feel that through genetics we're manipulating God. Is our role as humans to be caretakers of his creation, or do we perhaps exist as cocreators with God?* God gave us intelligence and expects us to use it so we can understand and appreciate the intricacies of his creation. As a scientist, on rare occasions, I have had the opportunity to grasp something that no human being has ever understood. This is an incredible experience.

In fact, this is a form of worship for the Christian in scientific research because he is seeing God's work firsthand. I agree with Copernicus when he said he didn't agree that ignorance was more devout than knowledge. I don't understand how scientists who are not of the faith avoid seeing God's beauty in their work. The experience can't be matched. The joy of discovery mixed with the joy of worship makes for a truly powerful moment.

I don't, however, think of myself as a cocreator. In fact, that term really bothers me. God is God. We are not God. The pursuit of knowledge is a way of recognizing a reverence for God and an appreciation for his creation.

*What should the Christian response to genetics be?* There's no point in throwing our hands up and saying, "This stuff is dangerous and we don't want anything to do with it." That would be the worst response the Christian community could have. Rather, it would be best to learn the facts and then begin to participate in a meaningful way in the many coming debates about the uses and misuses.

*What are some final thoughts you'd like to share about genetics?* It's becoming the central science of medicine. I think many are realizing the potential it has. And yet, to the clinician, genetics has barely become a significant part of his practice at all. So where is the disconnect? Up until now, genetics has been a research activity, but that's about to change.

The Christian physician should take advantage of this brief window of opportunity to seek out information on this topic from whatever sources are available. A good start would be the book, *Understanding Gene Testing*, published by the National Cancer Institute and the National Center for Human Genome Research. It can be obtained by calling 1-800-CANCER.

Also, Christian physicians can be salt and light in this arena. There are many wild and sensational ideas floating around about the dangers of genetics. The worst thing Christian physicians can do is play into those sensationalized concerns rather than seek out the truth of what's possible and what isn't.

As physicians, we need to remember our role as healers and keep in mind that the outcomes of genetic research are an extension of that tradition. We shouldn't be frightened of these advances.

*An Overview*

God has permitted science to uncover many of the mysteries that detail the delicate way in which the human body functions. These discoveries have helped to relieve much of the suffering that human fallenness or depravity has brought to bear on the human race. Further scientific and medical breakthroughs will inevitably result from the research of scientists who have been assigned to trace or identify the complete human genetic blueprint, i.e., the human genome. To avoid misuses of the valuable technology gained from the ongoing Human Genome Project, C. Ben Mitchell delineates six theological principles through which genetic research must be processed. He then identifies three current ethical issues that demand our immediate attention: prenatal screening and abortion, confidentiality, and discrimination. Without a theological framework, genetic technology would eventually and unfortunately be perceived as the catalyst for a humanly orchestrated paradise. If society chooses to pursue genetic research and technology without considering God's role in creation and society or the role that our sinful nature plays in human disease, it could fall victim to the potential abuses of such technological advancement and would most certainly embellish human arrogance—the result being that many more would be without God in eternity. The mysteries unveiled through the research conducted by the Human Genome Project should cause each of us to stand still and reflect on the incomprehensible greatness of God by whose hand we have been wonderfully made.

Chapter Two

# GENETIC ENGINEERING
*Bane or Blessing?*

## C. Ben Mitchell

WE ARE IN THE MIDST OF AN amazing biotechnological revolution. Technologies once thought only to be science fiction have become science fact. In the past, genetic manipulation was only possible through careful processes of breeding and crossbreeding plants and animals. Today the manipulation of genes or genetic engineering is not only possible for plants and animals but for humans as well.

Just because we *can* engineer humans, however, does not mean we *should* do so. While questions about what we can do scientifically must be answered by those who are actively engaged in scientific research, questions about what we should or should not do ethically must be answered by each of us. The ethics of genetic engineering is, in many ways, far more critical and demanding than the science of genetics. As evangelical Christians, we must bring all the tools at our disposal—science, biblical studies, hermeneutics, systematic theology, and so forth—to the task of grappling with the ethical issues that arise from the new genetics.

The expansion of scientific information and the multitude of treatment modalities presently available demand our utmost concern. The potential benefits of genetic therapies are exciting and enormous. The potential for evil uses of genetic technology is equally mind-boggling.

### THE BIG SCIENCE PROJECT

We are all aware of the power of our inherited genes. Eye color, hair color, and other physical characteristics are linked to our genes. Genetic factors also have been linked to a host of major health problems and birth defects. Conditions such as cystic fibrosis, Duchenne's muscular dystrophy, Down's syndrome, Huntington's chorea, Alzheimer's disease, diabetes, breast cancer, and perhaps some forms of mental illness, may each be traced genetically. To date, little or nothing can be done to treat, let alone cure, these diseases. But through a major science project, funded by U.S. taxpayer dollars, we may someday be able to offer treatments to help thousands of persons who suffer from these illnesses.

In 1990, the National Institutes of Health (NIH) and the Department of

Energy (DOE) officially began a jointly sponsored initiative known as the Human Genome Project (HGP). The HGP is a massive, fifteen-year project that has as one of its goals to identify the sequence of the three billion base pairs of DNA that together carry the complete human genetic blueprint. This genetic blueprint is known as a genome. "The information generated by the Human Genome Project is expected to be the source book for biomedical science in the twenty-first century and will be of immense benefit to the field of medicine. It will help us understand and eventually treat many of the more than 4,000 genetic diseases that afflict humankind, as well as the many multifactorial diseases in which genetic disposition plays an important role."[1]

The HGP, authorized by Congress in 1989, is divided into three five-year segments. The first third of the project seeks to: (1) map and sequence the human genome, (2) map and sequence the DNA of model organisms such as the fruit fly, (3) collect and distribute available data, (4) examine the ethical, legal, and social issues of the project, (5) train researchers, and (6) develop and transfer genetic technologies for the worldwide effort.[2] The budget for the HGP is more than $250 million per year, adjusted annually for inflation, or over $3 billion total. This is big science!

For the first time in a major government-funded science project, 3 percent of the first five years' budget was set aside to study the ethical, legal, and social implications (ELSI) of the technology. The ELSI component of the project is thought to be critical because of the tremendous social and ethical implications of studying and manipulating human genetic material. The ELSI working group—a committee of scientists, ethicists, insurance professionals, and others—has said:

> Any scientific endeavor of this magnitude must be developed in concert with a plan to ensure that the public has access to the benefits in improved health care, which should be the result of the research. It is also imperative to protect individuals and society from possible hazards which may be a consequence of our improved ability to detect and predict hereditary illness. The use of genetic information, for good or ill, has long been an issue in our society. But the quantity and complexity of genetic information that should become available requires that special precautions be taken.[3]

The committee on the ethical, legal, and social implications of the project has correctly identified the fact that the immensity of this initiative carries with it responsibilities of gargantuan proportions. It is imperative that each of us understands as much as possible about the implications of the HGP and seriously reflects on what the Bible informs us about the ethics of such an undertaking.

The HGP's accomplishments are already very promising. The genes have already been isolated for a number of devastating illnesses, including, amyotrophic lateral sclerosis (Lou Gehrig's disease), cystic fibrosis, Duchenne's muscular dystrophy, Fragile X syndrome, Huntington's disease, neurofibromatosis, retinoblastoma, retinitis pigmentosa, and Wilm's tumor.[4]

Announcements of the discovery of genes for other diseases are being made almost daily. Once the disease genes are identified, efforts can be made to find treatments or even cures for these diseases. Several genetic illnesses are already treatable through gene therapy.

The hope of being able to offer treatments and cures for more than four thousand genetically linked illnesses is absolutely wonderful. The relief of human suffering and the prospect of restoring health to those persons who are debilitated and who die from these diseases is sufficient to endorse the project. Indeed, we should applaud, encourage, and join scientists in their war against genetic illnesses.

## PROCEED WITH CAUTION

Is there a down side to the HGP? Are there precautions that should be taken? Should we scrutinize the technology or let it proceed unexamined? As with every technology, there are benefits and burdens, goods and evils. Sadly, the history of genetic experimentation and the use of genetic information is strewn with the wreckage of abuse. At the turn of the twentieth century in America, social reformers called eugenicists began a program to rid our nation of so-called genetic defectives.

*Eugenics* is a term "coined in 1883 by the English scientist Francis Galton, a cousin of Charles Darwin."[5] Galton saw eugenics as "the 'science' of improving human stock by giving 'the more suitable races or strains of blood a better chance of prevailing speedily over the less suitable.'"[6]

The American eugenicists, borrowing from Galton, pushed a social movement they hoped would rid the world of "heredity defectives" such as the feebleminded and criminal. At the Kansas Free Fair in 1929, an exhibit placard asked: "How long are we Americans to be so careful for the pedigree of our pigs and chickens and cattle—and then leave the ancestry of our children to chance or to 'blind' sentiment."[7] The impact of the eugenics movement led to a number of horrific efforts in social hygiene.

Charles Davenport, one of the founders of the American eugenics movement, defined eugenics as "the science of the improvement of the human race by better breeding." "Heredity," said Davenport, "stands as the one great hope of the human race, its savior from imbecility, poverty, disease, immorality."[8] Davenport pushed for so-called racial hygiene and worked to halt sexual reproduction between Americans and European, African, and Jewish immigrants. In an effort to prevent American genetic stock from "deteriorating," Davenport and other eugenicists supported statutes restricting immigration.

Sterilization was another method of "protecting" Americans from deleterious genes. By 1917, at least seventeen states had passed laws that made possible the mandatory sterilization of prison inmates who had been sentenced for crimes such as drug addiction, sexual offenses, and epilepsy. Included in most legislation were statutes permitting the sterilization and castration of the insane, deviant, and "idiots in state institutions."[9] It had been determined that the best means of preventing further corruption of the gene pool was to prevent those thought to be suffering from "bad genes" from reproducing. Justice Oliver Wendell Holmes Jr., put it most illuminatingly in the infamous Court case *Buck v. Bell* when he said: "Three generations of imbeciles is enough."[10] The decision of the Court was that the sterilization of a "mental defective" was within the police power of the state and did not constitute cruel or unusual punishment. (See Edward J. Larson, "Confronting Scientific Authority with Religious Values: Eugenics in American History" in this volume for a more detailed analysis of the early eugenics program in the United States.)

Eugenics lost popularity in the United States when it became apparent that human rights were being violated and human dignity assaulted through this kind of genetic engineering. Across the Atlantic, however, under national socialism in Hitler's Germany, the American experiment was taken ten steps further and became even more grotesque. "German racial hygienists throughout the Weimar period expressed their envy of American achievements in this area, warning that unless the Germans made progress in this field, America would become the world's racial leader."[11]

In 1923, Fritz Lenz, a German physician and advocate of sterilization, severely criticized his own countrymen for their hesitancy to adopt mandatory sterilization laws like those in the United States. He held up the American eugenics movement as a model for what ought to be done in Germany.[12] Thus was born one of the most notorious human tragedies of the century. An estimated four hundred thousand people were sterilized in Germany under the Law for the Prevention of Genetically Diseased Offspring, which was passed in 1934.[13] According to Robert Jay Lifton: "Only in Germany was sterilization a forerunner of mass murder."[14] That is, the sterilization program gave credence to the notion that justified the massive euthanasia program to follow; namely, that the "hereditarily sick" were living a "life unworthy of life" *(lebesunwertes Leben)*.

While no one is arguing that the Human Genome Project is anything remotely close to an extension of the Nazi atrocity or of the American eugenics movement for that matter, unless the lessons of the past are heeded, we may indeed repeat them. Human nature certainly has not changed since the turn of the century. The history of the abuse of genetic information and technology must not be permitted to devolve into a future of similar abuse.

Because we have a well-documented history and because the HGP is a big-science project involving many thousands of researchers around the globe, we can approach the project with cautious optimism. We, therefore, may be hopeful that the new genetics will result in the cure of thousands of diseases, but we must be careful not to violate the sanctity of human life along the way.

## WHERE IS GOD IN HUMAN GENETICS?

What does the Bible say about genetic engineering? While the writers of the Old and New Testaments did not envision a scientific project like the HGP, the omniscient God who inspired them certainly foreknew and gave humans the capacity for such knowledge. All truth belongs to God and is ultimately given to us for his glory and for our good. There are, no doubt, both good uses and evil uses of the knowledge God reveals or enables us to discover, and it is our responsibility as stewards of this knowledge to seek to use it in ways that will glorify God and bring good to humanity.

Are there precepts, principles, or examples in Scripture that should shape Christian ethics with respect to genetic issues? Since we do not find the words *gene, genetics,* or *genome* in a concordance of the Bible, what are some of the scriptural principles that ought to inform our thinking about the Human Genome Project?

First, we must begin where the Bible begins—at creation. Human beings, like all of the universe, are the result of the creative activity of a personal God: "In the beginning God created the heavens and the earth" (Gen. 1:1). The doctrine of creation is the foundation of the Christian theistic worldview. Christians may not agree about or fully understand all of the particulars, but we begin with the presupposition that the universe, including human life, is not the result of random events, the luck of the draw, or blind chance, but the purposive action of an omnipotent God.

Second, the Genesis account reveals that Adam and Eve, and all their progeny, were created in the image and likeness of God (Gen. 1:27). The human genome is, therefore, not only biologically unique, but spiritually (or metaphysically) unique. Human life has been invested by God with sacredness and has intrinsic value. Just as some ways of treating human life are clearly unethical and immoral, some ways of treating the most basic biological building blocks of human life are unethical and immoral.

Third, the Scriptures declare that when Adam and Eve sinned in the Garden of Eden, something tragic happened to the whole created order (Gen. 3:17–21; Rom. 6:12). Although theologians characterize differently the results of the Fall, it is obvious to anyone who is observant that this is not the best of all possible worlds. Sin has brought with it disease and death. Not only that, but the fact that we human beings are sinners means we often find ways to use good things for evil purposes.

Because disease is ultimately the result of the corruption of the world through sin, it is critical that we understand that genetics will not be a new "messiah" to redeem us from all bodily or mental ills. That is not to say, however, that we ought not use genetic technology for the purposes of curing human disease where possible. The genome project is not, in and of itself, open to the charge of "playing God" any more than are other medical therapies. Whenever we take advantage of medical therapies or interventions (even one so common as the flu shot) we are using technology as an intervention against human disease.

There is, though, a curious reductionism that sees every human ill— physical, mental, or spiritual—as curable through genetics. Reducing the human predicament to "bad genes" is tantamount to making the new genetics another utopian vision.[15] Paradise exists in "another world" and awaits only those who trust in Jesus Christ as Savior and Lord.

Fourth, what we are already able to accomplish through genetics is simply phenomenal. But genetic technology can be used as a potent weapon, as a means of eliminating the unwanted or nonuseful or persons who are living so-called lives not worth living. Genetic information may be used as a method of high-tech discrimination against persons based on their genomic characteristics. For instance, in the 1970s mandatory sickle-cell screening among African-American children became a method of discriminating against black children because they were merely carriers of the sickle-cell trait. Screening is currently being used in some cases for gender discrimination. Parents are using genetic information for sex-selection. If they determine they are going to have a girl baby and they wanted a boy, they may abort the baby and try again.

Fifth, and more optimistically, we must acknowledge that all of God's creation, especially we humans, are "fearfully and wonderfully made" (Ps. 139:14). Efforts to better understand the human body, the disease process, and the ways to fight those diseases should, all things being equal, be celebrated and encouraged. Discovering more about the profound complexity of the human body, mind, soul, and spirit points to the reality of the Creator and gives believers more cause to praise and worship him intelligently. That our great God has permitted us to discover ways to relieve physical human suffering, save lives, and cure diseases is certainly a manifestation of his grace and mercy. Every good and perfect gift comes from God (James 1:17). That fact makes it imperative that we not misuse or squander the gifts he gives, including the gift of genetic technology.

Finally, we must face squarely the limits of the new genetics and not think more highly of it than it deserves. Genetics will not ultimately save us from death and the grave. Human beings have an "illness" that permeates us more completely and is more deadly than any genetic disease. Our predisposition to sin is a result of who we are as fallen creatures. If left untreated, that fallenness will result in an eternity without hope and without God. The remedy for our sin is new life in Jesus Christ. He alone is Messiah. He alone is the Great Physician. Ultimately, in heaven, we will be cured of every disease, even our bent toward sinning. *Soli deo gloria!*

## ETHICAL ISSUES IN GENETIC ENGINEERING

Realistically, the Human Genome Project probably does not raise many new ethical issues. Centuries of medicine and research already have surfaced most of the dilemmas that face the project. The new genetics does, however, amplify and make more critical issues that earlier were thought of as exotic or extraordinarily rare. And the social power of genetic information is even more dangerous than in the past.

Although the ethical issues in human genome research are myriad, we will focus on only three: prenatal screening and abortion, privacy, and discrimination.

### Prenatal Screening and Abortion

Presently, there are two major kinds of genetic screening tests. On the one hand, prenatal screening, the more common application of genetic screening technology, aims at the early recognition of individuals who are affected by a genetic anomaly. Prenatal testing is done for a host of genetic illnesses, such as Down's syndrome, and neural tube defects, such as spina bifida.

On the other hand, carrier testing is done to identify individuals who are at risk of transmitting genetic diseases to their offspring. Screening for Tay-Sachs disease and sickle-cell anemia are classic examples of this form of genetic screening. Prospective parents who have a high probability of passing a genetic disease to their children may choose not to conceive children who will be at risk for such an illness.

Once a child is conceived and then diagnosed in utero to have a genetic illness, parents will have only one of three possible choices: (1) to bring the baby to term despite the illness, (2) to attempt a presently experimental treatment in utero (which is only possible in an extremely limited number of cases), or (3) to choose to abort the baby because of his or her genetic disease.

As Nancy Wexler, a geneticist and member of the ELSI committee has said, we must "keep in mind that more often than not, diagnostic information will become available well before any ability to act on it therapeutically."[16] In other words, through genetic screening, parents will be able to predict whether their children will be affected by a deleterious gene, but they will be impotent to do anything about it except to carry the baby to term or abort him or her. In many cases, genetic counselors may encourage abortion, "due to the anguish of carrying a fetus with a severe or lethal genetic disease."[17]

We do not wish to trivialize or underestimate the anguish involved in having a child with a radical deformity or lethal genetic disease. Christian compassion demands that we display utmost concern for, and minister to parents of, children who are devastated by such an event. At the same time, we should not condone or support technologies that encourage abortion, except to save the life of the mother.[18]

For many evangelical Christians, the issue of abortion has been at the forefront of concern for two decades. Since 1973, with the passage of *Roe v. Wade*, the number of abortions in America has consistently increased to the point where more than thirty million legal abortions have been performed. Information gained by genetic testing will increase the number of elective abortions unless parents are adequately informed and choose not to abort. "Until effective treatments become available, such tests offer little more than scientific guidance to inform the decision of parents who are willing to consider abortion to prevent the birth of a child who could be gravely ill."[19] As one sociologist has warned:

> Clearly, it is a just and meaningful desire to prevent fatal and debilitating diseases. Yet in pursuing this goal, we pay unobserved costs. In eliminating individuals with unwanted diseases, we also create a mind-set that justifies the process of human selection. We thus move into the questionable arena of human worth, and to some degree eugenic thought. We forego the idea of therapeutic change (i.e., dietary change or other forms of treatment) and

opt instead for elimination. Individuals are seen as flawed. It is easier and more desirable to prevent their existence than to work for their survival.[20]

Only a sanctity-of-human-life ethic will prevent our society from tumbling down the slippery slope into an even greater holocaust—that of abortion and eugenics. Genetic screening for diseases for which there are no treatments or cures will, no doubt, lead to a significant increase in the number of abortions performed in the United States. Furthermore, genetic screening for sex-selection purposes is an affront to the sanctity of all human life and is a peculiarly grotesque form of gender discrimination. We essentially agree with Christian ethicists and biologists at Calvin College who have said, "Where there is a safe and accurate test for a condition and where the test is related to available and effective treatment, we celebrate this new power to diagnose newborns, children and adults. Where such conditions are not met, we are more cautious than celebratory, and we are particularly concerned about the sort of mentality that would routinely screen for such conditions for which there are neither accurate tests nor effective therapy."[21]

We urge that, until we know more about the ethical, psychological, and social impact of prenatal and carrier screening, such screening for genetic diseases for which there are no treatments or cures be prohibited or highly regulated.

## Confidentiality

One's genetic information is the most personal and highly sensitive information one could possess. We can be separately identified from an unlimited number of persons through a DNA fingerprint. Our genetic information enables us and others to know, among other things, our predisposition to certain diseases. Our family heritage may be determined through genetic tests. In short, our genetic information is extraordinarily comprehensive.

Who has a right to know one's personal genetic information? Who wants to know? Certainly, you and your immediate family might want to know if you are predisposed to a genetic disease. But, do insurance carriers have a right to know? Would a genetic anomaly be classified as a preexisting condition and thus lead to the cancellation of your insurance coverage for a disease you *might* acquire? Some entire families have been refused health insurance because one member of the family had a genetic disorder (such as Tourette's syndrome).

As the HGP progresses, large data banks of genetic information will be stored. The government is already screening members of the Armed Forces and convicted sex felons. In these cases, information is being kept for identification purposes. What about information gathered on other persons? Will insurance companies, prospective employers, and government agencies have access to that information without asking permission or gaining consent? How might that information be used?

We cannot predict today what we will be able to detect or know in twenty years about an individual through genetic tests. As tests become more accurate and we are able to interpret the data more fully, it is impossible to discern what might be discovered in the year 2010 from a blood or tissue sample taken today. These facts have led some states to pass genetic privacy legislation, which aims to protect individuals against the misuse of that information.

Persons who are having genetic tests should: (1) inquire as to the nature of the test (What are you being tested for?), (2) be allowed to consent or not consent to the tests, and (3) be permitted to determine whether or not the results should be destroyed. Only then can genetic privacy be protected.

The Genetics, Religion, and Ethics Project of the Institute of Religion and Baylor College of Medicine in Houston, Texas, issued a "Summary Reflection Statement" concerning the Human Genome Project. Part of that statement says:

> Religious values mandate the defense of personal privacy, integrity of the family, and good social relations. Therefore, they support policies and methods of securing consent to have access to genetic information obtained through screening. Moreover, the use of confidential information must be carefully circumscribed to avoid embarrassment, social stigmatization, disruption of marital and familial relations, and economic discrimination. Care should be taken to avoid or prevent the unjust uses of an individual's genetic data in respect to securing and holding employment, insurance, and health care.[22]

## Discrimination

The uses of genetic information for the purposes of discrimination have already been mentioned. The American eugenics movement, the Nazi experience, and the sickle-cell public-policy disaster are potent testimonies about how genetic information can be used to discriminate against certain groups in a society.

Even though many denominations have not yet spoken specifically to the issue of genetic screening, it is relatively simple to translate Christianity's abhorrence of racism to an abhorrence of all forms of stigmatization and discrimination against individuals based on their genotype. The new genetics offers the potential, if abused, of using high-technology medicine as a weapon of discrimination. Individuals who were predisposed to Huntington's disease have been unable to secure jobs. In 1988, China passed legislation prohibiting the marriage of mentally retarded persons unless they were sterilized. Nobel laureate Linus Pauling suggested:

> There should be tattooed on the forehead of every young person a symbol showing possession of the sickle-cell gene or whatever other similar gene, such as the gene for phenylketonuria (PKU), that has been found to possess in a single dose. If this were done, two young people carrying the same seriously defective gene in single dose would recognize this situation at first sight, and would refrain from falling in love with one another.[23]

While Pauling's research in other areas has been discredited, in light of past abuses of genetic information, his suggestion no longer seems out of the realm of possibility. Think of the implications for discriminating against individuals who might be more highly susceptible to illnesses such as colon cancer, diabetes, or muscular dystrophy. It may well be the case that they will never come down with the disorder, or may be able to prevent its occurrence through changes in diet or lifestyle, yet their genetic profile marks them for life. Persons with disabilities are particularly interested in how the information gained through the Human Genome Project might be used, especially how that information might be used in a discriminatory way.

Again, the Institute of Religion's "Summary Reflection Statement" is apropos:

> A religiously based consensus on the full and equal dignity of all human persons is often contradicted in practice by discriminatory prejudice of one group against another. Ethnic and racial diversities among human beings are due in large part to genetic factors which must never be interpreted as indices of personal or social worth. Neither should the presence of physical or mental disabilities, whether or not they are due to genetic inheritance, detract from one's personal or social value.[24]

## CONCLUSION

It is too early to know whether the information discovered through the Human Genome Project will catapult us into a modern Eden or a Jurassic Park. Sadly, we may not know until after the fact. We are optimistic about the results of the project because of the potentials for healing and the relief of human suffering. At the same time, we are realistic in our view of the propensity of human beings to use good things for evil purposes. Christians call this propensity the sin nature. This predisposition to sin is clearly part and parcel of every human being. We must, therefore, guard against the abuse of genetic information for the purposes of abortion, the violation of privacy, and discrimination.

The psalmist declares that we are "fearfully and wonderfully made" (Ps. 139:14). To the extent that genetic engineering enables us to celebrate that fact, we can endorse it. But to the extent to which genetic technology is used to devalue the sacredness of human life, or as a means of discriminating against individuals, we must reject it. Furthermore, we should resist premature legislation that could jeopardize informed public debate on the merits or hazards of genetic technology.

## ENDNOTES

1. *Understanding Our Genetic Heritage, The U.S. Human Genome Project: The First Five Years FY 1991–1995* (Washington, D.C.: U.S. Department of Health and Human Services, U.S. Department of Energy, 1990), 1.
2. Ibid., 5.

3. Ibid., 65.
4. Lori A. Whittaker, "The Implications of the Human Genome Project for Family Practice," *The Journal of Family Practice* 35 (1992): 295.
5. Daniel J. Kelves, *In the Name of Eugenics: Genetics and the Uses of Human Heredity* (Berkeley and Los Angeles: University of California Press, 1985), ix.
6. Ibid.
7. Ibid., 63.
8. C. E. Rosenberg, *No Other Gods: On Science and American Social Thought* (Baltimore: Johns Hopkins University Press, 1976), 89.
9. Ibid., 100.
10. Ibid., 111.
11. Robert N. Proctor, "Nazi Doctors, Racial Medicine, and Human Experimentation" in *The Nazi Doctors and the Nuremberg Code*, ed. George J. Annas and Michael A. Grodin (New York: Oxford University Press, 1992), 21.
12. Robert Jay Lifton, *The Nazi Doctors: Medical Killing and the Psychology of Genocide* (New York: Basic Books, 1986), 23.
13. Proctor, "Nazi Doctors," 20–21.
14. Lifton, *The Nazi Doctors*, 22.
15. For a critical assessment of biological reductionism, including genetic reductionism, see R. C. Lewontin, *Biology As Ideology: The Doctrine of DNA* (New York: HarperCollins, 1991). Lewontin is a leading geneticist and holds the prestigious Alexander Agassiz chair in zoology at Harvard University.
16. Nancy S. Wexler, "Disease Gene Identification: Ethical Considerations," *Hospital Practice* (October 1992): 145.
17. Thomas D. Gelehrter and Francis S. Collins, *Principles of Medical Genetics* (Baltimore: Williams & Wilkins, 1990), 282.
18. See Larry Lewis, *What the Bible Teaches About Abortion* (Nashville: The Christian Life Commission, 1989).
19. David Suzuki and Peter Knudtson, *Genethics: The Clash Between the New Genetics and Human Values* (Cambridge: Harvard University Press, 1989), 166.
20. Marque-Luisa Miringoff, *The Social Costs of Genetic Welfare* (New Brunswick, N.J.: Rutgers University Press, 1991), 159–60.
21. Hessel Bouma III et al., *Christian Faith, Health, and Medical Practice* (Grand Rapids: Eerdmans, 1989), 245.
22. "Summary Reflection Statement," Genetics, Religion and Ethics Project, The Institute of Religion and Baylor College of Medicine, The Texas Medical Center, Houston, Texas, 1 June 1992, 2.
23. Linus Pauling, "Reflections on the New Biology," in *UCLA Law Review* 15 (1968): 269, cited in Troy Duster, *Backdoor to Eugenics* (New York: Routledge, 1990), 46.
24. Ibid.

*An Overview*

Four basic types of genetic therapy and three procedures for prenatal testing provide the backdrop for this critique of the secular principles that govern their application. Michael McKenzie expresses thoughtful concern over the suitability of *autonomy*, *beneficence*, and *justice* to provide an adequate safety net on which genetic therapy can safely be implemented into broader society. Biblical principles are discussed to encourage reflection among Christians while genetic engineering is still a young science. The numerous medical possibilities and the moral questions that they provoke demand that believers engage in this issue immediately. The science is new and advancing quickly, the principles are old and enduring; the application of these principles must not lag behind.

Chapter Three

# GENETICS AND CHRISTIANITY
*An Uneasy but Necessary Partnership*

## Michael McKenzie

IN THE PAST DECADE, the field of human genetics has undergone nothing short of a revolution. Under the vanguard of the Human Genome Project, the knowledge of genes and how they work in human development is growing at an exponential rate.[1] Disturbingly, this overwhelming growth in knowledge goes virtually unnoticed by all laypeople, including Christians.

### WHAT ARE THE STAKES?

To study human genetics is to study the very blueprints for life. As we learn more about the roles that DNA plays in our development and behavior, Christians will be pressed theologically to think through questions of morality and how those questions are influenced by both nurture *and* nature.

Moreover, few disciplines have within them so much potential for both good and evil. Many debilitating diseases such as Tay-Sachs, Huntington's, Lesch-Nyhan, and Adenosine Deaminase (ADA), are directly attributable to defective genes. Others are apparently the result of faulty genes working in concert with environmental factors. In any case, recent breakthroughs in identifying these genes for possible substitution with healthy genetic material offer nearly miraculous hope for those previously doomed to either an early death or lingering lives of agony.

As genetic knowledge increases, however, so do the possibilities that this knowledge may be misused. Will it be possible someday to clone colonies of humanoids simply for the task of organ harvesting? Given the human drive for the "new and improved," will genetics be harnessed to the engine of social improvement? One of the most dreadful mistakes we could make is to think that eugenics is an idea that died with the Nazis.[2]

This chapter is designed, not to swamp the reader with intricate details on cutting-edge genetic science, but to inform Christians of what's going on in genetics generally, and to sketch out a direction for a Christian response. Thus, there are few if any pat answers, and Christians should view this work as a starting point for their own research and reflection.

## GENETIC THERAPY

There are four basic types of genetic therapy, listed here in order of increasing complexity and moral difficulty.[3] First, somatic cell gene therapy involves the injecting of healthy genetic material into patients with genetic diseases. This has proven highly successful, and often provides the patient with a chance at complete recovery. Since the reproductive cells of the patient are not involved, the effects of the therapy—either bad or good—are not passed to the offspring.

The second type, germ line therapy, involves the rearranging of the patient's own replicating genetic material in such a way that he produces the healthy genes himself. This, too, has been tried, but the complexity of the procedure has made the procedure more risky. Likewise, since the patient's reproductive genetic material has been altered, any deleterious effects unintentionally introduced into the patient are likewise passed down to the offspring. Thus, until risk to both the patient and offspring can be more thoroughly assessed, it is proper to be more cautious about this type of procedure.

Third, enhancement therapy involves not the healing of disease, but the *improvement* of average or less than average characteristics. Hence, this is different in principle from the previous two therapies. No longer is it a case of "fixing a broken part," but of "adding something new to a normally functioning system."[4] Since the issue is not one of healing disease, there has been tremendous pressure both to redefine and widen the concept of disease to make this treatment more acceptable to the general public and to bring in the perceived psychosocial effects of being considered "less than perfect." For instance, most people may agree that it would be better to be of normal height; but is short stature a disease that needs a genetically altered cure? Or, should parents give genetically manufactured growth hormone to their normal sons to produce better candidates for basketball or football?

There are also scientific concerns as well. To correct a faulty gene presents little in the way of danger to the patient. But "to intentionally insert a gene to make more of one product might adversely affect numerous other biochemical pathways."[5] Such dangers are sharpened when enhancement therapy is joined with germ line procedures, thereby passing any deleterious effects to the offspring.

The last type of genetic therapy is, in reality, no therapy at all. Eugenic engineering involves the altering of extremely complex traits to *improve* a given gene pool. In the past, eugenicists have oversimplified how genes are linked with behavior, either ignoring environment altogether, or neglecting the polygenetic (many gene) character of most traits.[6] With the accelerated progress of the Human Genome Project, however, such polygenetic linkages may soon be identified; thus removing that scientific barrier.

Historically, there has never been a time when eugenics was severed from an accompanying social philosophy. Dorothy Nelkin argues persuasively that biological and genetic testing has always been linked with a social pressure to conform, and that there is a "tendency to reduce social problems to measurable biological dimensions."[7] Thus, whether it is the specter of Nazism, Marxism, or Social Darwinism, the political philosophy of the day, as much as the resultant science, deserves close scrutiny.

When surveying the different types of gene therapy, Christians must focus on questions of disease versus enhancement, the purpose(s) of medicine, and the dangers involved in possibly releasing new (and unintended) harmful genes into the human gene pool. The present author would argue that the primary purpose of medicine ought to be, in Nigel Cameron's words, "a tradition of healing."[8] This places both proper focus and limits on the art of medicine—focus, in that it gives proper place to the role of the physician; limits, in that it gives little or no place to the physician as either *enhancer* or eugenicist. Thus, as a corollary, it is not only possible but necessary to sketch a range of normal health and to keep genetics focused on *therapeutically* aiding people into that range.

## GENETICS IN THE WOMB

One of the fastest growing aspects in the broad field of genetics is prenatal testing, i.e., the attempts to detect the presence of chromosomal abnormalities before birth. As will be shown, prenatal testing is inevitably linked with both the larger issues of abortion and genetic testing in general. There are three different procedures used to examine the unborn baby for genetic defects.

*Amniocentesis* utilizes a hollow needle that penetrates the abdomen and uterine wall, extracting amniotic fluid surrounding the fetus for chromosomal, biochemical, and DNA analysis.[9] It cannot normally be performed before sixteen weeks of gestation; and coupled with the two or more weeks necessary for results to appear, the earliest a fetus can be diagnosed with a genetic abnormality would be eighteen weeks or more of gestation (well into the second trimester of pregnancy).[10]

*Fetoscopy* employs a fiber optic device that allows the physician to see the fetus directly. It is usually guided by ultrasonography, the technology that employs high frequency sound waves to create a picture of the fetus in utero. Often, ultrasound technology is used by itself to examine for certain disorders, but fetoscopy allows the obstetrician to make much more certain judgments in borderline cases.

The third method of fetal examination is called *chorionic villus sampling* and involves the extraction of membrane tissue adjacent to the fetus. This procedure is notable because, unlike amniocentesis, no incisions are necessary, and it is effective as early as twelve weeks into gestation.[11] In addition, there are other techniques for prenatal genetic diagnosis on the horizon that will likely make the preceding procedures obsolete and prenatal screening more common.[12]

Whatever type of prenatal screening is utilized, the purpose for the screening must be examined. Because prenatal genetic surgery is extremely limited in its current applications, the usual option offered the prospective parents, when it is learned that the fetus is suffering from a genetic malady, is to abort. Thus, how one feels about prenatal screening and testing is inextricably bound up with how one feels about abortion.[13] To sharpen the dilemma, it is not unusual for physicians to exert pressure to abort by refusing to perform prenatal screening *unless* the couple agrees to the abortion if the genetic anomaly is severe.[14] Insurance companies, hospitals, and HMOs can also exert their own pressure. It is not uncommon for such institutions to offer prospective at-risk parents the "choice" of either a paid abortion or the termination of their health-care benefits (forcing the parents to pay enormous costs of long-term care out of their own pockets).[15] Surely, when such individuals or institutions frame the choice in such a way, it is in reality no choice at all.

Thus, a host of tragic dilemmas arise because *our ability to diagnose genetic disease has far outstripped our ability to treat.*[16] If we start with the premise that real human life (or true moral personhood) begins at conception, should Christians opt for prenatal screening at all (knowing the options that will be presented)? Well, even if one considers abortion murder, there are some reasons for Christian parents to decide on prenatal screening. If the parents are at risk to produce a genetically diseased baby, they may want to know beforehand in order to financially, emotionally, and spiritually prepare for the delivery and the raising of the child. It is often a supremely difficult task to raise, for example, a Down's syndrome child, but, as columnist George Will can testify, often a supremely rewarding one. When parents know beforehand that a "special child" will be entering their world, it often gives a chance for their family, as well as the body of Christ, to come together and show support.

Deplorably, more and more parents are opting for abortion for a whole host of reasons, ranging from mild retardation to even sex selection. Attempts have been made to rank the different congenital conditions in terms of their severity, the least severe being the so-called Fragile X syndrome, and the most severe, anencephaly (in which the babies are born with no cerebral cortex and die within days or weeks).[17] It is morally unacceptable to argue from an evangelical standpoint that abortion is the proper option for any of the diseases, though I understand the difficulty of caring for a child born with anencephaly.[18]

However, those couples who are worried about being carriers for congenital disease may wish to *undergo their own genetic screening before conceiving* to assess their chances of a normal conception. The screening results may indicate that adoption is a viable choice for such couples, thereby avoiding the pressures and risks of the abortion dilemma. In any event, genetic knowledge is increasing at such a pace that genetic counseling is quickly becoming simultaneously more routine and extremely complex.

## SECULAR SAFEGUARDS: THE NEW MAGINOT LINE?

Before the outset of World War II, the French placed their country's security against Hitler's aggression in the Maginot Line, a line of defensive fortifications along their eastern frontier. They thought themselves safe from attack behind impregnable barriers. When Hitler attacked, however, he simply went *around* the Line, turning the vaunted defenses into bastions of irrelevancy. Paris fell in six weeks.

Likewise the present author has little confidence in the three principles that have been erected in secular bioethics to safeguard humanity against genetic abuses. While certainly helpful for general guidelines, and better than no principles at all, they suffer from serious flaws that will, I believe, render them nearly useless when applied to real cases. Two texts are squarely within the bioethical mainstream and are here utilized as the sources for these three principles.[19]

Bioethical textbooks cite either three or four principles that are used to guide bioethical decision making: *autonomy*, *beneficence*, and *justice*. Sometimes *nonmaleficence* (do no harm) is added as an additional principle, sometimes it is subsumed under beneficence. But whatever the number, all rules, ethical judgments, and actions must flow from the above three (or four) principles.[20]

*Patient autonomy*, currently the principle most in vogue, is defined when patients are simply able "to determine their own destiny" without being "subjected to controlling constraint by others."[21] Thus, there is little if any emphasis or concern as to the *content* of the patient's decision. As long as he or she is given enough information, the physician is normally obligated to abide by it.

*Beneficence* (and nonmaleficence) is concerned with the "doing of good and the active promotion of good, kindness, and charity," and may include "any form of action to benefit another . . . [and that helps] . . . others further their important and legitimate interests."[22] How terms, such as *good*, *kindness*, *charity*, *important*, and *legitimate* are to be defined is never explained, leaving patients to define such terms and concepts as they see fit.

Regarding *justice*, even the authors throw up their hands in dismay, saying that "it has proved an intractable problem to supply a single, unified, theory of justice that brings together our [the authors'] diverse views."[23] Thus, this principle suffers the same fate as the others: That which is just is never defined, leaving the physician and/or patient to again provide the meaning.

Thus, our principles are ripe to create more problems than they solve. What happens when a patient's autonomy conflicts with a physician's duty toward beneficence? There is simply no way to rank the principles in order to decide a case. The current stress on autonomy is primarily an indication of modern-day relativism: Because nobody knows what is right, the patient's decision is as good as any, and absolves the physician of any liability.[24] Thus, the principles are empty of any specific content, hopelessly vague, and powerless.

Consequently, no physician or secular ethicist can say if it is good or just to undergo a prenatal screening, nor can they say whether it is good or just to undergo an abortion. The entire question has been thrown into the laps of the patients—and this year in America there will be well over one million abortions.

## GENETICS AND MORALITY

Before suggesting how we Christians might develop our own theology of genetics, let us examine the emerging larger issue of genetics and morality.

In the last twenty years or so, there has been a huge paradigm shift in how we view behavior, disease, and morality in general. It is reflected in our modern vocabulary: Drunkenness is called alcoholism, gluttony is labeled compulsive overeating, promiscuity is titled sexual addiction. Slowly our society has shifted from a moral model to a medical or biological model to explain sinful behaviors. Sins are now complexes, phobias, syndromes, or addictions. Recently, a major weekly news magazine raised the issue of whether even adultery might be in our genes. There is indeed an obvious move to reduce social problems to measurable biological dimensions.

Genetics is one of the engines behind this new way of thinking. It is providing new challenges to the idea of human responsibility and morality. It is going beyond suggesting that our genetic makeup might *predispose* us to certain antisocial behaviors; now there are suggestions that our genes *cause* such actions.[25] That raises sharp questions, especially for those who favor all people's (both Christian and non-Christian) having a free will. Can behavior be morally wrong if it is genetically predisposed or even determined? Is free will necessary for a biblical view of morality? Many Christians, following the thinking of Martin Luther (e.g., *On the Bondage of the Will*) would say no. Instead, they would be quick to point out that the fall of a perfect creation is bound to have certain physical effects, and we should not be surprised if those effects propel us toward rebelling even more against our Creator. In other words, sin is still sin, whatever its proximate cause and source. This new flexing of muscles by geneticists will most certainly cause Christian theology to examine the entire relationship between sin, the will, and morality.[26]

## TOWARD A THEOLOGY OF GENETICS

We as Christians have what the secular world does not: infallible and unchanging principles on which to draw. However, it is not a simple matter of proving simple answers to complex questions. Instead, it is a time for urgent reflection—for fleshing out unchanging biblical principles that speak strongly to specific situations. Lest the wrong impression be given, it is not the case that all will be crystal clear and without gray areas. Nevertheless, Christians have much more to go on, much more certainty on which to rest than does the secular world.

As starting points, here are a few such principles, with their accompanying genetic applications:

1.  Humanity is, and will always be, both finite *and* sinful. It is, therefore, immoral and unwise to utilize genetic technologies such as human eugenics and human cloning.[27] Thus, a theology of health and disease (as opposed to enhancement) must also be developed in accordance with sound biblical guidelines.
2.  Human life, with the image of God and an accompanying unique ensoulment, begins at conception. We are also responsible for how we treat the most helpless in our society, i.e., "the least of these." Thus, there are important limitations for prenatal testing, and genetic diagnostics must not be used to pressure parents into abortion.

3. God's Word is clear that humankind—both corporately and individually—is fully responsible for actions labeled *sin*. Consequently, Christians should resist attempts to convert all antisocial behaviors into genetic diseases that carry no personal responsibility or accountability.
4. Humans are the apex of God's creation and are commanded to be good stewards of the earth and its resources. We are also directed "to love our neighbors as ourselves." Thus, we have a mandate to engage in genetic research and therapy, *when it is directed toward the healing end of medicine.*

The difficulty with these principles rests, of course, on their implementation in the secular world. It is a daunting task to dialogue in the public arena while keeping one's Christian values intact. The outright failure of certain secular projects—most notably the sexual revolution of the 1960s—may provide some openings, but making Christian ethics both acceptable (i.e., getting a hearing) and remaining true to Scripture is becoming increasingly difficult. Perhaps evangelical Protestants—long cool to the idea—may become more sympathetic to natural law as a legitimate way to translate biblical values. It may be that evangelicals will be forced to be more forthright in creating their own structures and institutions (e.g., hospitals) that will be more friendly to religious arguments.

Whatever the tack chosen, the history of science is crystal clear on one point: Genetic science will not wait for Christians to "catch up." By the time this work is published, new discoveries will have been made and new claims put forth. Under the flagship of the Human Genome Project, genetic information is accumulating at a staggering rate. Christians must first become genetically informed; then, with data in hand, be able to address highly technical issues with scriptural principles. Considering what's at stake, this task may be one of the most necessary—and one of the most difficult—ever faced by the body of Christ.

## ENDNOTES

1. The Human Genome Project (begun in 1990) has an ambitious goal: to identify and map all the genes of the DNA molecule that make up the chromosomes in each human cell. Because of the data-processing speed of so-called super computers, the Project is ahead of schedule, and should reach its goal ahead of the 2005 target date. The HGP is divided up amongst nine research centers across the country, and its total budget for the fiscal year 1994 was nearly 170 million dollars.
2. Dorothy Nelkin warns of the disturbing reemergence of eugenic thinking in "The Social Power of Genetic Information," in *The Code of Codes: Scientific and Social Issues in the Human Genome Project*, ed. Daniel J. Kevles and LeRoy Hood (Cambridge: Harvard University Press, 1992), 182. There are also distinctions made between positive eugenics, the enhancing of the genetic heritage of the species, and negative eugenics, the prevention of the deterioration of the gene pool. See Thomas Mappes and Jane Zembaty, eds., *Biomedical Ethics* (New York: McGraw Hill, 1986), 496. Speaking morally, such definitions function much

like two sides of the same coin: to speak of enhancing one trait is to speak of
the undesirability of others (i.e., the "deterioration" of the gene pool). Hence,
this work will treat eugenics as a unified concept embracing both aspects.

3. For an excellent discussion of the different types of gene therapy, see W. French
Anderson, "Human Gene Therapy: Scientific Considerations," in *Contemporary
Issues in Bioethics*, ed. Tom Beauchamp and LeRoy Walters (Belmont: Wadsworth
Publishing, 1989), 513–19.
4. Ibid., 518.
5. Ibid.
6. Daniel J. Kevles, "Out of Eugenics: The Historical Politics of the Human
Genome," in *The Code of Codes*, 8.
7. Nelkin, "The Social Power," 180–81.
8. Nigel M. de S. Cameron, *The New Medicine: Life and Death After Hippocrates*
(Wheaton: Crossway Books, 1992), 129.
9. J. Robert Nelson, *On the New Frontiers of Genetics and Religion* (Grand Rapids:
Eerdmans, 1994), 37. Also, see Laurence Karp, "The Prenatal Diagnosis of
Genetic Disease," in *Biomedical Ethics*, 496–502.
10. Nelson, *On the New Frontiers*, 37; and Karp, "The Prenatal Diagnosis," 497–98.
11. Nelson, *On the New Frontiers*, 38.
12. Ibid.
13. This relationship is acknowledged by Ruth Schwartz Cowan in "Genetic
Technology and Reproductive Choice: An Ethics for Autonomy," in *The Code
of Codes*, 246.
14. Karp, "The Prenatal Diagnosis," 502.
15. Nelkin, "The Social Power," 184.
16. Nancy Wexler, "Clairvoyance and Caution: Repercussions from the Human
Genome Project," in *Code of Codes*, 211, 223.
17. Nelson, *On the New Frontiers*, 39–40.
18. It is important to point out that this observation does not lessen the extreme
difficulty of the decisions involved.
19. One is the already cited Beauchamp and Walters, the other is by Beauchamp
and James Childress, *Principles of Biomedical Ethics* (New York: Oxford, 1989).
20. Beauchamp and Walters, *Contemporary Issues*, 28, or Beauchamp and Childress,
*Principles*, 15.
21. Beauchamp and Walters, *Contemporary Issues*, 29.
22. Ibid., 30, 194.
23. Beauchamp and Childress, *Principles*, 256.
24. Beauchamp and Childress admit that the principles are "equally weighted"
(*Principles*, 222).
25. Nelson, *On the New Frontiers*, citing the determinism of Edward Wilson, 105.
26. Nelson, *On the New Frontiers*, 102–3.
27. As the recent cloning of a sheep has indicated, the technological advances in
this area are startling. If, despite humanity's best wisdom, human cloning should
occur, it is critical to remember that such clones would be fully human, and
thus deserve to be treated as "ends in themselves," and not as means to other
ends, e.g., clones should never be created simply to furnish organs for others
or to perform dangerous tasks or functions.

*An Overview*

What role does justice play and can it really exist in a country that develops its direction through personal autonomy and popular opinion? Without a stable moral standard, our relationships with God and one another have no framework in which to operate and no ethical system of right and wrong from which to govern fairness and care. Dónal P. O'Mathúna looks at justice through the matrix of God's character to examine the values that are behind the concept of genetic essentialism. While genetic technology has much to offer, it must be distributed judicially through a process that is consistent with God's standard of righteousness to avoid unnecessary abuses and unwanted consequences. The welfare of a society can never be dependent on science and technology, but rather, on a transcendent system of justice that understands humanity's strengths and weaknesses and, therefore, can compassionately and fairly care for all its citizens.

# Chapter Four

# APPLYING JUSTICE TO GENETICS

Dónal P. O'Mathúna

## INTRODUCTION

Genetic technology has been fraught with ethical controversy. The role of justice in genetics is usually raised in connection with the privacy of genetic information. Fears of discrimination, if this information does not remain confidential, have led to some legislation on the use of genetic information in the United States.[1] However, concerns about justice and genetics deserve a broader and more thorough analysis.

The connection between justice and genetics could be explored by examining whether certain genetic practices are just in and of themselves. While this approach would be productive in certain cases, it will not be the primary approach in this chapter. Genetic practices are not specifically addressed in the Bible, but this is also the case with other types of practices that raise ethical concerns. Some activities and practices discussed in the Bible are viewed as legitimate in some places but are denounced elsewhere. This points to the importance of examining the motivations and attitudes underlying a person's use of specific practices.

For example, the Old Testament frequently commands the Israelites to celebrate a number of festivals, offer sacrifices to God, and praise him with song and music. Yet, at other times, God, through his prophets, rejected all of these practices. Frequently, the problem was that these activities were carried out to the neglect of justice and righteousness (Isa. 1:11–17; Amos 5:21–24). The biblical concept of justice can help evaluate the underlying assumptions and values that impact how people use, and will use, genetic technology. This evaluation is needed because the increased use of this technology will impact people's understanding of justice. Unless people's ethical stances are based on an objective moral standard, they will default to either arbitrarily chosen values or the changing status of scientific knowledge. The eternal character of God, as expressed in his concern for justice, provides the objective standard many seek.

Another reason for evaluating genetics in light of biblical justice is that genetic technologies raise ethical issues that run deeper than the specific practice. These technologies are proliferating within a culture that holds certain values and assumptions. Many discussions seem to assume that justice

51

is violated only when people deliberately discriminate on genetic grounds. They tend to ignore "the pervasiveness of stereotypes, unfounded beliefs, and prejudices fueled by genetic notions."[2] These beliefs strongly impact whether the technologies will be used justly or not.

Part of this belief system is a popular notion of the nature of genetics and what it can accomplish. Nelkin and Lindee, in their book *The DNA Mystique*, describe this view of genetics in detail, calling it "genetic essentialism." This view "reduces the self to a molecular entity, equating human beings, in all their social, historical, and moral complexity, with their genes."[3] Genetic determinism, or geneticism, are similar terms used by other authors that, although having some nuances, will be viewed as synonymous here. Elsewhere, Nelkin elaborates:

> Genetic essentialism posits that personal traits are predictable and permanent, determined at conception, "hard-wired" into the human constitution. If comprehensively known and understood, these inherent qualities would largely explain past performance and could predict future behavior. Standing in sharp contrast with the relational definitions of personhood observed in some societies, this ideology minimizes the importance of social context.[4]

Nelkin and Lindee expose the widespread acceptance of genetic essentialism through numerous cultural trends. The increased tendency to settle child custody disputes on biological rather than relational criteria is one such example. One highly publicized case involved a surrogate mother who refused to give the child to his biological parents. Eventually, the judge awarded custody of the child to the biological parents. This decision could have been supported by a number of well-established precedents. But instead, the judge defended his ruling on the ideas of genetic essentialism. He stated that the child's identity was primarily in his genes and assumed that a common genetic heritage was the most important aspect of human relationships.[5]

Many other examples are given by Nelkin and Lindee. Newspaper headlines have announced the discovery of genes for everything from a variety of diseases to obesity, alcoholism, infidelity, homosexuality, divorce, violence, and selfishness. One billion dollars is spent per year on infertility in America because of the high value placed on having one's own biological children. Groups opposed to adoption are growing, as are those helping adopted children find their biological parents. These groups equate the importance of knowing one's genetic roots with forming one's personal identity. Although many other examples could be given, these should suffice to demonstrate the widespread acceptance of genetic essentialism. *Our focus will be on the ethical implications of this view and how biblical justice provides a better alternative.*

Genetic essentialism is attractive to many Americans because it seems to validate and promote values deeply held in American popular culture, such as individualism and personal autonomy. Because of this, it has caught the American public's imagination. Yet genetic essentialism is, in many ways, scientifically inaccurate, and far exceeds medical science's present capabilities.[6] Flawed as they may be, these assumptions motivate many of the responses people have to genetic developments. As such, these ideas strongly influence what is seen as ethical.

This chapter will address the values underlying genetic essentialism and evaluate them in light of biblical justice. A description of biblical justice involves a number of elements that offer important alternatives to genetic essentialism. By contrasting biblical justice with genetic essentialism, even those who are not Christians might become more cautious in their willingness to implement some genetic technologies. When these technologies are put into practice in a culture infused with values contrary to biblical justice, ethical problems will inevitably result and already have started to arise. In contrast, genetic technology used within appropriate ethical guidelines has the potential to lead to much good and could even promote justice in our society.

## BIBLICAL JUSTICE

Justice is a central concept in the Bible. The Old Testament scholar, Gerhard von Rad, stated: "There is absolutely no concept in the Old Testament with so central a significance for all the relationships of human life as that of *sedaqah* [justice/righteousness]."[7] God declares that he loves justice (Isa. 61:1) and calls on people to be just and fair to everyone (Isa. 56:1). The concept of justice in these passages and others is integral to being good and right. The call to be just is found in important passages that summarize what God expects of people (Mic. 6:8; Amos 5:24). Jesus, too, declared that justice was one of the weightier provisions of the law (Matt. 23:23). The notion of biblical justice is so intertwined with goodness that many Old Testament passages treat both ideas together in the phrase *sedaqah mispat*, which means justice and righteousness.

Yet, there is controversy over precisely what biblical justice involves or requires. For example, Schoenfeld claims that while justice was a central ideal in the Old Testament, it is totally absent from the New Testament.[8] His conclusion arises from his definition of justice as the legitimate exercise of power by rulers. The Old Testament prophets critiqued the exercise of power by kings and religious leaders in the name of justice. However, according to Schoenfeld, Christians are not to critique political powers (based on his reading of Romans 13). Hence, he sees no call for justice in the New Testament.

However, Schoenfeld's definition of justice is narrow and neglects much of the biblical use of the term. The Bible presents justice as one attribute of God and hence a moral virtue expected in the followers of Yahweh or Jesus Christ. Biblical justice incorporates concern for legal issues such as the just execution of laws and governance. Justice also has an eschatological dimension in its concern for final vindication of good and judgment of evil in the end times. In the New Testament, the concept frequently deals with personal justification before God.

Biblical justice also incorporates concern for concrete actions on behalf of the underprivileged.[9] Throughout the Old Testament, justice required compassion and provision for the oppressed, the poor, widows, orphans, and strangers (Exod. 23:6; Deut. 10:17–19; Job 29:12–17; Ps. 82:2–4; Isa. 61:1–2). This same view of justice is carried over into the New Testament, though expressed in different ways and more often in terms of love (Luke 11:39–44). Nevertheless, Christians are similarly called to care for the oppressed (Heb. 13:3), the poor (Acts 2:45; 4:32–37; Eph. 4:28), widows (1 Tim. 5:3–16), strangers (Matt. 25:34–46), and orphans (James 1:27).

The dominance of this aspect of biblical justice has led Karen Lebacqz to propose that only the poor can determine the true nature of justice. "If justice is the restoration of right relationship, the rectification of injustice, then there must be an 'epistemological privilege' of the poor, for only they can judge the true character of injustice and hence the demands of justice."[10] She acknowledges the importance of biblical justice but guts it of divine authority by placing its definition in the hands of a group of humans, the "poor." She defines this group to include "minority groups, white women, those with disabilities, gay, lesbian and bisexual people, and anyone who is either economically disadvantaged or politically and socially disenfranchised."[11]

While Lebacqz's postmodern approach sounds like it empowers the oppressed, it actually returns the definition of justice to a group of humans who are as likely as any other to abuse their authority. This is why Christians must turn to the Bible for their definition of justice. The Bible instructs us on the nature of justice and provides examples of how God and others have acted justly. These accounts must be the basis of a biblical understanding of justice. The biblical teaching on justice, as with any other issue, can be viewed as authoritative only if its divine authorship is upheld.

As with many other concepts, however, justice in the Bible is not described in abstract terms. No ideal norm is given against which current practices should be measured. Abstract ideas of justice lead to questions of what it means for each person to receive fair treatment or a fair portion of limited resources. While many have sought a theologically based abstract notion of justice, these pursuits have yielded little fruit. The problem is that "ancient Israel did not in fact measure a line of conduct or an act by an ideal norm, but by the specific relationship in which the partner had at the time to prove himself true . . . the just man is the one who measures up to the particular claims which this relationship lays upon him."[12]

The relational basis of biblical justice is carried over into the New Testament. When the Hebrew Bible was translated into Greek, justice was described by a group of words based on the root *dikaios*. While Greek philosophy discussed justice frequently, the New Testament concept strictly follows the Hebrew view. "There is a deep gulf between the NT *dikaios* and the Greek ideal of virtue, which isolates man in independent achievement."[13] Like the Hebrew concept, New Testament justice is rooted in relationship with God and promotes faithfulness in people's relationships with one another.

Biblical justice is relationally based, as opposed to being concerned primarily with adherence to some ethical standard, or motivated solely by duty. "In general terms the biblical idea of justice can be described as fidelity to the demands of a relationship."[14] Being relational, biblical justice is motivated by deep compassion and mercy for others (Zech. 7:9–10; John 8:1–11; Heb. 13:1–3). Frequently, the notion of kindness is associated with biblical justice (Ps. 101:1; Jer. 9:23–24; Hos. 2:19; Mic. 6:8). In many of these verses, justice is equated with goodness and mercy. "We must therefore conclude that the word *sedaqah*, and especially the phrase *sedaqah mispat*, does not refer to the proper execution of justice, but rather expresses, in a general sense, social justice and equity, which is bound up with kindness and mercy."[15]

Biblical justice is complex and all encompassing. The Bible does not give a simple definition of justice, but reveals it gradually by describing how God acts to uphold justice. While defining justice concisely is difficult, we are forced to attempt to do so for the purposes of clarity. Justice is relating to others in the same ways that God relates to people. Just relationships should be characterized by all the attributes visible in God's relationships, such as his goodness, mercy, love, forgiveness, and so forth. The standards for justice are set by an external authority, and are not subject to individual autonomy. Hence, justice is not determined by one's circumstances or feelings, but by an authority focused on everyone's best interests. This definition reveals the central problem with justice based on human authority, even one such as the United States' Constitution. Any standard of justice designed by humans is fallible and changeable. In contrast, *God's standard of justice is infallible and unchanging*.

God's justice is revealed throughout the Bible by his faithfulness to his covenant with his people. Underlying this covenant is his deep compassion and love for people (Exod. 34:6–8). This leads to his continual concern and provision for humanity, culminating in the sending of his Son as Savior. "The justice of the One who is absolutely righteous is demonstrated in the atoning sacrifice of Jesus"[16] (Rom. 3:26; 1 John 1:9). God's justice is revealed in his activity on behalf of humanity and should inspire Christians to relate similarly toward others.

Justice is integral to the character of anyone who wishes to follow God because justice is one of his attributes. God declares that knowing him means doing justice/righteousness, which is seen when someone pleads the cause of the afflicted and needy (Jer. 22:16–17). The love of God is to emanate from all Christians in their concern for justice: "But whoever has the world's goods, and beholds his brother in need and closes his heart against him, how does the love of God abide in him?" (1 John 3:17 NASB). The remainder of this chapter will focus on how these ideas can be applied to the issues raised by developments in genetic technology.

## THE JUST DISTRIBUTION OF GENES

Discussions of justice in medical ethics frequently focus on either the just distribution of resources or the just treatment of people with diseases or disabilities. These same concerns are raised with the distribution of genetic technology and treatment of those with genetic diseases. One of the major concerns with genetic testing is whether those discovered to have genes associated with various traits or diseases will be treated differently and in unjust ways. Genetic information carries the potential for discrimination at the workplace, with health insurance, and in social status.

The view of justice underlying these discussions assumes a genetic lottery that randomly assigns everyone a genotype.[17] Some have been fortunate with the genetic "cards" they were dealt; others less fortunate. Justice would insist that people receive a fair share of the resources available to help them grow and develop within the limitations set by their genes. What constitutes a "fair share" would be evaluated differently depending on one's view of justice.[18]

Recent genetic technology, however, appears to make it possible to influence the genetic "lottery." Now, distribution of genes seems to come under the consideration of justice. Historically, justice was not applied to a person's genotype because this was not something people could influence. Having a certain set of genes was not a matter of justice but one of the realities of life with which a person had to learn to live. If anyone was at fault, it could only be God or nature, and humans had little recourse against either of them!

The early eugenic movement raised the idea that one's genotype was not inherited completely randomly. By choosing one's spouse carefully, one's children could inherit better genes. From this came the alleged responsibility, both to one's children and to society, to only conceive children of the best heritage. Much of the eugenics of the early twentieth century was based on simplistic notions of inheritance, and a lack of appreciation for the role of environment in determining phenotype traits. Many of these same assumptions underlie the recent promotion of genetic essentialism.

Genetic testing allows parents to detect a wide range of genes associated with various illnesses and traits. This gives parents the ability to determine whether they will bring a child into the world with a certain set of genes. It even gives the impression that parents have "the right to choose the particular genetic makeup of their child."[19] Wrongful life lawsuits are being filed against parents or physicians on the assumption that people have the right not to be born if their life involves some level of disability. Not only is it claimed that it is unjust for the disabled individual to have to live with the consequences of a genetic defect, but it is also said to be unjust for society to have to bear the financial consequences.

Claims that it is unjust for society to have to pay for the needs of a disabled child reveal the selfish priorities of modern Western society. The problem is not that society does not have the resources to pay for the care of these people. Society chooses to spend its resources in ways that reflect its values. For example, in 1993 the cost of all U.S. state-operated residential facilities for persons with mental retardation was $5.87 billion.[20] In the same year, Americans spent $29.6 billion on tobacco products, and $26.3 billion on jewelry and watches. Our citizens bet three times as much money on legal gambling as they give to charities, including churches and synagogues.[21] People choose to spend their money on things rather than on people. Candidly stated, America values things more than it values people.

Parents must be responsible in their reproductive decisions, but deciding to bring a disabled child into the world cannot be unjust in the eyes of God. He is perfectly just, and yet he permits every single disabled child to be born. He even declares that he is the one who makes people dumb and deaf and blind (Exod. 4:11). As difficult as these conditions may be for us to accept, they represent opportunities for people to depend on God (4:12). Blindness is not a punishment for past sins but is an opportunity for God to be glorified (John 9:1–5). All disabilities can be difficult to live with. Watching one's child deal with a disability and its consequences can be even more difficult. But this does not change what is just.

Biblical justice involves faithfulness in relationships. The physical process of conception creates new human life that God is faithful to from the beginning. He chooses to love people because of who he is not because of their abilities or righteousness (Matt. 5:43–44). He chooses to sustain and support all people, regardless of how good or evil they have been (Matt. 5:45). They are conceived in sin (Ps. 51:5), born alienated from him (Eph. 2:1–3), and yet he still chooses to be just toward them. Likewise, we are to act justly toward others because of who we are—God's children (Matt. 5:45).

Biblical justice flows out of a relationship with God and is enacted because of relationships with others. Conceiving a life initiates a relationship between parents and child that carries certain responsibilities and should be characterized by certain traits. Justice demands that the parents be faithful to the child by affording him or her the opportunities needed to accomplish the plans God has prepared beforehand (Eph. 2:10).

## GENETICS, JUSTICE, AND COMMUNITY

A community is not unjust because it allows the birth of people with disabilities. Injustices occur when the community fails to help disabled children reach their potentials. Assistance is needed from the immediate family and also from the whole community. Throughout the Bible, followers of God are called on to care for the needs of the weakest and most vulnerable in society. The challenges facing the disabled, which can be very difficult, should be the struggles and challenges faced by the community. The whole community, not just individuals, may have to learn to change from within to develop the character needed to truly help others.

Genetic essentialism fosters values and beliefs that work against community-based solutions. Society's problems are increasingly ascribed to individuals. When behavior is viewed as genetically determined, people are increasingly viewed as products; products, primarily, of their genes. Genetic essentialism pulls community apart by reducing society to its individuals and people to their genes. At its core, *genetic essentialism is driven by personal autonomy, not justice.*

Another implication of viewing behavior as predetermined by one's genes is that notions of moral responsibility must be radically revised. For example, if alcoholism is "defined as a genetically determined trait, neither society nor the alcohol industry appears responsible. And if behavior is completely determined—either by genetics or environment—even the addicted individual cannot really be blamed."[22] Defendants in recent court cases have tried to avoid culpability by using a defense that amounts to claiming, "My genes made me do it."

While genetic essentialism removes responsibility for behavior, it is a two-edged sword. If behavior is primarily determined by our genes, there is little hope we can change. We're stuck with our genes and, therefore, our behavior. To change and improve means our choices must be able to significantly impact our behavior and the environment. If this is so, others and the environment will have an important role in influencing who we are. This has important implications for determining public policy for social problems. Genetic essentialism calls for gene-focused solutions. Hence is born the fervent hope that gene therapy will cure some of society's most intractable ills, even criminal behavior.[23]

However, genetic solutions to social problems tend to draw attention away from more difficult and complicated issues. The focus again becomes the individual, not the community. "To focus on genetic marker studies for lung cancer rather than, for example, on cigarette billboard spending in black communities, is to avoid crucial social issues. To focus on genetic marker studies is to privatize what should be a public issue. To privatize genetics is to blind ourselves to harsh social realities that constrict private lives."[24] Finding wayward genes and fixing or eliminating them appears much easier than taking wayward persons and giving their lives meaning and direction.

Genetic essentialism makes social problems the responsibility of the medical community rather than the community at large. Having medicalized the problems, everyone else can go about their own business without having to worry about those with genetic problems. Since the problems are in their genes, there is nothing society can do anyway. In this way, *genetic essentialism desensitizes people to the plight and suffering of others in the community.*

Herrnstein and Murray, in their highly publicized book *The Bell Curve*, take genetic essentialism to its logical social policy conclusions.[25] If behavior is predominantly genetically determined, as they argue, educational and welfare assistance should no longer be provided to the poor. If problems are genetic, there is nothing more the state can do about them. They assume that social programs in the United States for the last couple of decades have removed all barriers to individual progress. Therefore, those who remain poor and undereducated are genetically inferior to those who succeed in the present system. As a result, they advocate the immediate abandonment of remedial education programs, the abolishment of social programs because they lead to poorer women having more children, and the encouragement of successful women to have more children.[26] In fact, it would be unjust to continue to use society's limited resources in ways that will never (in their view) yield results.

The biblical view of justice is very different because it places such great emphasis on community. Israel and the body of Christ are to be living examples of the priority God places on community. Christians are to be involved intimately in one another's lives, contributing to the needs of others and empathizing with them in their struggles (Rom. 12:9–15). The whole community needs to examine its role in causing the inequities in society. Sin and injustice are not only problems for individuals, they are social problems that span generations.

Even if certain problems do originate with individuals, the solution lies with much more than just their genes. The biblical position is that people have free will and are called to exercise control over their passions and behaviors (Gal. 5:19–23). Genetics and environment influence people, but we are ultimately responsible for our choices. No matter what role genetics plays in alcoholism and homosexuality, if it plays any role at all, the behaviors stemming from these genes are condemned in the Bible (1 Cor. 6:9–10). Yet, this is also a source of hope. With the condemning of a behavior comes the promise of the empowering of God to overcome those temptations (1 Cor. 10:13; Phil. 1:6).

Any attempt to correct problems without addressing the physical, emotional, spiritual, and moral aspects of individuals and the relational aspects of society will not succeed. However, these are bigger, more complicated problems without easy solutions. They require insight and resources not readily at our disposal. In fact, they require divine intervention. Genetic tests and therapies appear to be promising remedies, but they are only physical, external solutions. They will not get to the root of our problems that, according to the Bible, originate in people's hearts, and will only be dealt with when people repent and turn to God (Matt. 15:15–20).

The move away from community-based policies to individualism has other practical social-justice consequences. Genetic screening to determine insurability would not be as much of an issue if insurance companies based their policies on the more just policy of "community rating" rather than "experience rating."[27] The former method provided health insurance at the same premium for all persons in the same geographic region. However, in the competition for employer contracts, insurance premiums became based on the actual claims experienced by employees (experience rating). Because the working population tends to be healthier, insurance companies could offer lower premiums to employers than to communities in general. This created pressure both on insurance companies and employers to assess and minimize risks through prescreening, including genetic testing. In doing so, however, some people became uninsurable, or at least subject to higher premiums.

On an individual basis, experience rating results in lower premiums for the healthy and employers. While this makes sense economically, it forces "those in greatest need to shoulder their burdens alone."[28] As genetic screening becomes more widely available, and possibly required by insurance companies and employers, more individuals are likely to become uninsurable. A direct application of biblical justice would be for people to speak up for the weak, and offer to sacrifice some of their own gain for the good of those with genetic illnesses.

Insurance companies and employers can better serve justice by returning to a community rating where the costs of health care are more evenly spread across the community. This is clearly in keeping with the biblical pattern. Like those with genetic illnesses, orphans and widows in the ancient Near East were placed in precarious circumstances through no fault of their own. Survival without the help of others was very difficult. Similarly, those with genetic illnesses will find it very difficult to survive today's health-care system without some sort of insurance coverage.

One of the biblical motivations for sharing resources with others is the realization that we have already been given so much (2 Cor. 8:13–15). Those who do not have genetic illnesses are blessed through no action of their own. Gratitude for the gift of health should motivate them to provide for those less fortunate. When we remember that all of us carry some genetic anomalies, we should be less willing to allow discrimination against those whose genetic anomalies have been discovered. The day may soon arrive when the genetic anomalies of the apparently healthy are revealed.

## GENETICS AND CATEGORIZATION

As described above, biblical justice focuses attention on the underprivileged in society. It emphasizes the importance of each individual to the community as a whole. Genetic essentialism is based on conflicting assumptions. It assumes that some people are so useless to society, or such a burden on society, that they should be marginalized in some way. In accomplishing this, genetic essentialism becomes yet another way to categorize people so they can be treated differently from the privileged in society.

In the past, groups of people have been categorized to justify differential treatment. Eugenic programs in the early twentieth century encouraged "superior" people to have more children and tried to reduce the number of socially disadvantaged children. This was done by attempting to prevent (sometimes coercively) the birth of those deemed less useful to society. These practices were justified because "concerns about the economic dislocations and political upheavals caused by industrialization, immigration, and the changing ethnic composition of cities created a need for categorization and classification. Genetic labels satisfied this need."[29]

The history of this century shows that people tend to use genetic information (and misinformation) to categorize and discriminate. Patricia King gives examples from the eugenics movement, and also discusses the compulsory sterilization of people with mental illnesses and the screening of African-Americans for sickle-cell anemia. She concludes that "genetic information historically has been used to reinforce negative stereotypes about racial and ethnic groups and poor people, rather than to de-emphasize differences among groups in the United States."[30]

The question of how to relate to and treat others, especially those who are different, has long troubled humanity. A common method used to justify treating others differently is by categorizing "them" as somehow fundamentally different from "us." This usually justifies treating them in some way we would not approve of treating us. The underlying assumption is that the obligations owed to us are very different from those owed to them. The difficulty seems only in figuring out which criteria best distinguish them from us.

While many of these earlier categorizations were crude and phenotype related, recent developments allow more precise genotype-based distinctions. Genetic technology appears to offer a scientific, objective way to categorize humans. Those with a gene for a particular disease can then be treated differently from those without the gene. For example, insurance companies might want to determine who carries genes for certain illnesses so they can refuse coverage and thereby avoid higher claims. Genetic screening appears more justifiable since this decision is based on "objective" scientific tests, not arbitrary or prejudiced ideas.

However, genetic categorization is not objective and value free. The entire endeavor is value laden, and the appearance of objectivity hides inherently unjust values. "Similarly, condemning individual instances of genetic discrimination will do little to address systematic genetic categorization, a world view that seeks to sort people by their genetics, and the conviction that supposedly deviant genes merit different treatment."[31]

The problem with this whole approach is the desire to categorize and treat differently. Jesus was confronted with this same issue when the lawyer asked who his neighbor was (Luke 10:29–37). The assumption was that he could treat his neighbors one way and his nonneighbors differently.[32] Jesus' reply in the parable of the Good Samaritan puts the whole question in proper perspective. He tells the lawyer to focus on how he could act as a good neighbor, in particular by being merciful. Instead of focusing on how to distinguish between people genetically, we should focus on how to act justly toward everyone. All people are created in the image of God, and all are entitled to just treatment (Gen. 9:6; James 3:9).

## GENETIC TESTING AND THE UNBORN

While genetic categorization of children and adults opens the door for discrimination, genetic categorization of the unborn can lead to a death sentence. Genetic essentialism "involves creating genetic categories, actively looking for any kind of information about people in order to sort them into those categories, and harboring attitudes and prejudices that motivate such behavior."[33] Genetic testing is thus used to categorize the unborn into a class of those viewed as functionally worthy of being allowed to live. Ostensibly, this seems to mercifully save those who are not viewed as functionally worthy of being allowed to live from a life of suffering. Sometimes concern about the unnecessary suffering of a disabled child is really concern for the suffering this child might cause those around the child. These decisions reflect the assumption that some lives are not worth living. Genetic testing is thereby used to determine whether the unborn meet the genetic qualifications required to merit life. Genetic testing used for this purpose violates biblical justice.

The unborn are often categorized as nonpersons to justify embryo research and abortion. Most view it as unethical to allow humans to be experimented with in ways that cause their deaths. However, by denying that embryos and fetuses are persons, researching them to death, literally, is justified.[34] Mothers may not kill their children, but by labeling the unborn as nonpersons, abortion is justified. The underlying premise in these arguments is that some functional criteria make the unborn fundamentally different from the born and, hence, not entitled to the same rights or treatment.

This issue becomes even more problematic with genetic testing of fetuses. While only 39 to 47 percent of Americans favor legalization of abortion in general, 78 percent believe abortion of fetuses with Down's syndrome should be legal.[35] In the small number of studies available on this issue, the majority of women have abortions after their unborn children are diagnosed with genetic abnormalities. "These findings appear to indicate that genetic testing as a logical extension of eugenics is indeed being used as a means to screen for and then prevent the birth of persons with Down syndrome."[36]

Underlying these abortion decisions is a desire not to have children with disabilities. This is certainly understandable given the emotional and material costs of raising disabled children. No one wants children to have genetic disabilities, but once they are conceived, justice calls for them to be treated as human beings. Biblical justice calls for them to be given even more honor than healthy children (1 Cor. 12:22–24). Unfortunately, we see them treated with less honor.

The devaluing of disabled children was apparent even before fetal genetic testing became readily available. A 1975 survey asked pediatricians and pediatric surgeons if they would "acquiesce in parents' decision to refuse consent for surgery in a newborn with intestinal atresia."[37] This surgery is relatively straightforward and has a high success rate. If the newborn had no other anomalies, 2.6 percent of the pediatricians and 7.9 percent of the surgeons said they would acquiesce to this decision (which is certainly different from approving of it). However, if the only other complicating factor was that the newborn had Down's syndrome, 49.5 percent of the pediatricians and 76.8 percent of the surgeons said they would acquiesce to the parents' decision to refuse to allow surgery. These newborns would thereby die within a week or two.

Genetic testing of the unborn, followed by abortion, seems to offer a better solution by avoiding the slow death of these children. Certainly, fetal genetic testing can help parents plan for a future likely to be very different from one with a "normal" child. It can help the health-care team prepare for what may be a difficult pregnancy or delivery. Having time to reflect on the difficulties of raising a disabled child, and grieving the loss of "normalcy," has important advantages. But genetic essentialism makes this potentially useful tool for healing a weapon of destruction. The technology itself is not necessarily unjust. But in the hands of a society that does not value those who fall below certain functional or intellectual standards, genetic testing may promote injustice. For example, efforts are being made to promote respect and justice for the disabled. "However, there seems to be a contradiction to the notion that a person is more than his or her disability when termination of a pregnancy may be based solely upon this status. Society apparently considers mental retardation to be a disability of such magnitude that, by itself, it is sufficient reason for termination."[38]

Friedrich Nietzsche, whose philosophy influences much postmodern thinking, viewed the protection of the weak as the central weakness of Christianity. For him, "the invalid is a parasite on society."[39] Postmodernism strongly influences popular culture, especially its relativism stemming from its denial of objective truth. Hence, there are no objective standards to call everyone to act in certain ways toward the young, the weak, and the disabled. Instead, their vulnerability lessens their value because decisions are based on pragmatic, functional grounds.

For example, one couple could not obtain health insurance because they were "at risk" for having a child with a serious genetic disorder. They were willing to sign a paper promising to abort any child conceived with the disorder, yet they still could not obtain insurance.[40] While it is easy to criticize the parents for their willingness to agree to such a stipulation, they are responding to strong social pressures not to have children with genetic disorders. The underlying social value, which is part of genetic essentialism, is that an unborn child with a genetic disorder can be categorized as a child society does not need.

Biblical justice involves speaking on behalf of those who have no voice (Prov. 31:8–9; Isa. 1:17). It "is rooted in the nature of Yahweh himself who is defender of the oppressed."[41] Who are more vulnerable than the unborn? "They have no clothes, no money, no property, no power. They cannot speak or organize to defend themselves. If their right to life is not recognized and protected, then they are completely vulnerable to power and violence and death."[42] God frequently comforts anxious biblical writers by referring to his concern and protection when they were in their mothers' wombs (Job 10:2–12; 31:15; Ps. 139:13–15; Isa. 46:3–4) or infants at their mothers' breasts (Ps. 22:9–10). If God describes his relationship to the unborn and very young as one of protection, this should characterize our relations with them also.

Shedding the blood of the innocent was viewed as a violation of justice in Israel. Those who destroyed lives to acquire unjust gains for themselves were condemned (Ezek. 22:27–29). Those who sought to destroy the needy from off the face of the earth were viewed as wicked (Prov. 30:14). Infant sacrifice is repeatedly condemned in the Bible (Lev. 18:21; 2 Kings 3:26–27; Ps. 106:37–38; Jer. 32:35). Although part of the biblical prohibition of pagan idolatry, this demonstrates the abhorrence of killing innocent infants in an attempt to benefit society as a whole.

To "truly practice justice" incorporates a refusal to shed innocent blood (Jer. 7:5–6; 22:3, 17; Ezek. 22:12–13, 27–29). Justice demands that all people be comforted and nourished. According to the Bible, all people are images of God and thus should be treated with the same level of respect. Yet genetic essentialism categorizes people into those deserving of full respect and those deserving little or no respect. Some of the unborn are viewed as so genetically disadvantaged that their parents owe it to society not to bring them to term. These infants must be sacrificed on the altar of society's prosperity and the family's lifestyle. Some material things have become more important than life itself.

Biblical justice incorporates belief in the value and dignity of even the weakest members of the community. They, too, have an important role to play in society (1 Cor. 12:22–27). The Bible does not try to ignore or diminish the tragic reality of suffering, disease, disability, and death, but it responds by emphasizing the inherent value of the weak and vulnerable. It calls on all people to comfort those who suffer, not eliminate them. It offers the hope that even in the midst of disability and pain, people's characters can mature (Rom. 5:3–5; 2 Peter 1:5–9). Disability does not make life meaningless. As others respond to the weak and infirm with justice, they can learn more about themselves and develop a more godly character. Thus, 84 percent of mothers who chose to raise their children with Down's syndrome described their experiences as "rewarding overall."[43] People's lives are not destroyed when the disabled are allowed to live. God can use these difficult circumstances for good if we are prepared to respond to unwanted circumstances his way (Rom. 8:28).

## GENETICS AND DISEASE

In spite of the negative influences of genetic essentialism, genetic technology has the potential to do great good. "Genetic control could serve justice by improving the lot of the least advantaged in the distribution of natural assets."[44] We have focused on the values underlying our society that make the just use of this technology difficult. However, applications of genetic technology within biblical limits and with biblical values and motivations can serve humanity. An example of this sort of application is where genetic technology has made available recombinant human insulin. This corrects a deficiency that is clearly a disease and thus helps to relieve the suffering and incapacitation of many in a safer way than previous therapy allowed. The living who suffer are served; thus making this a just practice.

However, even this genetic technology raises new ethical problems. Products can be made in the same way that change other human characteristics. Questions arise about which traits should be open to manipulation. What should be regarded as diseases warranting genetic treatment, and on what basis will these decisions be made? Biblical justice provides guidelines for distinguishing between those traits that genetic therapy should legitimately treat as opposed to those that are not diseases and should not be treated genetically.

Biblical justice calls for the relief of oppression and discrimination against those who have been deprived, often through no fault of their own, of something God has declared good and valuable. Hence, orphans have lost their parents, the poor have lost all resources, and the sick have lost their health. Christians are clearly called to help the sick. However, genetic technology is opening a questionable route through which medical resources can be used for the relief of nonmedical problems. For example, human growth hormone therapy can be used to build strength for sports. Fetal genetic testing can be done for sex selection. Gene therapy may some day allow adjustments in intelligence or social skills before children are born.

While all new, high-tech, high-expense therapies run the risk of only helping the rich, genetic technology is particularly problematic in this area.[45] When genetic therapies are used to treat problems that are ultimately caused by nonmedical problems, like injustice in society, they will have the effect of exacerbating those underlying problems. For example, human growth hormone has been promoted as a way to help short children overcome the problems they experience from being teased, ridiculed, and discriminated against.[46] While some view shortness as a handicap, the underlying problems are social, not medical.[47] "Short stature is, to some extent, a natural variation and falls within the limits of normality. The associated psychological morbidity results from cultural prejudice. We do not usually call prejudice-induced conditions, which confer social disadvantages but have no intrinsic negative health effects, diseases."[48] Neither does society usually call on those discriminated against to bear the responsibility for dealing with the prejudice.

Little evidence exists for growth hormone's effectiveness except for children deficient in the natural hormone. Even if it did work, though, it raises ethical concerns. It shows how some genetic therapies could inherently violate biblical justice. If the shortest children in society were given growth hormone and grew taller, other children would become the shortest. The therapy would have done nothing to address the underlying prejudice and discrimination. Hence, the children now the shortest would suffer the same problems. Injustice would only be transferred to others.

Since human growth hormone is expensive and usually not covered by health insurance, only the wealthy can afford it. Thus, the shortest children would increasingly be poorer children. In this way, human growth hormone therapy for richer children would pass the "disease" on to poorer children. Also, since society will always have some who are the shortest, there will never be any overall reduction in the incidence of this so-called disease. Contrast this with a genetic cure for cancer. If effective, the therapy will eliminate or reduce cancer, which is always laudable. The poor may never be able to afford an expensive cure for cancer, but at least they would not suffer more because others have access to this therapy. The elimination of cancer in one person does not promote cancer in another.

The condition for which a therapy is used must be carefully chosen. The Bible gives a clear mandate for involvement in healing. God alone was Israel's Healer (Exod. 15:26) and Jesus' ministry involved much physical healing (Luke 4:18). The disciples were told to heal as part of their ministry (Mark 6:13; Luke 9:2; Acts 5:15–16). Throughout its history, the church has been actively involved in providing health care. In biblical times, little other than prayer was available (1 Kings 8:37–40; Ps. 35:13–14; James 5:13–16); however, medical interventions available at the time were pursued (2 Kings 20:1–7; 1 Tim. 5:23; James 5:14).

Healing in the Bible involves restoring people to health. They were not being made taller, faster, or more beautiful. In fact, the Hebrew term for healing means to restore something to its original condition, or make it whole again.[49] This implies that something intrinsically wrong or dysfunctional was being corrected.

Thus, overcoming the groaning and suffering of this present age is one way people can be faithful images of God (2 Cor. 1:3–7). Medicine in general, and genetic technology in particular, should be used to prevent or relieve suffering and disease. However, only those traits that are inherently dysfunctional or themselves cause pain and suffering should be treated. Having a trait that falls outside normalcy or that is not valued by society, does not justify its medical manipulation. In other words, *genetic therapy should treat only consequences of the Fall, not the results of genetic diversity.*

Arthur Caplan proposes that "we restrict the definition of disease to cover only those mental or physical states of human beings that are abnormal, dysfunctional, *and* disvalued" (emphasis added).[50] With the inclusion of the term *disvalued*, this definition does not appear very restrictive. Treating shortness and similar traits as diseases creates the idea that attributes that society disvalues and sees as below normal should be eliminated. In the same way, when intelligence, beauty, strength, skin color, and so forth fall outside society's limits of normalcy, their modification may be desired. If society comes to believe (whether correctly or not) that these traits are genetically determined, their modification will be demanded. As genetic essentialism becomes more pervasive, the elimination of the trait will be equated with elimination of the carrier, as we have seen with the unborn. People will become less sensitive to the needs of those less fortunate than themselves. In the current climate it would be a small step to view these unfortunates as candidates for euthanasia.

## CONCLUSION

If genetic essentialism is true, society can do very little to influence people's behavior. Hence, social programs to educate or care for the underprivileged will be of little use and should be abandoned. The root of the problem lies in genes. Social programs will have little or no impact on those genes anyway. While this places the burden on individuals to cope with their problems alone, genetic essentialism also undermines any hope these individuals have for change. If behavior is genetically determined, there is little these individuals can do about their own genes. They are left alone in a hopeless situation.

If society's problems are fundamentally genetic, only genetic solutions will improve the situation. If an individual's life and behavior is determined by his or her genes, those genes must be changed to improve the situation. Present technology does not allow us to manipulate the genes of those who are alive. This only leaves the unacceptable option of ensuring that those who have genetic defects are not born.[51] Hence the prevalence of fetal genetic testing to find those traits that parents do not want in their children. Because people are equated with their genes, eliminating the defective gene requires eliminating the person. Society is thus spared another problem.

*Genetic essentialism has the capacity to turn the womb into a symbol of humanity's ability to categorize and destroy those it deems useless and worthless. God uses the womb as a symbol of his protection.* God's justice and faithfulness commit him to comfort and bless all people, regardless of their functional abilities. People should likewise commit themselves to protecting the weak and vulnerable in society, regardless of their functional abilities. This is part of what it means to live out biblical justice.

Genetic testing could identify the causes of people's suffering and ameliorate or eliminate some of that suffering. But this assumes that the problem is distinct from the one with the problem. Genetic essentialism assumes that the problem is the genes that are the person. The Bible assumes that people are valuable, made in the image of God, but still have problems. In spite of how disabled or dysfunctional people may be, they remain valuable in the eyes of God. One of the ways God reveals this is through his faithfulness to every person and his desire for a meaningful relationship with each one (1 Tim. 2:3–4).

In response to God's just ways with us, we should be just in how we relate to others by defending the weak and vulnerable, relieving suffering wherever possible, and by sharing our resources with those in need. Hence, biblical justice could be promoted by the proper application of genetic technology. Yet tragically, there is a great danger that some aspects of genetic engineering will be used to benefit only a few and may even further widen the gulf between those who have and those who have not.

Finally, biblical justice gives us a way to deal with life in an unjust world. It is not fair that some suffer more than others through no fault of their own. Just like Job, we all have to come to the point of seeing that the tragedies that befall us will not be explained to our satisfaction in this life. But we can come to see them differently by viewing life through the lens of biblical justice. "To live justly is to rejoice in the good things of life and at the same time to be able to recognize that life is a gift even in the face of loss and destructiveness. To be just is to be open to the world as gift and God as mystery."[52]

If we refuse to accept the way God has created some people, maybe even ourselves, we are rejecting a gift God has bestowed on society. We are claiming to know better what it takes to be a valuable member of our society. But God's plans for each person are, to some extent, a mystery. We can accept his plans for us and for everyone else as part of the way he is providing for society in general. Or we can use genetics to guess which people with which traits are best suited for the society we want to build. Justice applied to genetics demands that people not be rejected for failing an arbitrary genetic test. Instead, they should be given what they need to become all that God intends them to be. While this path still leaves many tough decisions to be made, it is the only hope we have for a just society.[53]

## ENDNOTES

1. Karen H. Rothenberg, "Genetic Information and Health Insurance: State Legislative Approaches," *Journal of Law, Medicine, and Ethics* 23 (1995): 312–19.
2. Susan M. Wolf, "Beyond 'Genetic Discrimination': Toward the Broader Harm of Geneticism," *Journal of Law, Medicine, and Ethics* 23 (1995): 346.

3. Dorothy Nelkin and M. Susan Lindee, *The DNA Mystique: The Gene as a Cultural Icon* (New York: W. H. Freeman, 1995), 2.
4. Rochelle Cooper Dreyfuss and Dorothy Nelkin, "The Jurisprudence of Genetics," *Vanderbilt Law Review* 45 (March 1992): 320–21.
5. *Johnson v. Calvert*, No. X 63 31 90 (Cal. Super. Ct. 22 October 1990).
6. John Horgan, "Eugenics Revisited: Trends in Behavioral Genetics," *Scientific American* 268 (June 1993): 122–31.
7. Gerhard von Rad, *Old Testament Theology*, vol. 1, trans. D. M. G. Stalker (New York: Harper, 1962), 370.
8. Eugene Schoenfeld, "Justice: An Illusive Concept in Christianity," *Review of Religious Research* 30 (March 1989): 236–45.
9. Moshe Weinfeld, "'Justice and Righteousness'—*sedaqah mispat*—The Expression and Its Meaning," in *Justice and Righteousness: Biblical Themes and Their Influence*, ed. Henning Graf Reventlow and Yair Hoffman (Sheffield, England: Sheffield Academic Press, 1992), 228–46.
10. Karen Lebacqz, "Genetic Privacy: No Deal for the Poor," *Dialog* 33 (winter 1994): 41.
11. Ibid., 41.
12. von Rad, *Old Testament Theology*, 371–72.
13. Gerhard Kittel, ed., *Theological Dictionary of the New Testament (TDNT)*, vol. 2, trans. and ed. Geoffrey W. Bromiley (Grand Rapids: Eerdmans, 1964), 187.
14. John R. Donahue, "Biblical Perspectives on Justice," in *The Faith That Does Justice: Examining the Christian Sources for Social Change*, ed. John C. Haughey (New York: Paulist Press, 1977), 69.
15. Weinfeld, "Justice and Righteousness," 238.
16. Kittel, *TDNT*, 188.
17. Daniel R. DeNicola, "Genetics, Justice, and Respect for Human Life," *Zygon* 11, no. 2 (June 1976), 115–37.
18. Gene Outka, "Social Justice and Equal Access to Health Care," *Journal of Religious Ethics* 2 (spring 1974): 11–32.
19. DeNicola, "Genetics," 133.
20. U.S. Bureau of the Census, *Statistical Abstract of the United States: 1995*, 115th ed. (Washington, D.C., 1995), 135, 458.
21. Bread for the World Institute, *Hunger 1997: What Governments Can Do* (Silver Spring, Md.: Bread for the World Institute, 1996), 3–4.
22. Nelkin and Lindee, *The DNA Mystique*, 94.
23. For example, much controversy surrounded the recent conference on the role of genetics in criminal behavior sponsored by the National Institutes of Health. David L. Wheeler, "The Biology of Crime," *Chronicle of Higher Education* (October 1995): A10–11.
24. Lebacqz, "Genetic Privacy," 47.
25. Richard J. Herrnstein and Charles Murray, *The Bell Curve: Intelligence and Class Structure in American Life* (New York: Free Press, 1994).
26. Ibid., 548–50.
27. Nancy E. Kass, "Insurance for the Insurers: The Use of Genetic Tests," *Hastings Center Report* 22 (November–December 1992): 6–11.
28. Ibid., 11.
29. Dreyfuss and Nelkin, "Jurisprudence of Genetics," 340.
30. Patricia A. King, "The Past As Prologue: Race, Class, and Gene Discrimination,"

in *Gene Mapping: Using Law and Ethics as Guides*, ed. George J. Annas and Sherman Elias (New York: Oxford University Press, 1992), 95.

31. Wolf, "Beyond 'Genetic Discrimination,'" 47.
32. Dónal P. O'Mathúna, "The Bible and Abortion: What of the 'Image of God'?" in *Bioethics and the Future of Medicine: A Christian Appraisal*, ed. John F. Kilner, Nigel M. de S. Cameron, and David L. Schiedermayer (Carlisle, U.K.: Paternoster, 1995), 199–211.
33. Wolf, "Beyond 'Genetic Discrimination,'" 347.
34. For example, see National Institutes of Health, *Final Report of the Human Embryo Research Panel* (Bethesda: National Institutes of Health, 1994).
35. Noreen M. Glover and Samuel J. Glover, "Ethical and Legal Issues Regarding Selective Abortion of Fetuses with Down Syndrome," *Mental Retardation* 34 (August 1996): 208.
36. Ibid., 209.
37. Anthony Shaw, Judson G. Randolph, and Barbara Manard, "Ethical Issues in Pediatric Surgery: A National Survey of Pediatricians and Pediatric Surgeons," *Pediatrics* 60 (October 1977): 588–99.
38. Glover and Glover, "Ethical and Legal Issues," 207–8.
39. Friedrich Nietzsche, *The Twilight of the Idols and the Antichrist* (London and N.Y.: Penguin, 1990), 98; cited in Stephen N. Williams, "Bioethics in the Shadow of Nietzsche," in *Bioethics*, 112–23.
40. Lebacqz, "Genetic Privacy," 45.
41. Donahue, "Biblical Perspectives," 74.
42. Mary Meehan, "More Trouble Than They're Worth? Children and Abortion," in *Abortion: Understanding Differences*, ed. Sidney Callahan and Daniel Callahan (New York: Plenum Press, 1984), 151.
43. Glover and Glover, "Ethical and Legal Issues," 211.
44. DeNicola, "Genetics, Justice, and Respect," 132.
45. Council on Ethical and Judicial Affairs, American Medical Association, "Ethical Issues Related to Prenatal Genetic Testing," *Archives of Family Medicine* 3 (July 1994): 633–42.
46. Dónal P. O'Mathúna, "The Case of Human Growth Hormone," in *Genetics and Ethics: Do the Ends Justify the Genes?* ed. John F. Kilner, Rebecca D. Pentz, and Frank E. Young (Grand Rapids: Eerdmans, 1997), 203–17.
47. David B. Allen and Norman C. Fost, "Growth Hormone Therapy for Short Stature: Panacea or Pandora's Box," *Journal of Pediatrics* 117 (July 1990): 16–21.
48. Erwin Bischofberger and Gunnar Dahlström, "Ethical Aspects on Growth Hormone Therapy," *Acta Pædiatrica Scandinavica Supplement* 362 (1989): 16.
49. Michael L. Brown, *Israel's Divine Healer* (Grand Rapids: Zondervan, 1995), 28–31.
50. Arthur L. Caplan, "If Gene Therapy Is the Cure, What Is the Disease?" in *Gene Mapping: Using Law and Ethics as Guides*, ed. George J. Annas and Sherman Elias (New York: Oxford University Press, 1992), 134.
51. Council on Ethical and Judicial Affairs, "Ethical Issues," 633–34.
52. Donahue, "Biblical Perspectives," 68–112.
53. I would like to express my appreciation to the Summer Science Institute at Capital University, Columbus, Ohio, and in particular to Heather Smith and Jeff Holtzlander for the research support provided for this chapter.

*An Overview*

Advances in technology often precede society's ability to determine how such advances can or should be used. Advances in cloning technology appear to be doing exactly the same. When a technology's impact has the potential to alter the way a society views each of its citizens, further advances and implementation of that technology may have to be temporarily suspended—society needs time to evaluate the technology's various applications and to initiate guidelines within which safe application of the technology can be made. Physician and scientist, Frank E. Young, combines compassion and a genuine love for knowledge as he examines issues related to the sanctity of human life, advances in cloning technology, and the religious and ethical concerns that require thorough consideration. He offers policy options that respect the concerns of both scientists and the general public. Scientific research and advancement is a critical part of life, but its efforts must always benefit and never harm the public it serves.

Chapter Five

# WORLDVIEWS IN CONFLICT
## Human Cloning and Embryo Manipulation

### Frank E. Young, M.D.

UNDERSTANDING THE MEANING OF life is a basic human quest. Accordingly, each of us searches for the meaning of life using a variety of methods. A worldview, according to David Clark and Norman Geisler, is the conclusion we reach when we seek to explain the sum total of things.[1] Our approaches to developing a worldview are strongly influenced by culture, education, experience, and our fundamental frame of reference. In his provocative book, *Creating God in the Image of Man*, Geisler analyzes seven basic ways of understanding the world or reality: theism, deism, finite godism, pantheism, panentheism, polytheism, and atheism, and he contrasts these with an emerging neotheism.[2] For the purposes of this discussion, I will focus on the two views that have the greatest disparity: theism and atheism.

The conflict among worldviews is distorted by the tendency of contemporary culture to elevate science to the status of a god. The development of the scientific method, the dramatic changes from simple traditional medicinal therapies in the seventeenth century to the major interventive procedures of the twentieth century, the explosion of genetic information that began with the observation of genetic transformation of bacteria in 1928 by Griffith,[3] the discovery of deoxyribonucleic acid (DNA) as the transforming principle in 1943,[4] the ability to manipulate DNA in vitro leading to guidelines on the use of recombinant (rDNA technology),[5] and the Human Genome Project have markedly altered the technological landscape of the debate but not the basic issue of the meaning of life. Whether one has a theistic or atheistic worldview, one is bombarded daily by an array of new scientific "factoids." These discoveries need to be harmonized with one's view of the significance of life. Thus, the scientific imperative is a strong influence in today's debate on the sanctity of life as noted by Dubos:

> [T]oday, however, science and the technologies derived from it constitute the forces which affect most profoundly the environment in which men have

Acknowledgment: The excellent editorial assistance of E. Meadowcroft, who helped prepare this chapter, is greatly appreciated.

to function and to evolve. Either by choice or from necessity, the cultural evolution of man will be molded in the future by scientific concepts and technological forces. Even more important probably is the fact that science is accelerating the rate of environmental and conceptual change.[6]

When the genetic sequence of the human genome becomes available in 2004, there will be an intense examination of the significance of the meaning of life.[7] This contribution is offered as a framework for the coming debate on the sanctity of life as it relates to the fundamental issues of human cloning and embryo manipulation.

## SANCTITY OF LIFE

The understanding and application of the principles that shape the sanctity of life in relation to human cloning and embryo manipulation is influenced in large measure by one's worldview. In a theistic worldview, human life is made sacred by a holy Creator. Man is created in the image of a personal God who is self-existent, immutable, omnipresent, all-powerful, and the maker of all things *ex nihilo* (from nothing).[8] In creating humans in his image, God endowed humanity with a special status and with the responsibility to "fill the earth" (i.e., procreation) and exercise dominion over creation.[9] The sacredness of human life is emphasized by the condemnation that Cain received following the premeditated murder of his brother, Abel.[10] The very blood of Abel cried out to God. In the Ten Commandments, God commanded that humans should not kill, thereby establishing a prohibition against murder. Additionally, God prescribed a death penalty for murder based on the concept that humans are made in the image of God (Gen. 9:6).[11] As Murray stated: "The sanctity of human life resides in the fact that man was made in the divine image. This sanctity underlies the prohibition of murder, and validates and necessitates capital punishment for the crime of murder."[12]

The fall of humanity into sin is an integral part of the Christian worldview.[13] This sin is universal: "for all have sinned and fall short of the glory of God" (Rom. 3:23). Creation is flawed and must be redeemed from the consequences of this sin. Humanity, its relationship with God now severed by disobedience, is unable to restore itself to God's favor by its own efforts. Therefore, the Christian worldview includes the redemption of human life through grace. "For it is by grace you have been saved, through faith—and this not from yourselves, it is the gift of God—not by works, so that no one can boast" (Eph. 2:8–9).

Sanctity of life and grace are closely linked. It is the unmerited grace of God that offers redemption to humanity. The ethical system of the Christian worldview reflects God's unmerited favor and love for humanity and the command from God for people to love one another. Jesus clearly taught these ethical principles: "'Love the Lord your God with all your heart and with all your soul and with all your strength and with all your mind'; and, 'Love your neighbor as yourself'" (Luke 10:27). It is one's love for God that drives a person to love and to cherish one's own life and the life of another. Thus, life is sacred because each is made in the image of God and because God has determined that one's own life, as well as the life of one's neighbor, is equally priceless. The practical result of holding to this view is the protection of all human life.

In contrast to the Christian worldview of humanity as created, sustained, and redeemed by a loving God is the secular or atheistic worldview that contends that human life is neither special nor derived from a creative act of God. Instead, the atheist views all life as an accident, a mere chance of evolution, with no ultimate meaning and destined only for death. Life is neither sacred nor valuable; it is merely there. In the absence of God, as Geisler quotes Jean Paul Sartre, "[n]othing happens while you live. The scenery changes, people come in and go out and that is all. There are no beginnings. Days are tacked on to days without rhyme or reason, an interminable monotonous addition."[14]

Because life has no ultimate purpose, it is the right of each individual to use whatever means are available to extend or to end life based on the "usefulness" or "quality" of that life. The individual has only general "moral" guidelines with no absolute point of reference in making decisions about the value of life. In the absence of God, there is simply no absolute or transcendent standard of right or wrong. Individual morality becomes dependent on one's own feelings of rightness. Ultimately, societal decisions are made by an "ethical consensus." Under such circumstances, one might posit that any cell, somatic or germ,[15] embryo or fetus, could be used and manipulated for any purpose, if enough people agree that it is the "right" thing to do. One could also justify the ending of a life at any stage, if society generally agrees that this life lacks sufficient quality, potential quality, or usefulness. When people begin to talk of life in terms of its value, degrees of usefulness are then established—a person's worth is judged by subjective standards of potential and productivity.

This devaluing of human life stands in stark contrast to the purpose of humans as described by Paul: "For we are God's workmanship, created in Christ Jesus to do good works, which God prepared in advance for us to do" (Eph. 2:10). The Christian worldview portrays life in its broadest sense—there is life beyond the physical life we now experience. Our earthly or "good works" have as much, if not more to do with faithfulness and character than with mere productivity and have eternal consequences as well (1 Cor. 3:6–15; 2 Cor. 5:10; James 3:13–18). How we treat our neighbors, despite their economic or physical deficiencies, is more important than the positions or jobs we hold or perform (James 2:2–9, 15–17). God determines human worth; humanity does not.

## WHEN DOES LIFE BEGIN?

The very essence of the debate regarding the application of scientific and technological advances in the new genetics is embedded in the definition of life. What constitutes a human being? Is life more than the sum of the biological components encoded in DNA? Do people have a soul and a spirit in addition to a body, and if so, when is each imparted? Is there a point at which life begins or is it a gradual process? While theology helps to shed light on some of these questions, they remain largely unanswered and unanswerable scientifically, at least, at this time. Yet, if we are to find any resolution to the debates on the use of genetic technology, we must come to some agreement on what we mean by the term *human life*.

We can all agree that once it has left the womb, even prematurely, a fetus has reached the status of a baby (i.e., a living human being). The argument has been made that a fetus does not have the full status of human life until it reaches the point of viability outside of the womb. In fact, from a legal standpoint, a fetus of any age lacks the rights accorded an individual following birth, as evidenced by the legal status of partial-birth abortion. One problem with such a position is that there is no precise moment in time at which a fetus becomes viable because, with advances in medical care for premature infants, the survival rate of even the most premature babies has increased. Although the fetus may not yet be able to survive outside of the womb without the support of advanced medical technology, it is still clearly and recognizably a living human. Obviously, life begins some time before birth.

One could posit that life begins when the organs of the embryo are differentiated at approximately twelve weeks. It is at this point that the developing embryo becomes distinctively human. The effect of viral infections can be used to illustrate the vulnerability of fetal differentiation during the formation of the organs that occurs within the first three months of gestation. For example, in the first two months of pregnancy, rubella virus infections (German measles) result in a 40 to 60 percent chance of multiple congenital abnormalities that cause spontaneous abortion, while such an infection in the third month of gestation is associated with 30 to 35 percent chance of congenital heart disease.[16] Because the immune system is formed around the twelfth week of pregnancy, any gene therapy done on fetuses needs to be accomplished before that time. Thus, the advances in stem cell[17] transplantation may require the establishment of life beginning at a minimum of twelve weeks because the transplantation of genetically modified stem cells needs to be accomplished prior to the stage when the fetus begins to become immunologically competent.

The medical and legal considerations of informed consent and liability may result in establishing the beginning of life at an earlier period. For example, if in utero genetic therapy is considered for correction of a genetic abnormality, is the fetus legally alive at eleven weeks of fetal age? Who gives the informed consent, one or both parents or a separate advocate for the fetus? If there is an error, can a malpractice suit be brought on behalf of the unborn child? It is plausible that the attendant medical and legal concerns support the position that life begins some time between the fourth and the eighth week, a time when neurulation (the formation of the primitive nervous system) is complete and organs are rapidly differentiating. But can we really say that there is no life before then?

Research with in vitro fertilization, in which the egg is fertilized by sperm outside of the womb in a petri dish, has lead to the suggestion that life begins upon successful completion of the neural tube at fourteen days followed by fertilization and implantation on the fifteenth day. By this time, a number of vital differentiation steps have occurred: the division of the fertilized egg into a solid mass of cells (approximately thirty-two cells) followed by the development of a blastocyst characterized by an outer layer of cells called the trophoblast that will develop into the placenta, a hollow center, and an inner cell mass that will develop into an embryo. Subsequently, the embryo develops into a two-layered (bilaminar) mass of cells with a well-defined amniotic cavity and the development of a primitive neural tube. Within this mass of cells that constitute the bilaminar or two-layered embryo, neural cells differentiate at approximately fourteen days. At this time the preimplantation phase is complete and the differentiation of the various organs begins. Subsequently gastrulation occurs in which the bilaminar embryo is converted into a trilaminar embryonic disc.[18] Based on the absence of a nervous system until after gastrulation or neurulation and the certainty that the preimplantation embryo cannot experience pain, has no brain activity, and is not conscious or self-aware,[19] the Panel on Human Embryo Research concluded that the preimplantation embryo does not merit the same degree of moral protection given to children or adult human beings. They did not speculate when life began, but the Panel implied that human life could not begin prior to this time. However, if all of the complex events leading to differentiation of the fertilized egg to form an individual occur successfully, a new person will be born. The recent birth of a baby boy following the implantation of an embryo frozen for seven years not only demonstrates that embryos can be frozen for a long time but that the very essence of life resides in such embryos.[20] Some argue that these embryos do not invariably lead to humans, since 60 to 70 percent of the fertilized eggs undergo early spontaneous abortion. This, however, only signifies the fragility of life, not that life does not exist in the preimplantation stage.

The Bible contains a number of passages that establish personhood before birth (Ps. 139:13–16;[21] Isa. 44:24; 49:1). "Before I formed you in the womb I knew you, before you were born I set you apart; I appointed you as a prophet to the nations" (Jer. 1:5). Thus, since Jeremiah's life and vocation were determined by the Lord not only before his birth but before he was formed, inescapably he was viewed by God as a living person within the womb and a potential person before he was even conceived. These passages clearly teach that God knows each person prior to birth, that there is a purpose to one's life even before birth, and that every life is precious.

Therefore, I contend that life begins upon successful fertilization. Of all the points that could be chosen as the moment when life begins, the most clear-cut and conservative choice is upon fertilization of the egg by a sperm. It is at this time that the essential step to initiate life occurs and differentiation begins. Furthermore, this view is consistent with Scripture. Although the arguments cited above could result in the arbitrary legal definition of life at later stages, I have chosen the most conservative definition because of the biblical passages, the ancient medical principle of do no harm, and the inability to unequivocally establish a point for the beginning of life after the initial point of fertilization.

## SCIENTIFIC CONCERNS ABOUT HUMAN CLONING

No single experiment can be identified as the breakthrough that enabled cloning of mammals. Instead, as with all advances in basic science, there are a variety of studies and at times unexpected experimental results that culminate in the change of a field. As noted in the Report and Recommendations of the National Bioethics Advisory Commission, there have been studies over the last forty years exploring the question of whether a somatic cell still had the genes necessary for differentiation into a new adult. Additionally, the techniques that were required to harvest eggs, enucleate eggs,[22] and culture embryos were perfected as part of the development of methods for in vitro fertilization. The convergence of these fields, and explosive development of molecular techniques through the revolution in molecular genetics set the stage for the cloning of Dolly, the sheep. Some of the most critical advances are shown in Table 5–1.

**Table 5–1: Seminal Advances Leading to Somatic Cell Nuclear Transplantation**

| TECHNIQUE | IMPACT |
|---|---|
| Cloning of tadpoles | Nuclei from adult frog cells could be implanted into enucleated frog eggs |
| Techniques to harvest, enucleate, and transfer nuclei from embryos into enucleated eggs | Development of requisite technology |
| Harvesting, enucleating, and successful transfer of two-cell stage embryo nuclei in mice | Successful development of the blastocyst stage demonstrating pleuropotency of the cells |
| Capacity to develop viable offspring in sheep with enucleated eggs and blastomers at the eight-cell stage | Demonstration of ability of cells to be reprogrammed to produce an animal |
| Electrofusion of cells and egg activation | Ability to fuse cells and produce animals using all of the components of both cells, cytoplasm as well as nuclei |
| Nuclear transfer from late-stage embryos | Demonstration that nuclei from sheep and cow embryos at the 120-cell stage can be reprogrammed and implanted in enucleated eggs to produce calves |
| Studies on the mechanism of nuclear reprogramming | Elucidation of events that occur when a nucleus is introduced into an enucleated egg and activated usually by electrofusion |

| Use of nuclei from embryo cell lines to produce live lambs | Established the technical requirements to synchronize the nuclei at the gap phase (GO) to facilitate chromosomal replication |
| --- | --- |

The study by Campbell and colleagues resulted in the development of the techniques necessary to transfer nuclei from cell lines of early embryos into enucleated eggs.[23] Subsequently, Wilmut and colleagues[24] were able to develop lambs from enucleated eggs and nuclei synchronized at GO (the resting stage of chromosomes prior to replication) from late embryo, fetal, and mammary gland cell lines. The results with embryo mammary gland cell lines are summarized in Table 5–2.

**Table 5–2: Nuclei at GO Fused with Enucleated Activated Eggs**

| TYPE OF NUCLEUS | BLASTOCYSTS | LAMBS |
| --- | --- | --- |
| Early sheep embryo lines | 14% | 12% |
| Adult mammary gland* | 11% | 3% |

*Twenty-nine blastocysts were obtained in 277 attempts at somatic cell nuclear transplantation. One of these developed into a live lamb.

It is essential that this experiment be confirmed and careful genetic analysis be conducted to determine that the animal was the result of an activation of an enucleated egg by a somatic cell nucleus rather than the result of an unexpected normal pregnancy. (See Raymond G. Bohlin, chapter 17, pages 268–69.) Assuming that the experimental results reported by Wilmut were valid, there are a number of safety questions that must be addressed. First, will mutations accumulated during the life of an adult be passed on to the offspring and produce more inborn genetic errors than occur with normal conception by fertilization of an egg by a sperm? The answer to this question will not be known for many years. Second, will genetic imprinting[25] be altered so that a different array of genes are expressed from the maternal and paternal set of chromosomes? Normally certain genes, for unknown reasons, are expressed from each of the maternal and paternal chromosomes. Will the pattern of expression be altered? Third, will the aging that occurred in the transplanted somatic cell nucleus alter the life span of the cloned individual and influence the onset of cancers? Fourth, will the process of somatic cell nuclear transplantation influence the function of mitochondria thereby introducing an increased incidence of mitochondrial induced disorders? These obvious safety concerns in themselves require caution in the application of this methodology to humans. New medical technologies are assessed by two primary methods, safety and effectiveness, with safety being the initial concern. Regulatory management (i.e., oversight procedures) will need to be established for this technology. The cloning of Dolly sounded a wake-up call for those dealing with the regulation and ethics of human cloning and embryo manipulation.

## RELIGIOUS CONCERNS ABOUT HUMAN CLONING

Scientific or technological developments that affect personhood raise significant religious concerns. The conflict between science and religion is somewhat of an irony since it was the Western Judeo-Christian heritage during the Renaissance that encouraged scientific inquiry. However, at that time, science was viewed as a way to elucidate God's creation. Eventually, the controversy surrounding Darwin's evolution hypothesis lead to a discordant clash between theistic and atheistic worldviews and created a greater separation of science from religion. At the center of the debate is the question of whether humanity was created by God or whether it evolved. The development of a theology of evolution later led to conflict within the church itself.

More recently, medicine has changed from simple supportive measures to high-tech interventions. Medical technology has introduced procedures to extend, end, and manipulate life to such an extent that ethics committees have been established in most hospitals. However, in the absence of an absolute or transcendent standard, advice on the maintenance of life is offered on the basis of the subjective moral consensus of medical, sociological, and philosophical professionals. As Arthur Leff points out:

> We are never going to get anywhere . . . in ethical or legal theory unless we finally face the fact that, in the Psalmist's words, there is no one like unto the Lord. If He does not exist, there is no metaphoric equivalent. No person, no combination of people, no document, however hallowed by time, no process, no premise, nothing is equivalent to an actual God in the central function as the unexaminable examiner of good and evil.[26]

When there is no scriptural teaching that *directly* relates to a particular scientific question, we face a dilemma of how to apply God's Word. Two major approaches can be used to address the technological concerns of those with deep religious beliefs. The first approach undertakes a normative analysis in which one searches the Scriptures for principles that may apply. The second approach uses the concept of moral justice to evaluate the technology in light of the medical practices embraced by the religious community. This second approach returns us to a consensus of finite human opinion rather than an absolute standard.

A normative analysis of the Scriptures leads us back to the image of God or *imago Dei* (see Eugene Merrill's chapter in this volume). For example, Genesis 1:27 and Genesis 9:6 establish that one should not kill another human being because each is created in the image of God. Jesus extends this prohibition against killing to include hatred.[27] Thus, the respect for human life and the importance of responsible interpersonal relationships are based on the biblical principle of *imago Dei*. This concept of the image of God shapes the beliefs and actions of those who hold to a literal interpretation of the Bible as the Word of God and influences many of them to recommend a moratorium on all research leading to the cloning of humans.

God also gave humanity dominion over creation (Gen. 1:28). Scientific research can be viewed as a legitimate aspect of this dominion. As humanity attempts to harmonize the findings of science with Scripture, it struggles with the question of whether there should be any prohibitions on scientific inquiry. The conflict between the Inquisition and Galileo Galilei in 1615 illustrates the problem of ecclesiastical interpretations of scientific observations. While the question of whether the sun revolved around the earth or the earth around the sun had implications for the interpretation of Scripture, it did not influence the health and well-being of people. By contrast, today's decisions regarding the application of scientific advances, especially in genetic and medical technology, profoundly affect the way human life is perceived.

Recognizing the number of diverse religious beliefs in the United States, C. S. Campbell examined the literature of various religions and supplemented these with interviews to determine the prevailing feelings about cloning research in general and the cloning of humans specifically.[28] She developed a signal system based on the color of traffic lights to report her findings. *Red* indicates a preference for a full stop to any further research. The policy implication for red is permanent moratorium or prohibition. *Flashing red* indicates a desire for a temporary moratorium on research to assess the impact and risks before deciding whether or not to proceed. The policy implication for flashing red is a temporary moratorium until risks are evaluated and social questions addressed. *Amber* indicates a need to slow down and proceed with caution. The policy analog for this is regulation and adoption of guidelines by relevant professional bodies. *Green* indicates permission for cloning research and/or human cloning, assuming responsible behavior on the part of researchers. The results of her analyses are summarized in Table 5–3. While there is some divergence of views in cloning research, most of the religious groups favor a temporary or permanent moratorium.

**Table 5–3: Analysis of Various Religious Beliefs**

| RELIGION | RECOMMENDATION | |
|---|---|---|
| | Cloning Research | Human Cloning |
| African American | flashing red | red |
| Buddhism | flashing red | amber |
| Hinduism | flashing red | flashing red |
| Judaism | amber | amber |
| Native American | flashing red | flashing red |
| Orthodox Christianity | red | red |
| Protestant "Conservative Evangelical" | red | red |

| Protestant: mainline | green/amber | amber |
| Roman Catholic | red | red |

## ETHICAL CONSIDERATIONS

In addition to these concerns, there are a number of ethical issues that plague those responsible for developing policy. First, will this technology usher in a new eugenics? While the first forays into this brave genetic world are less threatening, the technology does raise the possibility of a new determination of who will live and who will not. Without ethical restraint, new technologies have the potential for being used to establish a standard for what a human being should look like.

Second, is it possible to develop embryos for use as spare parts? Associated with this concern is the question: Does the woman who donated the egg and the somatic cell nucleus own the embryo or does the embryo have inherent rights of its own? A case now before the New York Supreme Court will address this question. If the embryo has no rights, will scientists be permitted to develop eight cell embryos, disaggregate the cells, and use them for spare parts or to produce embryos and sell them for research?

Third, can chimera embryos (embryos composed of two or more genetically distinct tissues) be made from closely related species? Is it ethical to form cells at an early stage from human and baboon lines and introduce the resulting embryo into an enucleated egg? A patent was recently applied for by Stuart Newman, a New York biologist, on a method for making animal-human chimera embryos. Although this application was intended to precipitate debate on the legality of patenting life forms,[29] such possibilities demand caution and careful analysis.

Fourth, does the advent of somatic cell nucleus transplantation influence the value of human uniqueness? There is already conflict between parents and children. Would the quest for identity be intensified in clones?

Fifth, are there limits to be imposed on scientific inquiry? In his exposé of the grotesque and scientifically flawed Dachau hypothermia experiments, Berger stated that it is good science that usually involves ethical debate. As Berger noted, "inferior science does not generally come to the attention of the ethicists because it is discarded by scientists. Ethical dialogues deal with work of sound scientific but controversial moral content, and the fact that a debate is conducted implies that the subject under consideration has scientific merit."[30] The constraint of science is a delicate question. As a scientist, I instinctively abhor restrictions on scientific inquiry. Yet as Robertson noted:

> Science is not an unmitigated blessing. It is expensive, and its discoveries like the tree of knowledge in Eden expand man's capacity for evil as well as good. More knowledge is not a good in itself, nor is it necessarily productive of net good. Society, as the provider of the resources, the bearer of the costs, and the reaper of the benefits, has an overriding interest in the consequences

of science, hence an interest in the direction and the routes that research takes.[31]

Furthermore, it is questionable whether humanity can successfully deal with making right decisions without an absolute frame of reference for the judgment between right and wrong. As Arthur Leff notes:

> I want to believe—and so do you—in a complete, transcendent, and immanent set of propositions about right and wrong, *findable* rules that authoritatively and unambiguously direct us how to live righteously. I also want to believe— and so do you—in no such thing, but rather that we are wholly free, not only to choose for ourselves what we ought to do, but to decide for ourselves, individually and as a species, what we ought to be. What we want, heaven help us, is simultaneously to be perfectly ruled and perfectly free, that is, at the same time to discover the right and the good and to create it.[32]

This view is profoundly different from the idealist goal of science that I enunciated earlier: "[W]e stand as pygmies on the shoulder of giants sifting our observations through the grid of our prejudice in an attempt to approximate truth not merely to sacrifice it on the altar of our ego but to serve humanity. Let us pursue our research with the humility that a historical perspective demands."[33]

Finally, the greater good must be sought through the appropriate balance between high-tech medicine and preventative public health. Should we spend monies on expensive transplantation technology, for example, at the expense of low cost, but highly effective immunizations? Thus, in the midst of these many ethical concerns, the government is responsible to make appropriate policy decisions.

## POSSIBLE POLICY OPTIONS

During my career in government, I have learned that policy is formed on the basis of societal consensus. The policy makers endeavor to develop an appropriate compromise among discordant views, influenced strongly by public opinion, special-interest groups, the state of technology, and competing political agendas. In the case of the evaluation of scientific advances, the policy makers rely on scientific and medical experts. Yet, it is important to emphasize that there is an inherent conflict of interest within the scientific community that is more difficult to detect than the conflict within commercial interests of industry. The scientific community is innately and strongly opposed to the regulation of scientific research and may seek protection through consensus or under the first amendment. While there must be great care given to protect the legitimate rights of scientists, the reproductive rights of individuals and the rights of a pluralistic society in general must be carefully considered. In a comprehensive analysis of the legal status of cloning, Andrews concluded that "[i]t would be constitutionally permissible to enact a federal ban on creating individuals through human cloning. There is widespread public support for such a ban."[34] Therefore, all options are available, from an outright ban to federal regulations administered by the Department of Health and Human Services to voluntary guidelines.

Two major approaches are plausible at this time. First, legislation could be passed that would impose a moratorium or ban on human cloning. The comprehensive legislative hearing held by Senator Friske is a good example of how the legislative hearing and formulation of a bill occurs.[35] Alternatively, regulations or guidelines can be formulated by an administrative agency such as the Food and Drug Administration (FDA) or the National Institutes of Health (NIH) and implemented with the force of law as a regulation or as guidelines for voluntary compliance. The experience from the NIH guidelines on recombinant DNA research should serve as an effective guide to both the advantages and disadvantages of such an approach. Because this technology and the attendant studies involving human embryo manipulation strike at the very essence of personhood, the religious community must join the debate with others who are involved such as ethicists, scientists, physicians, special-interest groups (e.g., the pharmaceutical industry and patient advocacy organizations), and politicians.

## WHERE DO WE GO FROM HERE?

Today, science and medicine have progressed from observation and supportive therapies to intervention. While some have contended that humanity is empowered as cocreators, there is no scriptural evidence that the concept of dominion involves creation *ex nihilo*. Instead, the Bible focuses on humanity's stewardship and management of the biosphere. This concept of stewardship has fueled the expansion of medical advances under the principle of promoting health and well-being. Most human experimentation is done under carefully controlled conditions prescribed by the FDA. In the infamous case of the Dachau hypothermia experiments, however, bad science was conducted under an ideological imperative. As reported by Berger, these experiments were not only cruel and inhumane, but there were "critical shortcomings of scientific content end credibility."[36] Further, one of the principal experimenters, Dr. Rascher, collected human skin for making saddles, riding britches, ladies handbags, and other items. While everyone would rightly decry such brutalization of living people, we must also be careful to ensure protection for living embryos from brutalization that might take place in the name of science. While humanity was given free will, that free will must exist within boundaries.[37] The dilemma is the establishment of these boundaries.

Despite the initial goodness of God's creation (Gen. 1:31), the conflicts of the twentieth century clearly illustrate humanity's propensity to sin.[38] Fifty years after the Holocaust, "ethnic cleansing" reared its head again. Warfare continues, terrorism is a threat everywhere, and humanity's inhumanity seems to be the default policy. As Leff keenly observes: "It appears that if all men are brothers, the ruling model is Cain and Abel."[39] Therefore, humanity's ability to use technology for good cannot be blindly accepted. As noted by

Campbell: "[F]inally, although creation is 'good' and human beings are 'very good,' over the course of history humans have displayed an irremediable propensity to use their divinely authorized dominion for unauthorized dominion, to violate their covenant of partnership with God, and to create after their own image rather than the divine image."[40] In other words, all humanity is under the sentence of sin and, therefore, all humans, even scientists, are imperfect fallen creatures with a natural propensity to do great harm to one another.

It is possible to use the argument of dominion to both support and detract from human cloning. For example, it could be argued that once humanity justified, for the purposes of dominion, the use of technological advances such as the wheel, light, sources of energy, and interventive medicine, then human cloning can and should also be justified to fulfill humanity's responsibility for dominion. Besides, one could argue that it potentially offers a new procedure for a few infertile couples who want to avoid using surrogate mothers and donated sperm or eggs. This argument flounders on two grounds. First, there is no direct medical benefit to the individuals seeking to use this technology other than the desire to procreate. Therefore, the burden of proof for the need of this technology should be on its proponents. Second, God established marriage and ordained the unique "one flesh" union of man and woman (Gen. 2:24; Mark 10:7–9) within which children are to be born. One can seriously question whether human cloning would change the intimate relationship of procreation to mere replication, wherein the ideal parental responsibilities are replaced by a technological manipulation that bypasses the "ordained" method of reproduction. Moreover, there is a possibility that these children are more likely to be regarded as possessions and replicas of oneself rather than individual persons produced by the classical method of procreation.

At this time, the rapid rate of technologic advances are outstripping society's capacity to determine the appropriate legal, ethical, and religious positions. The potential cloning of humans and the manipulation of embryos, including interspecies chimeras, raise many questions about the very nature of human beings.

Therefore, a temporary moratorium on such research is necessary to enable societal concerns to catch up to state-of-the-art technology. To this end, I propose a five year moratorium on human somatic cell nuclear cloning and human embryo manipulation, including the development of animal and/or human preimplantation embryos, to enable the theological, ethical, legal, scientific, and societal issues to be addressed. To ensure a careful study, I recommend that Congress establish an independent commission composed of theologians, ethicists, scientists, physicians, and public representatives. In addition to addressing broad policy issues, potential legislation, regulations, and/or guidelines, the commission should hold public forums to ensure that all sectors of society are heard. Additionally, the Commission could undertake special studies as remanded by Congress. To do less, at such a time of uncertainty, would undermine the integrity of debate in our Republic and lead to the erosion of confidence in biomedical science. This is too important a decision to be left only to those scientists who are involved in and have a vested interest in the technology.

## CONCLUSION

The report of Dolly, a cloned mammal, has awakened the primal fears of humanity that were kindled during the debates on expanded reproductive technologies, recombinant DNA technology, in vitro fertilization sparked by the birth of Louise Brown, and the manipulation of human embryos. Following the example of the moratorium on recombinant DNA technology, it is appropriate to have a national moratorium on human cloning and embryo manipulation until the ethical, religious, and safety concerns are resolved. The implications of this technology force us to examine the very nature of personhood and the relationship between creator and creature. There must be meaningful, courteous, and professional discussions among all parties. I strongly recommend that those with deep religious beliefs become knowledgeable about the scientific, medical, and ethical concerns and contribute to the debate. As I have noted previously: "Christians must be prepared to bring the truths of God's word into the contemporary technological debates, confident that God is the Creator and the Redeemer. Otherwise, the Christians will be 'missing in action' in one of the more important engagements of the twenty-first century."[41]

## ENDNOTES

1. David K. Clark and Norman L. Geisler, *Apologetics in the New Age* (Grand Rapids: Baker, 1990), 139.
2. Norman L. Geisler, *Creating God in the Image of Man* (Minneapolis: Bethany, 1997), 15–22.
3. F. Griffith, "Significance of Pneumococcal Types," *Journal of Hygiene* 27 (1928): 113–59.
4. O. T. Avery, C. M. MacLeod, and M. McCarty, "Studies on the Chemical Nature of the Substance Inducing Transformation by a Deoxyribonucleic Acid Fraction Isolated from Pneumococcus Type III," *Journal of Experimental Medicine* 79 (1944): 137–58.
5. For more information see National Institutes of Health, Department of Health, Education, and Welfare, "Recombinant DNA Research Guidelines," *Federal Register*, 7 July 1976, 37902–943.
6. René Dubos, "Science and Man's Nature," in *Science and Culture*, ed. Gerald Holton (Boston: Beacon, 1965), 252.
7. The genome project will enable scientists to determine the complete genetic sequence of the functioning genes within human chromosomes. For more information, see Francis S. Collins, "The Human Genome Project" in *Genetic Ethics*, ed. John F. Kilner, Rebecca D. Pentz, and Frank E. Young (Grand Rapids: Eerdmans, 1997), 95–103.
8. Genesis 1:26–27: "Then God said, 'Let us make man in our image, in our likeness, and let them rule over the fish of the sea and the birds of the air, over

the livestock, over all the earth, and over all the creatures that move along the ground.' So God created man in his own image, in the image of God he created him; male and female he created them."

9. Genesis 1:28: "God blessed them and said to them, 'Be fruitful and increase in number; fill the earth and subdue it. Rule over the fish of the sea and the birds of the air and over every living creature that moves on the ground.'"

10. Genesis 4:10–12: "The LORD said, 'What have you done? Listen! Your brother's blood cries out to me from the ground. Now you are under a curse and driven from the ground, which opened its mouth to receive your brother's blood from your hand. When you work the ground, it will no longer yield its crops for you. You will be a restless wanderer on the earth.'"

11. Genesis 9:6: "Whoever sheds the blood of man, by man shall his blood be shed; for in the image of God has God made man."

12. J. Murray, *Principles of Conduct: Aspects of Biblical Ethics* (Grand Rapids: Eerdmans, 1957), 115–16.

13. Genesis 3:17–19: "To Adam he said, 'Because you listened to your wife and ate from the tree about which I commanded you, "You must not eat of it," Cursed is the ground because of you; through painful toil you will eat of it all the days of your life. It will produce thorns and thistles for you, and you will eat the plants of the field. By the sweat of your brow you will eat your food until you return to the ground, since from it you were taken; from dust you are and to dust you will return.'"

14. Geisler, *Creating God in the Image of Man*, 20.

15. A somatic cell is one of the many cells that compose the body *other* than the germ cells, which are involved in reproduction. A genetic change in a somatic cell is not passed on to the next generation, whereas a change in a germ cell may be inherited.

16. Lewis Markoff, *Principles and Practices of Infectious Diseases*, ed. G. L. Mandell, J. E. Bennett, and R. Dolin (New York: Churchill Livingston, 1995), 1461.

17. Stem cells are the earliest hemopoietic cells that form the various cellular components of blood. For a more detailed explanation, see F. E. Young, "Genetic Therapy" in *Genetic Ethics*, 177.

18. National Institutes of Health, "Report of the Human Embryo Research Panel," vol. 1 (Washington, D.C.: National Institutes of Health, 1994), 8.

19. Ibid., 37.

20. Frederic Golden, "The Ice Babies: Long-Lost Frozen Embryos Are Popping Up All Over," *Time*, 2 March 1998.

21. Psalm 139:13–16: "For you created my inmost being; you knit me together in my mother's womb. I praise you because I am fearfully and wonderfully made; your works are wonderful, I know that full well. My frame was not hidden from you when I was made in the secret place. When I was woven together in the depths of the earth, your eyes saw my unformed body. All the days ordained for me were written in your book before one of them came to be."

22. Enucleation is the process by which the nucleus containing one copy of each chromosome from the mother is removed from the egg. Normally upon fertilization the nucleus of the egg fuses with the nucleus of the sperm producing a fertilized egg with two copies of each chromosome. In somatic cell nuclear transplantation, the normal process of fertilization is bypassed by introducing a somatic cell nucleus from an adult cell into an egg from which the nucleus has been removed, producing two copies of each chromosome. Such an egg, under appropriate conditions could develop into a baby.

23. K. H. Campbell et al., "Sheep Cloned by Nuclear Transfer from a Cultured Cell Line," *Nature* 380 (1996): 64–66.
24. I. Wilmut et al., "Viable Offspring Derived from Fetal and Adult Mammalian Cells," *Nature* 385 (1997): 810–13.
25. Each of us inherits a chromosome from our father and our mother. Genetic imprinting is the mechanism by which one of the pair of genes from either the father or mother is expressed in an individual. For more information see: A. Chess, "Expansion of Allelic Exclusion Principle?" *Science* 279 (1998): 2067–68.
26. Arthur Allen Leff, "Unspeakable Ethics, Unnatural Law," *Duke Law Journal* 6 (1979): 1232.
27. Matthew 5:21–24: "You have heard that it was said to the people long ago, 'Do not murder, and anyone who murders will be subject to judgment.' But I tell you that anyone who is angry with his brother will be subject to judgment. Again, anyone who says to his brother, 'Raca,' is answerable to the Sanhedrin. But anyone who says, 'You fool!' will be in danger of the fire of hell. Therefore, if you are offering your gift at the altar and there remember that your brother has something against you, leave your gift there in front of the altar. First go and be reconciled to your brother; then come and offer your gift."
28. C. S. Campbell, "Religious Perspectives on Human Cloning," *Cloning Human Beings: Report and Recommendations of the National Bioethics Advisory Commission* (Washington, D.C.: U.S. G.P.O., 12 June 1997), D11.
29. Rick Weiss, "Patent Sought on Making of Part-Human Creatures," *Washington Post*, 1 April 1998, A12.
30. R. L. Berger, "Nazi Science—The Dachau Hypothermia Experiments," *New England Journal of Medicine* 322 (1990): 1435–40.
31. J. A. Robertson, "The Scientists Right to Research: A Constitutional Analysis," *Southern California Law Review* (1978): 1278.
32. Leff, "Unspeakable Ethics," 1229.
33. F. E. Young, "Reflections on Transformation: A Half Century Through the Looking Glass," in *Transformation 1978*, ed. S. E. W. Glover and L. O. Butler (Oxford: Cotswold Press, 1978), 455.
34. L. B. Andrews, "The Current and Future Legal Status of Cloning," in *Cloning Human Beings*, F53.
35. "Ethics and Theology: A Continuation of the National Discussion on Human Cloning," Hearing before the Subcommittee on Public Health and Safety of the Senate Committee on Labor and Human Resources, 17 June 1997.
36. Berger, "Nazi Science," 1435–40.
37. Genesis 2:15–17: "The LORD God took the man and put him in the Garden of Eden to work it and take care of it. And the LORD God commanded the man, 'You are free to eat from any tree in the garden; but you must not eat from the tree of the knowledge of good and evil, for when you eat of it you will surely die.'"
38. Romans 3:23: "For all have sinned and fall short of the glory of God."
39. Leff, "Unspeakable Ethics," 1249.
40. Campbell, "Religious Perspectives on Human Cloning," D11.
41. Young, "Genetic Therapy," 180.

*An Overview*

Although the evangelical Christian response to genetic engineering is mostly favorable, especially when it concerns itself with therapeutic applications, the issue over whether or not living organisms should be patented remains controversial even among many physicians, scientists, and genetic counselors. Who actually owns living organisms? Can a researcher manipulate a living organism and then claim to be its creator? C. Ben Mitchell provides a brief history of patenting in the United States, which has progressed from the patenting of living organisms, such as bacteria, to the patenting of both animal and human organisms. Present guidelines for patenting are carefully examined and theological concerns are raised that shed important light on whether or not it is appropriate to patent living organisms, especially living human organisms.

Chapter Six

# PATENTING LIFE
## An Evangelical Response

## C. Ben Mitchell

*The heavens declare the glory of God; the skies proclaim the work of his hands.*
—Psalm 19:1

*The earth is the LORD's and everything in it, the world, and all who live in it; for he founded it upon the seas and established it upon the waters.*
—Psalm 24:1–2

WHEN REPRESENTATIVES FROM MORE than eighty faith communities and religious denominations signed the "Joint Appeal against Human and Animal Patenting," on May 18, 1995, a number of evangelicals were among them. The fact that the Joint Appeal was organized by Jeremy Rifkin's Foundation on Economic Trends probably generated more controversy than the substance of the statement itself. Nevertheless, the press conference spun off a host of meetings and symposia focused on the issues at stake in the debate on patenting living organisms, tissues, cells, cell lines, and genes. A workshop on the ethics of gene patenting was held by the American Enterprise Institute a year later. About the same time, the American Association for the Advancement of Science (AAAS) began a dialogue on gene patenting issues. Similarly, in October of 1996, the Institute for Theological Encounter with Science and Technology (ITEST) in St. Louis held a workshop on the patenting of biological materials. During this same period, the Hastings Center convened a series of discussions on religion and biotechnology, targeting gene patenting. It is unlikely that such discussion would have taken place were it not for the response to Jeremy Rifkin's involvement.

There are a host of concerns about biopatents including social, legal, ethical, and religious concerns. As a person committed to the proposition that all truth is God's truth, I am convinced that every issue, including issues of science, has a religious dimension. That is to say, there is no sphere of human life and experience that falls outside a Christian worldview. The following account of my own views on biopatenting should be understood against this general background. What I will do in the following pages is attempt to address some of the biblical-theological concerns that I believe are at stake in this debate.

## REASONS BEHIND THE JOINT APPEAL

The affirmation of the Joint Appeal was extraordinarily succinct: "We believe that humans and animals are creations of God, not humans, and as such should not be patented as human inventions." This affirmation makes no claim about genetic engineering or biotechnology. While there may have been other signers of the Joint Appeal who oppose all forms of genetic manipulation and biotechnology, that is certainly not the case with most evangelicals. A number of evangelical groups are on record for their qualified support of the Human Genome Project in general and therapeutic uses of genetic technology in particular.[1] Moreover, they are generally supportive of the development of biotechnology. Biopatenting, however, is a separate issue.

The patenting of nonplant living organisms by the United States Patent and Trademark Office (PTO) is of fairly recent origin. Prior to 1980, the PTO refused to grant patent protection for living organisms, "deeming them to be 'products of nature' and not statutory subject matter defined by 35 USC 101,"[2] the patent provisions of the U.S. Code. On June 16, 1980, however, the United States Supreme Court broke new ground in its narrowly decided five-to-four ruling in *Diamond v. Chakrabarty*.[3] To be decided in the case was, according to Chief Justice Burger, whether or not "a live, human-made micro-organism is patentable subject matter." In 1972, Ananda Chakrabarty, a microbiologist at the University of Illinois, filed for a patent on behalf of General Electric Corporation for a novel bacterial strain capable of degrading components of crude oil. A genetically altered form of *Pseudomonas*, the bacteria was thought to be useful in cleaning up oil spills. After a lengthy appeals process, the Court granted the patent opining that Chakrabarty's "discovery is not nature's handiwork, but his own; accordingly it is patentable subject matter under § 101."[4]

As the applications of biotechnology continued to expand, increasing numbers of patents were applied for on living organisms. Because these patents were controversial and because the interpretation of the patent statutes was still undergoing revision, many of these patents were rejected by examiners and were, thereby, thrust into the domain of the courts or the Patent and Trademark Office's Board of Appeals and Interferences.

In 1988, in *Ex parte Allen*,[5] patent protection was extended to multicellular living organisms, namely, to a variety of genetically engineered oysters. Arguing that polyploid oysters were, once again, "nonnaturally occurring manufactures or compositions of matter" the Board of Appeals and Patent Interferences granted the patent. Donald J. Quigg, at that time Assistant Secretary and Commissioner of Patents and Trademarks, issued a statement elucidating the Patent and Trademark Office's policy on patenting animals. According to the statement, the PTO would, from that time forward, examine "claims directed to multicellular living organisms, including animals."[6] Also, the statement declared that "a claim directed to or including . . . a human being will not be considered to be patentable subject matter"[7] on the grounds that the right to own a human being is contrary to the Thirteenth Amendment to the United States Constitution. Quigg maintained that the Board of Appeals and Patent Interferences relied on the opinions in *Diamond v. Chakrabarty* and *Ex parte Hibberd*, "as controlling authority that the Congress intended statutory subject matter to 'include anything under the sun that is made by man.'"[8] Importantly, the phrase, "anything under the sun that is made by man," derives from the 1952 Committee Reports accompanying Congress's recodification of the patent law in 35 U.S.C.

Less than a year after *Allen*, on April 12, 1988, U.S. Patent 4,736,866 was granted to Philip Leder and Timothy Stewart for a mouse whose genome had been altered to make it useful in cancer research. These Harvard scientists had isolated a gene that causes cancer in mammals, including humans, and then injected the gene into fertilized mouse ova. One-half of the resulting female mice developed cancer within ten months after birth.[9] By introducing the cancer gene into the animal's germ cell, the cancer would be passed from the mother to her progeny.

With remarkably broad scope, the patent for the Harvard mouse covered any "transgenic nonhuman eukaryotic animal (preferably a rodent such as a mouse) whose germ cells and somatic cells contain an activated oncogene sequence introduced into the animal . . . which increases the probability of the development of neoplasms (particularly malignant tumors) in the animal." In essence, then, Harvard (in the names of Leder and Stewart) received a patent on any mammal whose genome had been altered to produce cancerous neoplasms. On December 29, 1992, Harvard received a patent on a second mouse. This time the mouse had been altered genetically to develop an enlarged prostate gland.

Even though human beings are not patentable under the existing protocols of the Patent and Trademark Office, human body parts have been patented. In an interesting California Supreme Court case, *Moore v. Regents of the University of California*,[10] John Moore brought suit against physicians who patented a cell line from his diseased spleen. In October 1976, shortly after learning that he had hairy-cell leukemia, Moore consulted physicians at the University of California at Los Angeles Medical Center. The attending physician, David W. Golde, informed Moore that his condition could be fatal and that a splenectomy was indicated. His spleen was removed October 20, 1976.

Either from Moore's diseased spleen or from tissues retrieved during follow-up treatment, Golde established a cell line from Moore's T-lymphocytes. Without the patient's knowledge or consent, Golde, and colleague Shirley G. Quan, applied for a patent on the cell line. Based on University policy, any royalties or profits arising out of patents obtained by employees in their function as employees would be shared by the University. The patent, issued on March 20, 1984, named Golde and Quan as inventors.[11] According to the record of the court, reports in biotech periodicals estimated the potential commercial value of products made from Moore's lymphocytes to be in excess of $3.01 million by 1990.[12] None of these dollars accrued to Moore because, according to the court, he did not own the lymphocytes. *Moore v. Regents of the University of California* both demonstrates that patents are issued on human body parts and illustrates the ways the courts typically treat matters of biological ownership vis-à-vis patents.

The history of patenting life was recently impacted by the effort of the National Institutes of Health, an agency of the United States government, to patent Expressed Sequence Tags (ESTs). ESTs are clones of small segments of DNA. These copies, called cDNA (complementary DNA), may be useful in the production of therapeutic products such as human growth hormone and EPO (erythropoietin). To be used for therapeutic benefit, the particular cDNAs must not only be identified, but their function in the gene must also be known. Once researchers have identified the function of cDNA, they can determine if and how it may be used to treat illnesses.

NIH researchers developed a technique to rapidly sequence genes using cDNA, making it possible to identify thousands of ESTs in a very brief span of time. While the ESTs had been sequenced, their use remained unknown. That is, even though researchers at NIH had identified the ESTs, they did not know how to use them to produce therapeutic tools.

Craig Venter and his colleagues at NIH filed for patents on several thousand ESTs in 1991.[13] In doing so, presumably NIH was hoping to protect their investment in developing the technology to identify ESTs. Once the attempt to patent ESTs became known, another cloud of controversy surrounded the United States Patent and Trademark Office and the patenting process. In November 1991, the American Society of Human Genetics, a professional society of over forty-five hundred U.S. and Canadian physicians, scientists, and genetic counselors, maintained that "the issuing of patents for ESTs is likely to do far more harm than good."[14] Much of the controversy focused not so much on the fact that patenting ESTs of unknown biological function violated the utility requirement of the patent statutes but on the patenting of human genes qua human genes. The debate made international headlines, leading to, for instance, an editorial in the *Financial Times of London*, calling for the NIH to cease and desist in their efforts to patent ESTs. In that editorial, the French Minister of Science, Hubert Curien, is quoted as saying: "A patent should not be granted for something that is part of our universal heritage."[15] Bernadine Healy, at that time director of the NIH, said in response to Curien's comments: "In fact, human and other genes have been patented by scientists of many countries. Indeed, most scientists and most governments of industrialized nations are arguing not against the patenting of genes, but rather against their being patented "prematurely"—that is, before their biologic function and commercial potential are adequately defined."[16] In December 1992, the Patent Office rejected the patent claims of NIH on ESTs. The PTO did so on the basis of the utility and nonobvious requirements of the patent statutes. Since, by definition, ESTs had unknown biological functions, the usefulness of ESTs could not be known. Moreover, since ESTs were identified by what amounts to a mechanical process, the identification of ESTs was deemed obvious to anyone skilled in the art.

HUGO, the Human Genome Organization, an international consortium of genetic scientists, issued its statement on patenting ESTs in January 1995. HUGO's position is that "the patenting of partial and uncharacterized cDNA sequences will reward those who make *routine* discoveries but penalize those who determine biological function or application."[17] The controversy over patenting ESTs is hardly over. In a recent meeting of the American Association for the Advancement of Science (AAAS), Lawrence J. Goffney, J.D., Assistant Commissioner of the Patent and Trademark Office, said that ESTs would be patentable by the PTO.[18]

Finally, in March 1995, the Patent and Trademark Office granted a patent on a cell line derived from a member of the Hagahai tribe of Papua, New Guinea.[19] The cell line was thought to be useful in a similar manner as John Moore's cell line. That is to say, the Hagahai cell line was derived from a person who was infected with human T-cell leukemia. The fact that the tribesman was not suffering from symptoms of leukemia gave researchers hope that his cell line would be helpful in treating the disease. The dispute over patenting the genetic materials of an indigenous tribe became so heated that on October 24, 1996, NIH filed paperwork to "disclaim" the patent.[20] Opponents of patenting genetic materials of indigenous peoples worry over not only the patenting of human genes but also the commercial exploitation of people groups in the Southern Hemisphere by the industrialized nations of the Northern Hemisphere. The Rural Advancement Foundation International (RAFI) has labeled this and similar practices as a new form of "colonialism."[21] RAFI charged that private ownership of human biological materials raises many profound social, ethical, and political issues. Industrialized nations are lobbying vigorously for "harmonization" of intellectual property laws worldwide with the ultimate goal of imposing patenting laws worldwide. In the South, issues of development and national sovereignty are at stake. Fundamental human rights are jeopardized everywhere.[22]

There are both good theological and prudential reasons why the policies of the PTO and the decisions of the courts with respect to biopatents warrant scrutiny. Biotechnology is expanding exponentially, and patents on human and animal biological materials continue to proliferate. Unless we institute a moratorium on biopatents to allow society to revisit the issue, we may do untold damage. Others in this volume have dealt with some of the prudential issues at stake in biopatents. In the following section, I will focus on specific theological concerns.

## THEOLOGY AND PATENTING

Although as University of Virginia ethicist John Fletcher has said: "You don't have to be religious to realize that there ought to be a debate about patenting,"[23] I argue that theological concerns are at the heart of the debate. While the law has been revised four times since 1790, the present patent provision states: "Whoever invents or discovers any new and useful process, machine, manufacture, or composition of matter, or any new and useful improvement thereof, may obtain a patent therefore, subject to the conditions and requirements of this title."[24] Patentable materials or processes must meet three primary criteria: novelty, utility, and nonobviousness.[25] Although the patent holder obtains the right to exclude others from making, using, or selling the patented invention, once the patent is granted, the patented item or process becomes public knowledge by being placed on record with the Patent and Trademarks Office in Washington, D.C. Patent rights confer exclusionary ownership or limited property rights for the term of the patent, including entitlements to royalty fees and judgments against others for infringement.[26] "It is common practice for a patent holder to permit others to use an invention upon payment of a royalty or licensing fee. In the absence of an agreement with a patent holder, a person who makes, uses, or sells the invention is liable to the patent holder for infringement."[27]

Composition of matter patents on living organisms are problematic from a theological perspective. Because a composition of matter patent grants an exlusionary property right in the subject matter of the patent, as in the case of patenting living organisms, the patent regards the patent holder as the inventor (or creator) of the living organism and grants to him or her the right to exclude others from the production, sales, or use of the subject matter.

The first affirmation in the Hebrew Scriptures is that "God created the heavens and the earth" (Gen. 1:1). As Creator, God is the Inventor of every living creature. The animals that are the subject matter of patents were already in existence prior to manipulation by human researchers. That Chakrabarty altered *Pseudomonas* and that Leder and Stewart manipulated oncomouse is undeniable. Neither Chakrabarty nor Leder and Stewart, however, were creators. Most Jews and Christians affirm that God made the universe *ex nihilo* (out of nothing). Chakrabarty and Leder and Stewart did not create *ex nihilo* but altered previously existing living creatures. Both the Court and the PTO regard the altered organisms to be, in Chief Justice Burger's words, "human made" and "not nature's handiwork." Regarding living organisms as objects of human invention is an affront to the Creator.

The oncomouse was not a human creation. The oncomouse was first a mouse created by God. Leder and colleagues did not invent the mouse, they merely inserted an oncogene into the mouse. The *process* for doing so may well warrant patent protection, but the mouse should not be patented as a composition of matter, much less should all mammals with the oncogene be patented (as is the case with this particular patent). "Everything under the sun made by man," simply does not include preexisting biological materials. The notion that a biological organism can be a human invention is not only an example of scientific and legislative hubris, but it is a blatant form of scientific and philosophical naturalism that should be repugnant to any theist. The exclusionary property rights conferred in patents redefine the locus of creatorhood. Oliver O'Donovan gets at this point when he says: "By virtue of the fact that there is a Creator, there is also a creation that is ordered to its

Creator, a world which exists as his creation and in no other way, so that its very existence points to God."

Why is this so important? In theological terms, patenting biological materials as though they were the stuff of human artifice risks blurring the revelation of God in the created order. This revelation is sometimes described by theologians as general revelation. Note the following formulation by the Reformer John Calvin:

> There are innumerable evidences both in heaven and on earth that declare [God's] wonderful wisdom; not only those more recondite matters for the closer observation of which astronomy, medicine, and all natural science are intended, but also those which thrust themselves upon the sight of even the most untutored and ignorant persons, so that they cannot open their eyes without being compelled to witness them. Indeed, men who have either quaffed or even tasted the liberal arts penetrate with their aid far more than enough of God's workmanship in his creation to lead him to break forth in admiration of the Artificer. To be sure, there is need of art and of more exacting toil in order to investigate the motion of the stars, to determine their assigned stations, to measure their intervals, to note their properties. As God's providence shows itself more explicitly when one observes these, so the mind must rise to a somewhat higher level to look upon his glory. Even the common folk and the most untutored, who have been taught only by the aid of the eyes, cannot be unaware of the excellence of divine art, for it reveals itself in this innumerable and yet distinct and well-ordered variety of the heavenly host. It is, accordingly, clear that there is no one to whom the Lord does not abundantly show his wisdom. Likewise, in regard to the structure of the human body one must have the greatest keenness in order to weigh, with Galen's skill, its articulation, symmetry, beauty, and use. But yet, as all acknowledge, the human body shows itself to be a composition so ingenious that its Artificer is rightly judged a wonder-worker.[28]

Notice that Calvin is not antiscience or antimedicine.

What I am arguing is that by claiming exclusionary property rights in a genetically altered composition of matter, the human manipulator is assuming a place that belongs alone to God, the divine Artificer. Thus, God's revelation of himself as Creator is blurred by the granting of a composition of matter patent.

The same argument should be applied to genes, cell lines, and organs. That the biological materials are altered in some way does not constitute a legitimate theological claim for "invention" and the exclusionary property rights that attach to inventions under patent law. That is how I understand the import of the phrase, "not humans," that follows the credo in the Joint Appeal statement: "We believe that humans and animals are creations of God, not humans, and as such should not be patented as human inventions." God created human and animal life; humans did not.

On this view, the *process* for altering genes, cells lines, organs, or organisms is patentable because the process certainly is "inventive" or novel. In fact, from my own perspective, the ethic of stewardship may endorse process patents. Philosopher Bruce Reichenbach and geneticist Elving Anderson, in their volume *On Behalf of God: A Christian Ethic for Biology,*[29] maintain that the divinely ordained stewardship responsibilities granted to human beings include three administrative functions: (1) to fill the land (reproduction), (2) to rule the land (as God's representatives on earth), and (3) to tend the earth (to cultivate and preserve the land). Under the aegis of the dominion (or stewardship) mandate, we are required to appropriately regard, care for, and cultivate the created order. But that is far different from assuming the mantel of the Inventor of living things and their parts.

Patenting human beings is doubly problematic. Not only does patenting human body parts (including genes, cells, cell lines, and other tissues) shift inventor status from God to the human manipulator, but patents on human body parts also violate human dignity. As Richard Land and I argued in an article in *First Things:* "Opposition to patenting *Homo sapiens* and their genetic parts is grounded in the unique nature of human beings. Human beings, alone among living organisms, bear the *imago Dei.*"[30]

In Scripture, humanness is not defined functionally. That is to say, human beings are ontologically distinct from nonhuman animals. Genesis 1:27; 5:1; and 9:6 all affirm that human beings bear the image of God. Genesis 9:6–10 demonstrates clearly that it is the image of God that distinguishes human beings from nonhuman beings. As theologian P. E. Hughes has said: "It is the image of God in which man was created, rather, which pervades his existence in its totality and is the cause of his transcendence over the rest of creation."[31] We thus learn from scriptural revelation that human life possesses a uniqueness, sacredness, or sanctity not possessed by other kinds of living beings. Thus, human beings are declared to be "made a little lower than the heavenly beings and crowned . . . with glory and honor" (Ps. 8:5).

By granting patents in human body parts, patent regimes revalue human beings. E. Richard Gold has argued just this point in his book, *Body Parts: Property Rights and the Ownership of Human Biological Materials.*[32] Gold maintains that "the advent of biotechnology creates a setting in which to value the body and its components as commodities."[33] Furthermore, he says, "to have a property right to the body or to a component of the body is to have the power to make decisions about the fate and use of the body or component."[34] Patent regimes, by definition, attend to economic values, focusing on the market for patentable subject matter. A patent permits the holder to produce, sell, or use the subject matter of the patent commercially. Thus, patents treat human beings and their parts as commodities to be bought and sold in the marketplace. So, in a much too real sense, the patenting of human beings and their parts is a form of biological slavery. Human tissues, genes, cells, and cell lines become marketable commodities. Such has been the case with John Moore's splenic cell lines. Moore's tissues became patentable subject matter useful not just for human healing but for marketable pharmaceuticals.

Interestingly, Gold points out that one of the judges in *Moore v. Regents of the University of California* was concerned about just this problem. Observes Gold: "Justice Arabian claimed that property discourse, and the commodification that he feared it represented, did not permit a wide-ranging discussion on the values inhering in human biological materials; in fact, he worried that by submitting these materials to property discourse, we would lose some of the sanctity with which he valued the body."[35] As I have just argued, human beings and human body parts are valued by God and should be valued by us in other than market values.

Furthermore, patent regimes assign rights of control. Control of the production, sale, or use of patentable subject matter is recognized by the law as a form of ownership right. Admittedly, there are different types of ownership.[36] Nevertheless, patents, by definition, assign a limited monopoly right in the patented subject matter. "Therefore," opines Gold, "if the current conception of property is not changed in the very near future, we risk allocating rights to human biological materials on the basis of an unchanged property discourse that ignores significant noneconomic values."[37]

The right to own one part of a human being is *ceteris paribus*—the right to own all the parts of a human being. The present position of the Patent Office is that a whole human being may not be owned because the Thirteenth Amendment disallows slavery. Kevin D. DeBré, writing in the *Hastings Constitutional Law Quarterly*, challenges this widely held judgment and correctly summarizes the Patent and Trademark Office's current stance:

> Given the Supreme Court's statement that statutory subject matter includes "anything under the sun that is made by man," human inventions would seem to be patentable subject matter. The PTO, however, has stated that "a human being will not be considered patentable subject matter under 35 U.S.C. 101" because "[t]he grant of a limited, but exclusive property right in a human being is prohibited by the Constitution."[38]

DeBré proceeds to argue, however, that the PTO's position is not consistent with either the role of the PTO or constitutional law. "Given the Supreme Court's statement that statutory subject matter includes 'anything under the sun that is made by man,' human inventions would seem to be patentable subject matter."[39] Thus, if it can be shown that patenting human genotypes does not result in the subjugation proscribed by the Thirteenth Amendment, it might well be the case that human genotypes are, legally speaking, patentable.

The Thirteenth Amendment provided Congress with broad enforcement powers to prohibit subjugation of one person by another, including the elimination of private and state actions that constitute "badges of slavery." "Under the Thirteenth Amendment, Congress is empowered to secure freedom, which may be described as the absence of restrictions, whether imposed by governments, by private individuals, or by environmental conditions."[40]

According to DeBré, subjugation would result through genetic engineering, "when the manufacture of a patented genotype creates inferiority in the resultant being."[41] Furthermore, subjugation of an individual with a manufactured genotype would include "disabling conditions ranging from highly visible restrictions on external autonomy (e.g., genetically engineering a person to be born of low intelligence) to subtle intrusions upon internal autonomy (e.g., mass-producing the same genotype throughout the population, leading to an erosion of the sense of individuality in one possessing the genotype)."[42] Additionally, a patent on a human life-form can be a badge of slavery where subjugation is a direct result of the patent. "For example, the property rights conveyed in a patent may give rise to constraints in the patented individual's external or internal autonomy."[43] Property rights granted under a patent, maintains DeBré, are limited to those rights prescribed by Congress. The patentee may recover damages from infringers of the patent. And although the patentee may manufacture, use, or sell the patented product, or assign or license others to do so, patents do not confer possessory rights in the article in which the inventor has patent rights.

Therefore, a holder of a patent in a human invention does not have rights in the physical manifestation of the patented genotype, in the trait expressed by the genetic manipulation, nor in any altered genotypes possessed by the recipient of the patented gene. An inventor holding a patent on a new form of human genotype would have an exclusive right only to practice the patent—that is, to make, use, or sell the patented genotype itself. The inventor would have the right only to enforce actions to exclude others from manufacturing, using, or selling the patented genotype. Once the patented genotype is sold and implanted, the patentee impliedly licenses the recipient to use the product.[44]

Since the patent holder does not have "possessory rights" over the genetically altered life form—in this case, a human life form—DeBré maintains that there is no necessary violation of the Thirteenth Amendment. "The patent holder's exercise of his right to exclude others from manufacturing, using or selling the human invention would not by itself give rise to socially imposed inferiority in patients of genetic therapy."[45]

While that may be the case, one wonders if DeBré's legal distinction is a distinction without a moral difference. That is to say, even though the patent holder is not entitled to possessory rights, does not the exclusive right to practice the patent and, thereby, exclude others from doing so, impose substantial limitations on the person whose genome has been altered? For instance, the person with the altered genome is, as DeBré seems to grant, a "human invention" and thus, a subspecies—namely, *Homo sapiens* plus the modified genome. Will this not negatively impact the psychology of either the modified individual or the culture in which he or she lives? Furthermore, if it were germ cell manipulation that took place, would the person's reproductive rights be threatened by the competing entitlements of the patent holder?[46] To the first question, DeBré answers: "One possessing the patented gene would feel no less human in relation to others than would one possessing an artificial limb or a transplanted organ."[47] DeBré may underestimate the psychosocial impact of amputation and organ failure. Women who have mastectomies, for instance, often complain of "feeling less than whole." To the second question DeBré responds that "It is unlikely . . . that any court would impose infringement liability under these circumstances, since the Supreme Court has recognized a fundamental right of privacy in certain personal decisions" and "has recognized procreation as 'a basic liberty.'"[48] Of course, who would have imagined that the Supreme Court would have granted a patent to Harvard for all oncomammals or that all the profits from the use of John Moore's splenic cell lines would accrue to someone other than the person whose spleen it was?

## SOCIAL JUSTICE ISSUES

In addition to explicit theological concerns, biopatenting also raises substantial social justice concerns. The Council for Responsible Genetics (CRG) highlights some of these social justice issues in announcing its opposition to biopatents.[49] According to the CRG:

*Patents make important products more expensive and less accessible.* While the biotechnology industry claims that patents are necessary to secure adequate funding for research that will result in marketable products, in fact, it can be argued that patents enable biotechnology and pharmaceutical companies to create monopolies in their products and, thereby, lead to artificially high prices.

*Patents in science promote secrecy and hinder the exchange of information.* Even though one of the requirements of the patenting process is the disclosure of the patentable product or process, the secrecy during the period of time between the filing date of a patent and the date the patent is granted tends to hinder the free flow of ideas. Furthermore, the fact that the PTO is significantly behind in processing patents extends this period of nondisclosure.

*Patents exploit taxpayer-funded research.* Because most basic research begins in university laboratories and patent rights are often licensed to biotechnology firms, taxpayers are effectively charged twice for pharmaceuticals and other products—once when they pay their taxes and once when they must purchase the final product.

*Patents promote unsustainable and inequitable agricultural policies.* We are just now beginning to appreciate the role that biodiversity plays in our environment. By holding overly broad patents on animal and plant species, biotechnology companies encourage farmers to grow genetically altered varieties with the promise of increased disease resistance and greater yields. The proliferation of so-called improved crops may well lead to the loss of diversity of traditional crop varieties.

*First World patenting of Third World genetic resources represents theft of community resources.* Corporations in the industrialized Northern Hemisphere are raiding the genetic resources of the underdeveloped and poorer Southern Hemisphere, patenting those resources, and manufacturing products that are then sold back to the South at significant profit. Some have argued recently that this practice is a form of biopiracy.

*Patents on living organisms are morally objectionable to many.* Not only some religious groups, but many others find biopatents and the commodification of living organisms endemic to patent regimes problematic.

Each of these objections to biopatents demands an essay of its own. There are many reasons to question the wisdom of biopatents. Nevertheless, the PTO continues to grant patents on living organisms and their parts.

## CONCLUSION

The call for a moratorium on biopatents was never intended to be the end of the story. There is still a great deal of discussion to be arranged between proponents and opponents of biopatenting. In my view, those who called for a reexamination of the practice of biopatenting were being courageous. In essence, they were functioning as a moral conscience in an age that is increasingly driven more by proceduralism than moral reflection. A blind frenzy of biopatenting is far more dangerous than a moratorium. If the history of research on human subjects has taught us anything, it is that we cannot be too cautious in considering the potential impact of our practices, especially in an era of rapidly expanding technologies.

The recent symposia and dialogues on biopatenting have improved understanding of both the potential benefits and the burdens that patents might impose when applied to living organisms. Most of our time has been spent in translation, helping one another understand and interpret the other's concerns. There is still much work to be done.

One area that warrants deeper exploration is the possibility of alternatives to biopatents. Perhaps there are other mechanisms through which biotechnology can continue to develop important products without resorting to a patent regime which, in my view, was never intended to cover human and animal biological materials. Surely there are ways to maximize incentives for pharmaceutical research and protect the investment of biotechnology companies without resorting to the devaluation of those organisms and parts of organisms that we believe transcend economic values. If, in fact there is not, then to use a biblical metaphor, we should refuse to sell our souls and our biological materials for a mess of pottage.

## ENDNOTES

1. See C. Ben Mitchell, "Genetic Engineering: Bane or Blessing," chapter 2 in this volume.
2. U.S. Congress, Office of Technology Assessment, *New Developments in Biotechnology: Patenting Life—Special Report*, OTA-BA-370 (Washington, D.C.: U.S. Government Printing Office, 1989), 7.
3. *Diamond v. Chakrabarty*, 447 US 303, 65 L Ed 2d 144, 100 S Ct 2204.
4. Ibid., 447 US 310.

5. *Ex parte Allen*, 2 USPQ2d 1425.
6. Statement by Donald J. Quigg, "PTO Policy on Patenting of Animals," *New Developments in Biotechnology*, 93.
7. Ibid.
8. Ibid.
9. *New York Times*, 13 April 1988, A1, A22.
10. *Moore v. Regents of the University of California*, 793 P.2d 479 (Cal. 1990).
11. U.S. Patent No. 4,438,032 (20 March 1984).
12. *Moore v. Regents of California*, 793 P.2d 482.
13. NIH had submitted patent applications on 347 fragments in 1991, another 2,375 fragments in early 1992, and 3,400 fragments later in the year. See Bernice Wuetrich, "All Rights Reserved: How the Gene-Patenting Race Is Affecting Science," *Science News* 144 (September 1993): 155.
14. "American Society of Human Genetics Position Paper on Patenting of Express Sequence Tags" (November 1991).
15. Cited in Bernadine Healy, "Special Report on Gene Patenting," *New England Journal of Medicine* 327 (August 1992): 666.
16. Ibid.
17. "HUGO Statement on the Patenting of DNA Sequences" (January 1995). Emphasis added.
18. Lawrence J. Goffney, "Notebook," *The Scientist* 11 (March 1997): 23.
19. "Patent Blather," *The Economist*, 25 November 1995, 87.
20. See *GeneWatch*, 10 (February 1997), Center for Genetic Responsibility, 6–7.
21. "Patent Blather," 87.
22. "The Patenting of Human Genetic Material," *RAFI Communique*, January–February 1994, 1.
23. Richard Stone, "Religious Leaders Oppose Patenting Genes and Animals," *Science* 268 (May 1995): 1126.
24. U.S.C. § 101 (1982).
25. 35 U.S.C. §§ 101–3 (1982).
26. According to the PTO, "a patent for an invention is a grant of a property right by the Government to the inventor (or his heirs or assigns), acting through the Patent and Trademark Office" (U.S. Department of Commerce, *General Information Concerning Patents* [Washington, D.C.: U.S. Department of Commerce, 1994], 2). Under the provisions of the General Agreement on Tariffs and Trade (GATT), the lifetime of patents was extended from seventeen years from the date of the granting of the patent to twenty years from the original filing date.
27. U.S. Congress, Office of Technology Assessment, *New Developments in Biotechnology*, 122.
28. John Calvin, *Institutes of the Christian Religion* (Philadelphia: Westminster, 1975), 1.5.2.
29. Elving Anderson and Brice Reichenbach, *On Behalf of God: A Christian Ethic for Biology* (Grand Rapids: Eerdmans, 1995), chapter 3.
30. Richard D. Land and C. Ben Mitchell, "Patenting Life: No," *First Things: A Monthly Journal of Religion and Public Life* 63 (May 1996): 20.
31. P. E. Hughes, *The True Image: The Origin and Destiny of Man in Christ* (Grand Rapids: Eerdmans, 1989), 19. For other significant evangelical treatments of the image of God, see G. C. Berkouwer, *Man: The Image of God* (Grand Rapids: Eerdmans, 1962); Anthony A. Hoekema, *Created in God's Image* (Grand Rapids:

Eerdmans, 1986); Charles Sherlock, *The Doctrine of Humanity* (Downers Grove, Ill.: InterVarsity, 1996); and see Eugene Merrill, "What Is Man?" *A Study of Old Testament Anthropology,* chapter 15 in this volume.

32. E. Richard Gold, *Body Parts: Property Rights and the Ownership of Human Biological Materials* (Washington, D.C.: Georgetown University Press, 1996).

33. Ibid., 2.

34. Ibid.

35. Ibid., 38.

36. Weil and Snapper point out that "the notion of property is further complicated by the variety of very different sorts of things that we claim to own. We may own a plot of land, or the trees on the land, or the fruit that we expect the trees to bare, or access to the space above the land. We may own a corporation including all its real assets, or the name and reputation of a corporation. We may own a book of poetry (that is, the material item consisting of paper and ink), or the poems contained in the book and none of their particular inscriptions. Obviously, these very different sorts of things are owned in very different sorts of ways. A car owner decides who may move the car and whether to destroy it in a steel compactor. A plot of land can be neither moved nor destroyed, but the owner decides who may occupy it. A poem can neither be moved or destroyed nor occupied, but the owner decides where it may be inscribed. Different sorts of things demand different notions of ownership.

"Although there is no single form of control over objects that characterizes ownership, philosophers often say that there is a 'bundle' of rights that are associated with property relations" (Vivian Weil and John W. Snapper, eds., *Owning Scientific and Technical Information* [New Brunswick, Conn.: Rutgers University Press, 1989], 3–4).

37. Gold, *Body Parts,* 168.

38. Kevin D. DeBré, "Patents on People and the U.S. Constitution: Creating Slaves or Enslaving Science?" *Hastings Constitutional Law Quarterly* 16 (winter 1989): 221.

39. Ibid.

40. Ibid., 230.

41. Ibid.

42. Ibid.

43. Ibid., 231.

44. Ibid., 232.

45. Ibid.

46. Noam Chomsky cites one cynical researcher who "remarked that as government-industry efforts are proceeding, some day parents might have to pay royalties for having children" (Noam Chomsky, *Year 501* [Boston: South End Press, 1995], 113).

47. Ibid., 235.

48. Ibid., 239.

49. Council for Responsible Genetics, *No Patents on Life!* (Cambridge, Mass.: Council for Responsible Genetics, n.d.), 1–4.

## An Overview

Today's rhetoric is latent with pleas to the religious community to refrain from imposing its moral will on the political life of America. Some in the evangelical world are succumbing to this rhetoric and removing themselves from the political discourse. Edward J. Larson discusses the history of religious involvement in Louisiana and Alabama and the role it played in preventing legalized sterilization of the feebleminded, the mentally ill, and the deviant. Though eugenics in the form of sterilization was overcome, new research has brought the discussion of genetic determination back into the public eye. Although genetic research offers great medical potential, our religious heritage must be represented in the political arena as a moral "check and balance." Our faith in God should not become so personal and passive that it has no more influence than a bystander at a congressional hearing. The Christian response belongs on the stage of philosophical and political discourse.

# Chapter Seven

# CONFRONTING SCIENTIFIC AUTHORITY WITH RELIGIOUS VALUES

## *Eugenics in American History*

### Edward J. Larson

SHORTLY AFTER THE RELIGIOUS RIGHT began reasserting influence in American politics with the election of Ronald Reagan as president in 1980, conservative Lutheran cleric Richard John Neuhaus critiqued mainstream efforts to marginalize the new activists in *The Naked Public Square*. On the one hand, this book denounced the secular "political doctrine and practice that would exclude religious and religiously grounded values from the conduct of public business."[1] On the other hand, it rejected the legitimacy of efforts by religious conservatives "to enter the political arena making claims on the basis of private truths."[2] Neuhaus's defense of a role for religiously grounded but rationally articulated arguments in public-policy debates appealed to many conservatives but had little apparent impact on mainstream culture—perhaps because of the author's political conservatism and religious position.

A decade later, following the political shift signaled by the election of Bill Clinton as president in 1992, liberal Yale law professor Stephen L. Carter took up the issue in *The Culture of Disbelief*. In this best-selling book, Carter asserted that Neuhaus was "surely correct to point out that the rules of our public square exist on uneasy terms with religion." Carter explained, "We are troubled when citizens who are moved by their religious understanding demand to be heard on issues of public moment and yet are not content either to remain silent about their religions or to limit themselves to acceptable platitudes."[3] He then related the story of two Notre Dame law students who were "mocked" by classmates for opposing abortion rights on religious grounds. "Had they but reached their moral positions with no reference to their religious beliefs, these students believed, they would have been welcomed into the classroom's version of the public square. But since they were accused of invoking, in effect, a forbidden epistemology, they were not."[4] Carter lamented this situation, and cited the standard historical examples of abolition and civil rights as instances where political movements founded on religiously grounded values triumphed.

According to Carter, religious arguments face the stiffest resistance in the public square when they challenge accepted scientific authority. Here, as he described it, a particularly suspect epistemology encounters a uniquely trusted epistemology, and he used the legal and political battles over creationism in public schools as an example. Elaborating on this point, Carter quoted Kent Greenwalt's observation, "The scientists are relying on premises that have so far been confirmed by common human experience," while the religionists rely on ones that "are less securely rooted in common human experience."[5] Yet, even in this least-favored battleground for religiously grounded values, there are encounters where, in retrospect, the religionist position triumphs over the scientific one. America's flirtation with eugenics during the first half of the twentieth century offers a prime example—one that should stand with the triumphs of abolitionists and the civil-rights movement.

## EUGENICS OF THE PAST

Eugenics grew out of turn-of-the-century developments in genetics, suggesting that human evolutionary development could be advanced through the selective breeding of people. According to its supporters at the time, eugenics "is closely parallel, in essential nature, to the improvement of domestic plants and animals; but it is clear that in man the methods of mate-selection, and of reproducing the best and forbidding reproduction by the most inferior, must be different from the methods employed in plant and animal breeding."[6] In short, scientists offered a means to breed better people just when urbanization and industrialization was creating an apparent increase in urban poverty, crime, mental illness, and mental retardation. Surely, the progressive response called for the application of scientific expertise to these problems, even if it meant the compulsory sexual sterilization of the unfit. The resulting eugenic sterilization movement carried the unqualified approval of the growing American scientific community. The United States Supreme Court added its blessing in *Buck v. Bell*, a 1927 decision by the great progressive jurist Oliver Wendell Holmes. Thirty-two American states enacted compulsory eugenic sterilization statutes during the years from 1907 to 1937. Opposition centered in a few religious groups, particularly Roman Catholics and fundamentalists.[7] Case studies of Catholic dominated Louisiana and fundamentalist leaning Alabama exemplify how these religious opponents challenged a scientific solution to a pressing social problem.

### Louisiana's Fight Against Sterilization

Louisiana became the site of protracted legislative skirmishes over sterilization from 1924 to 1932, during which time determined proponents led by the state mental-health establishment and Jean Gordon, an influential local progressive reformer and founder of a model institution for mentally retarded females, clashed with state Roman Catholic clergy and lay leaders. Long before the issue surfaced in the Louisiana legislature, the Catholic Church had emerged as the first major organization in America to oppose eugenic sterilization. This stance reflected both the Church's historic opposition to birth control as contrary to the "natural law" that linked sexual activity with procreation and its religious commitment to the sanctity of all human life regardless of eugenic "fitness." Social factors and self-interest reinforced this stance in the United States where church membership included large numbers of immigrants and the poor, two groups often targeted for eugenic restriction.[8]

At Gordon's request, freshman state senator Julius G. Fisher stepped forward in 1924 to introduce legislation providing for "the eugenical sterilization of inmates of State hospitals for the insane, of inmates of institutions for the feebleminded and of inmates of institutions for epileptics."[9] Senate committee amendments trimmed the proposal to the point where it only covered "persons committed in any public or private institution for the care of the feeble minded by the courts or legal guardians." Even though this left out patients at mental-health hospitals, it still included residents at Gordon's private Milne Home for mentally retarded females at a time when most compulsory sterilization statutes in other states only applied to patients at public institutions. Further, the authority to compel a patient's sterilization was entrusted solely to "the responsible head of the institution," acting with simply the "co-operation and advice" of the local coroner, the institution's doctor, and a psychologist. For the Milne Home, this meant Jean Gordon. The legislation omitted many standard procedural devices designed to protect patients, such as notice to the family and of hearings.[10] Nevertheless, it sailed through the Senate by a two to one margin. "Breeding of incurable feeble minded has become so rapid the asylums are being overloaded and the tax burden becoming increasing heavy because of it," a proponent argued on the Senate floor. "The operation merely sterilizes both male and female without otherwise affecting the normal sex inclinations."[11]

Such explanations of the measure, coupled with the prospect of its imminent passage by the House of Representatives stirred a prompt response from the local Catholic clergy. "The proponents of this act apparently believe that such a law will bring about a reduction in taxes and the practical elimination in time of the feeble minded," New Orleans' Archbishop John W. Shaw asserted. "And then we should have the millennium of supermen and superwomen as perfect specimens of the human animal, bred and reared according to the latest eugenic rules." He countered this elitist vision with a biting environmentalist explanation for social ills, stating that "if the poor were properly housed and protected against the profiteer who is fattening on their life's blood by charging exorbitant prices for the barest subsistence, we would not hear so much talk about the feebleminded being a menace to society." Shaw then turned his attack onto Gordon. "And the pity is that women should be numbered among the champions of such unnatural legislation," he declared. "But what can we expect of women who have abandoned the sanctuary of the home, and are fast becoming the arch-home wreckers, unlike their gentle sisters of other and happier days, who were noble home makers."[12] Following the archbishop's lead, priests throughout the state denounced compulsory sterilization as immoral mutation and urged their parishioners to stand against the bill. This had a significant political impact in a state where half the voters were Catholic.

Gordon fought back in a dramatic appeal before the House committee considering the bill. "If something of this sort is not done soon, our nordic [sic] civilization is gone," Gordon proclaimed in classic eugenic style, "and race preservation is the highest form of patriotism." Drawing on her experience at the Milne Home, she then told of "feebleminded" women producing "idiot" sons and "prostitute" daughters. One such daughter, Gordon declared, "is today in Charity hospital in New Orleans, and, I hope, dying as the result of a criminal [abortion] which is the only reason there is not a third generation of feebleminded persons already started." She then read a series of endorsements collected from prominent Louisiana physicians, including the president of the state medical society and two Tulane professors. "Shout from the housetops that I am in favor of this most needed legislation," one doctor wrote. Another described the measure as vital "for maintaining the purity of the white race in Louisiana." Directly challenging Catholic opponents of the bill, Tulane gynecologist S. D. M. Clark added, "This issue is not a clerical but a scientific one. The operation is not mutilation, simply sterilization."[13]

New Orleans' leading progressive newspaper, the *Times-Picayune*, pitched in with a series of editorials defending the legislation. Denying charges that it represented "some wild eugenic scheme to breed a race of supermen," one editorial described the measure as "simply a step to protect the community and the human race against the . . . unfit." Noting the logical connection between eugenic sterilization and earlier efforts to institutionalize the unfit, another editorial asked why no one objected to shutting up "these unfortunates" in institutions, but now some opposed performing "a painless minor operation" that could lead to the same results at lower cost and with less restrictions. "Which is the greater hardship? Which is the greater deprivation of 'inalienable human rights?'" the *Times-Picayune* asked.[14]

These efforts on behalf of the bill failed. With Gordon watching from the wings of the chambers, the full House voted to kill the measure by a slender four-vote margin. Both physicians then serving as state representatives supported the proposal, with one literally pleading for its passage, but key Catholic lawmakers rose in opposition. "Let nature take its course," one leading opponent declared on the House floor, adding his opinion that sterilization was "fundamentally wrong."[15]

Gordon rose to the challenge of this defeat with her characteristic resolve. Two years later, she returned to the next session of the state legislature with a new proposal for sterilizing both the feebleminded and the mentally ill. She then brought in a leading national speaker for eugenics, Judge Harry Olson, to help present the case for compulsory sterilization. "Formerly many believed that environment was everything, but science has repudiated that view today," the Chicago jurist told his New Orleans audience. "Surely the criminal is not an environmental product." Instead, he blamed criminal behavior on heredity in the form of mental defects. "The American child of the future must be well born," Olson declared. "We must drop out of the future blood stream the defective streams at present pouring into it."[16] Louisiana health official John Thomas chimed in with statistics and case studies about patients at the state mental-health hospitals. "The figures," Thomas asserted in a talk apparently presented several times during the year, "show conclusively that the care and treatment of this unfortunate class of people is an increasing economic problem and one that reaches the hearthstone of every taxpayer. The solution to the problem lies in the hands of the lawmakers of the state."[17] Those lawmakers refused to rise to the bait. Even though Gordon's 1926 bill contained somewhat greater procedural protection than her previous one, it suffered a similar fate.

Fisher again introduced Gordon's proposal, and it sailed through the upper chamber. This bill "passed the senate by a substantial majority in 1924," Fisher explained during floor debate. "Many more states now have this law in operation and find it is effective in lowering the percentage of defective persons." Specifically, he noted that "more that 6000 persons have been sterilized in the state of California during the last three years." Now, he claimed, Louisiana should catch up with California and other progressive states.

The leading Senate opponent of the bill, Grandy Cooper, interrupted Fisher at this point by asking about the mortality rate from these operations in California. When Fisher placed it at two percent, Cooper shot back, "Then do you realize that 120 persons have been killed in that state during these three years, all of them operated on against their wills? What right had the state to take their lives?" Later, Cooper raised a second fundamental objection to the proposal when he rhetorically asked Fisher, "And how are you going to determine just who is the proper person to sterilize?" Cooper then answered his own question by stating, "If we set the so-called mental standard even reasonably high and enforce the bill, there would not be another cotton picker born in this state—virtually all of our laborers are morons, or they would not be laborers." He obviously intended this backhanded objection to the bill because he then observed that "some of this state's most useful citizens are feebleminded." Denouncing eugenics as "a fanciful, theoretical, unproven theory," Cooper concluded, "My mind revolts at the whole theory of eugenic breeding of the human race."

The chairman of the Senate Committee on Health and Quarantine defended the proposal in purely eugenic terms. "At present there are estimated to be more than 8000 feeble-minded persons in this state, while our institutions can accommodate only about 400. For this reason the remainder must wander at large over the state, scattering the seeds of feeble-mindedness for the future generations," he stated. "Although they [could] be self-supporting, [sic] 400 are retained in confinement because their release would be a menace to the intelligence of the unborn children." Seeking to clarify this crassly eugenic argument, one opponent asked of these patients, "And you would make them sterile and release them, bringing others in to replace them until the 8000 you refer to have been operated on?" The chairman did not flinch: "Yes, this is just what he advocated, and what was contemplated by the authors of this bill—they wanted to reach them all." To justify this approach with a specific example, he made the implausible claim that "one feeble-minded man now living in Louisiana has been found to have over 100 feeble-minded descendants, and most of them have criminal tendencies. Without injustice or injury to anyone, these might have been eliminated by the operation of this bill a few years ago." According to this Senate leader, the "Feeble-minded have no god-given right to propagate."[18]

Louisiana's Catholic clergy held quite a different view on this point, however, and their followers waited to ambush the bill in the lower chamber. A correspondent for a local newspaper reported on the events unfolding on the House floor. "Like a bolt from the blue came the onslaught upon the sterilization bill," he observed. "The storm of opposition had gathered so quietly no one noticed its forming. Dr. Harrison Jordon of Rayville moved the [bill] be adopted, when like a shot Mr. Hebert moved that it be indefinitely postponed and Mr. Prophit laughed a broad smile from the floor."[19]

"God created these poor unfortunates just the same as he did legislators," declared Rep. Julius P. Hebert, who also served as Grand Knight of the Knights of Columbus, a Roman Catholic service organization. "This is one of the most vicious measures ever introduced in the legislature," fellow Catholic legislator R. L. Prophit added. "I hope that the House will go on record as opposed to making slaughter houses out of our feeble-minded asylums." Other opponents eagerly joined in the assault. One denounced compulsory sterilization as "morally and fundamentally wrong" and suggested, "We should kill this bill without mercy." Another described it as "humbug" and pleaded with his colleagues, "Don't make experimental white rats or guinea pigs out of these poor unfortunates." The reporter for the *New Orleans States* suggested that the fine hand of Archbishop Shaw lay behind this onslaught. Certainly the archbishop had sent an open letter to all legislators asking, "What man in Louisiana would want to feel guilty of having recklessly and wantonly voted in favor of a law that cruelly mutilates a citizen and thus robbed him of his God-given rights?"

Proponents valiantly tried to stem the tide. Jordon read telegrams from national experts praising the success of eugenic sterilization in other states. A colleague decried "the vast injustice that was being done by permitting thousands and thousands of feeble-minded children to be born in Louisiana simply through the failure of the state to take precautions to see that the feeble-minded do not reproduce." Another advocate stressed "the vast economic waste to the state through the absence of a sterilization law," and noted that "the operation was simple and without danger and there is no ill effect in 98 percent of the cases." He betrayed his own view of the mentally retarded and of the scant value of having a "defective" child by adding that, under the measure, "no one is deprived of his rights or pleasure except the right to reproduce."[20] Outside the legislature, many state medical and mental-health leaders offered their support through letters and articles.[21] The *Times-Picayune* appealed to lawmakers in an editorial, "Louisiana should take post with the humane and progressive commonwealths that are moving thus to relieve the coming generations of the menace of inherited insanity and feeble-mindedness and the crime and vice prolifically bred by these infirmities."[22] These entreaties failed. With Gordon again waiting in the wings of the chamber, the House defeated the bill by the slenderest of margins, forty-eight against to forty-six for.[23]

This vote marked the high-water mark of legislative support for eugenic sterilization in Louisiana. Gordon's 1928 proposal fell one vote short of passage in the state Senate, and was never considered by the House of Representatives.[24] In 1930, her fourth bill managed to clear the Senate, but failed to receive a vote in the house.[25] Before she could mount a fifth attempt, the grand dame of Louisiana eugenics died from a sudden attack of appendicitis suffered while attending a masked ball during the 1931 Mardi Gras festivities. In describing her remarkable achievements, the Associated Press obituary noted, "Principle among them were the child labor law passed in 1908 and the proposed sterilization act for the mentally incompetent which three [sic] times was lost and which she again was planning to propose to the next legislature."[26] When a modified version of that bill was offered in the 1932 session, it lost without debate on a tie vote in the Senate.[27] No further proposals for eugenic sterilization appeared in the Louisiana legislature.[28] The institutional opposition of the Catholic church had outlived Jean Gordon's best efforts. The issue was still very much alive in other states, however, and soon arose in Alabama.

### Alabama's Fight Against Sterilization

From the time that his institution opened, Superintendent William Partlow of Alabama's Partlow State School for Mental Defectives maintained a policy of sterilizing all patients released from the school. The law authorizing the procedure, however, only applied to this one state facility.[29] Partlow had long favored a more far-reaching eugenics program, however. After 1923, when he assumed the superintendency of the Alabama Insane Hospitals in addition to his responsibilities at the State School, Partlow took a particular interest in the role of sterilization in preventing mental illness and promoting public mental health. For example, in a 1928 address on ways to combat the mental stress of life in a modern industrial society, he observed, "A creed which includes high standards of living with temperance in all things for the normal, and a program of sterilization of the insane, mental defective, repeating criminal, drug and alcoholic addicts would go a long way in the right direction."[30] The Medical Association of Alabama (MAA) endorsed this approach the same year, when its president recommended sterilizing "all convicted criminals and insane cases committed to the State insane asylum." In a classic eugenic affirmation, the MAA president concluded, "It is not humane to allow the insane to propagate his species to the injury of himself and the public."[31]

Partlow strove to generate support for an expanded state sterilization program by writing and speaking about the social and economic cost of hereditary degeneracy.[32] Reporting largely on the fruits of his own labors, he asserted in a 1934 official report, "There is a growing, popular demand for a more comprehensive sterilization law in Alabama."[33] By the following year, Partlow and his fellow eugenicists were ready to seek such a statute. The proposal reflected the big plans of a big man. By 1935, Partlow had built an empire in Tuscaloosa as superintendent, first of the Partlow State School, and later of the Alabama Insane Hospitals. He had developed a statewide power base during multiple terms presiding over the MAA and several of its key committees, and he reached beyond Alabama through his involvement in regional and national professional organizations that would culminate in his election as president of the Southern Psychiatric Association for 1936–37.[34] Partlow also had become the Deep South's leading eugenicist and one of the few who walked on a national stage. He clearly had grown frustrated with Alabama's limited sterilization program.

Although Partlow could (and did) sterilize every patient departing the Partlow State School, this only reached a small fraction of those whom he considered eugenically unfit.[35]

Indeed, in this respect, Alabama's existing law covered fewer people than did any of the sterilization statutes then on the books in thirty-one other American states. Even though those other statutes typically included greater procedural protection than the Alabama law, they applied to inmates at a broader range of state institutions than simply a single small facility for the mentally retarded.[36] But even the efforts of these other states were inadequate for Partlow. Indeed, only the plan recently announced by Nazi Germany was sufficiently bold for some in Partlow's camp. Partlow's colleague and fellow eugenicist, Alabama State Health Officer, J. N. Baker, expressed this clearly to the state legislature early in its 1935 session, when he praised Germany's "bold experiment in mass sterilization" that he predicted would reach "some 400,000 of the population." After comparing the cost of sterilizing this many people with the cost of custodial care, he then estimated "that, after several decades, hundreds of millions of marks will be saved each year as a result of the diminution of expenditures for patients with hereditary diseases." Baker went on to call for a similar program in Alabama, and specifically to endorse legislation toward that end drafted by Partlow.[37] Endorsements for the proposal also came from the MAA, the Alabama Division of the American Association of University Women, and the state Society for Mental Hygiene.[38] Tuscaloosa's two young state legislators, Representative Aubrey Dominick and Senator Hayse Tucker, introduced the bill at the beginning of the 1935 session.[39]

Partlow's proposal would cover more individuals and offer less procedural protection than any sterilization program in the United States. First, it gave unlimited discretion to the superintendent of any state institution for the mentally ill or retarded to sterilize any or all patients upon their release. Next, it empowered a three-member board composed of the Superintendent of the Alabama Insane Hospitals (Partlow), the State Health Officer (Baker), and the Chief Medical Officer of the state prison, acting by majority vote, to sterilize "any sexual pervert, sadist, homosexualist, masochist, sodomist, or any other grave form of sexual perversion, or any prisoner who has twice been convicted of rape" or thrice imprisoned for any offense. Finally, it authorized county public-health committees to sterilize inmates of local custodial institutions, such as reform schools, and individuals who were either a "mental deficient of any grade," or "habitually and constantly dependent upon public relief or support by charity." In each instance, the decision to sterilize required "evidence of mental or moral degeneracy liable to be inherited," but only individuals facing sterilization by order of county health committees could appeal, and then only to the Superintendent of the Alabama Insane Hospitals (Partlow) and his staff. No right of judicial review existed: Mental-health experts made all decisions.[40]

Not surprisingly, given its broad sweep, the proposal was front-page news throughout the state and, according to one observer, generated "the longest and most intense debate of the entire 1935 legislative session."[41] Leading proponents included the state medical community and public-health officials, Partlow's state legislators (who led the floor fight in both the Senate and House of Representatives), and two major newspapers, the *Montgomery Advertiser* and the *Birmingham News*.[42]

Their arguments for the measure stressed scientific authority and common sense. "It is a rule of biology that excellence derives from excellence, that viciousness derives from viciousness," the *Advertiser* declared in one representative editorial, adding "that there is not a tenant farmer in Alabama who does not know that no exceptionally gifted man is ever born of imbeciles, and that no good man is born from a long line of vicious forebears."[43] With Partlow at his side, a University of Alabama biology professor warned in a public lecture "that the destruction of the human race is almost as certain as the dying out of the great dinosaurs of past ages, unless mankind does something about overproduction of people who are mentally and physically defective."[44] The *News* editorialized that, by adopting the bill, "Alabama will have taken a long step toward the social, mental and physical betterment of its people, which ought in time to be reflected in economic improvement for the State."[45] It later added that "the law would work no physical injury upon anyone. It would merely prevent the mentally unfit from reproducing their kind."[46] Although, by this comment, the *News* intended to reassure legislators and the public that sterilization did not diminish a person's sexual pleasure, it betrayed the eugenicist's typical disregard for the value of procreating a defective child.

Opponents of the measure focused on its broad reach and lack of procedural safeguards. State trade-union leaders, for example, objected "that there is nothing in the bill to prevent a labor man from being 'railroaded' into an institution where he could be sterilized on 'suspicion' of insanity or feeble-mindedness."[47] The national American Civil Liberties Union (ACLU) registered its opposition to the bill's sweeping authorization for sterilizing criminals.[48] After cautioning that "the modern science of Eugenics has yet to prove its efficacy," the state's Baptist newspaper editorialized that "the proposed bill gives too much power to the superintendent of any state eleemosynary institution [an institution that depends upon donations or charity]."[49] In a private letter to Governor Bibb Graves, the editor of the *Alabama Herald* wrote that "seeing how many elements, some in favor of sterilization, are bitterly opposed to the bill's great authority and loose language, I called Doctor Partlow on the telephone and asked him if he would be willing to save you any embarrassment by releasing the Senators he has pledged to vote for the bill."[50] When Partlow refused this request, the battle gained intensity.

The stiffest opposition came from Alabama's small Roman Catholic community, then centered in Mobile and Birmingham. Describing the bill as "the most far-reaching" legislation ever introduced in Alabama, the state's Catholic newspaper commented, "we wonder what our civilization is coming to when medical, political and economic leaders of a great state such as Alabama could have their viewpoint warped to the point where they could in good conscience and without shame introduce a measure fraught with such vicious, such inhumane, such criminal possibilities."[51] Prominent Alabama Catholics, including physicians, attorneys, and educators, expressed their opposition to their lawmakers in public hearings and private letters.[52] Father William F. Obering, a philosophy and sociology professor at a small Catholic college in Mobile, helped set the tone for this resistance in a series of articles and speeches articulating the moral arguments against compulsory sterilization, which he denounced as violating "the natural rights of man."[53] The Alabama Council of the Knights of Columbus crudely expressed this position in a resolution branding the sterilization measure as "unchristian, unnatural, ungodly and therefore pagan."[54] The Mobile legislative delegation, which included the state's only Catholic legislators, raised the issue in both the Senate and House of Representatives.[55] Some Protestants voiced similar concerns, such as the Baptist lawmaker who claimed to find "in the Bible all the warrant he required to vote against the bill."[56] Indeed, editorials in the state's Baptist and Methodist newspapers objected to the legislation, but the vociferous Catholic resistance prompted the greatest response.[57] For example, in the heat of the floor debate, one senator lashed out at the Roman church for opposing sterilization, as it "had ever opposed scientific progress." As he began recounting various historical episodes to support this allegation, Mobile's senator reminded him that the father of modern genetics, Gregor Mendel, was a Catholic monk.[58]

Both religious and nonreligious opponents cited the growing body of academic evidence against eugenics, which was just then beginning to accumulate as leading social scientists and geneticists began turning from nature to nurture and from simple Mendelian factors to complex genetic relationships in explaining human behavior. Obering, for example, cited leading national authorities ranging from sociologist Franz Boas and psychiatrist Abraham Myerson to biologist H. S. Jennings for the basic proposition that "the sterilization proposal as a measure of social betterment not only does not attain this objective, but is socially harmful."[59] This was not enough to overcome the support of local physicians and public-health officers, however, as both houses of the State legislature overwhelmingly passed the measure and sent it to Governor Bibb Graves for his signature.[60]

Both proponents and opponents of eugenic sterilization expressed surprise when Governor Graves vetoed the bill.[61] A delegation of Catholics from Mobile had visited the governor to urge his veto but that probably had little impact.[62] The popular, strong-willed Graves first won the governorship in 1926 with the backing of the militantly anti-Catholic Ku Klux Klan and once served as a Grand Dragon in that racist organization. Even though he later distanced himself from the Klan and became an ardent New Deal progressive, this shift does not explain the veto because progressives typically favored eugenics. Graves, however, always defied simple categorization. He had the blue blood of earlier Alabama governors flowing through his veins and a Yale law degree but won the governorship as an outsider opposed by every major newspaper in the state. One biographer compared the man to a "colossus, his feet firmly planted on the opposite foundations of a new progressivism and a close association with the most reactionary terrorist organization ever to appear in America."[63] Perhaps as a result, Graves had a mind of his own on many matters and often played his cards close to his vest.

After the bill passed, Graves asked the Alabama Supreme Court for an advisory opinion regarding its constitutionality. The court promptly and unanimously opined that the proposal violated the Due Process Clauses of both the state and federal constitutions. "We think that the sterilization of a person is such an injury to the person," the court wrote, "that this cannot be done without a hearing [or] notice before a duly constituted tribunal or board, and, if this is not a court, then with the untrammeled right of appeal to a court for a judicial review from the finding of the board or commission adjudging him a fit subject for sterilization."[64] Graves then convened a public hearing where proponents led by Partlow and opponents led by church leaders from Mobile presented sharply conflicting testimony regarding the scientific evidence for eugenic sterilization.[65]

Up to the last minute, Dominick believed that Graves would sign the bill, and the legislator spent several days working with the governor's legal advisor preparing executive amendments designed to deal with the constitutional issues raised by the court's advisory opinion.[66] Even Partlow expressed confidence only days before the veto, when he wrote Graves, "Knowing your views and beliefs in the need for such legislation . . . I am inclined to congratulate you upon this sterilization legislation as being one of the most forward-looking, progressive and constructive measures of your present administration."[67] In the end, however, the independent-minded governor concluded "that until the scientists themselves reach further agreement and until we are in a position to supply all concerned such legal and medical and court expenses as would be necessary for the protection of their individuals rights, this is not a wise policy for Alabama to adopt."[68]

Rather than attempt to override this veto simply to enact an unconstitutional statute, Dominick immediately reintroduced a virtually identical bill with added provisions for decisions by an expert Medical Board of Sterilization and appeals to the state supreme court.[69] Again the measure passed both houses of the legislature by overwhelming margins, only to be vetoed by the governor.[70] This time, Graves penned an emotional veto message stressing the physical risks in sterilizing women. "We know that the enforcement of the provisions of this bill as to girls and young women will entail major operations upon many thousands," he wrote. "Those who will die are innocent and pure, have committed no offense against God or man, save that in the opinion of experts they should never have been born." Sexual segregation, Graves maintained, was the better, albeit more costly, way to protect society.[71] After counting the votes of administration loyalists committed to back the governor, Dominick gave up the fight without attempting to override the veto.[72]

A clue to explain Graves's action may lie in the letters that he received prior to vetoing the measure. Nearly all of those supporting the bill were from physicians and experts, while those opposing it came from a broad spectrum of individuals ranging from lawyers and business owners to an anonymous "Citizen of Mobile" with a husband temporarily in a state mental-health hospital due to a head injury. "We are both in our twenties," the anonymous Mobilian pleaded, "and such an act [of sterilization] would simply ruin the lives of us both."[73] Twenty-five years earlier, Partlow had dismissed the idea of sterilizing habitual criminals as impractical because "maybe the criminal would out-vote us when we vote on such a matter as that."[74] Perhaps Graves appreciated this crude political calculus, especially when it involved a measure as far-reaching as Partlow's 1935 proposal. Privately, Partlow attributed the veto to the governor's "religious and political scruples," which also suggests some connection to Graves's membership in the small, fundamentalist Church of Christ denomination and longtime support from organized labor, which opposed the bill.[75]

Whatever the explanation for it, the governor's veto, coupled with the state supreme court's advisory opinion, curtailed the practice of involuntary sterilization in Alabama. The 1919 statute authorizing the sterilization of inmates at Partlow State School remained on the books, but it was undermined by the governor's strong stand and the court's position on judicial review. Shortly after his second veto, Graves assured the national ACLU that there would be no need to repeal this statute because "I do not think that the Superintendent will ever exercise the authority."[76] This was confirmed by an unrepentant Partlow in the School's next annual report that noted that, due to constitutional concerns, we have "positively discontinued the practice of sterilization, which will of necessity effect [sic] our previous liberal policy of granting paroles."[77] Even though Partlow persuaded his state representatives to reintroduce his compulsory sterilization proposal during the next two regular sessions of the state legislature in 1939 and 1943, the time had passed for such legislation in Alabama.[78] Both of these bills died in committee without ever reaching the House floor, which a bitter Partlow attributed to the "pressure of Catholic influence."[79]

The defeat of the Alabama sterilization bill roughly coincided with the decline of the eugenics movement in the United States as a whole. Leading historians of the movement point toward a 1936 report from the American Neurological Association critical of compulsory sterilization and a 1939 pronouncement by the International Genetics Congress denouncing Nazi eugenic theories as decisive events in that process.[80] No further state eugenic sterilization statutes passed after these events and utilization of existing laws gradually began to decline. Certainly a shift in scientific opinion on the inheritance of mental diseases and defects contributed to this process, as did the specter of Nazi eugenics. But in taking a stand against eugenic sterilization on scientific and political grounds, scientists simply adopted a position already held by many Catholics and conservative Protestants on religious grounds. For years, the loudest voices raised in the public square against eugenics came from speakers motivated solely by their religious convictions. In states such as Louisiana and Alabama, this protected countless individuals from the excesses and mistakes of a policy based squarely on the authority of science.

## THE NEW EUGENICS IN THE PRESENT AND BEYOND

America's past experience with eugenics gives good reason for caution as we, as a people, face a new era when scientists again hold out the promise of enhancing humanity through genetics. Indeed, some leaders of the current revolution in human gene therapy have hailed it as "a new eugenics." We have been there before, and it proved a false promise. But this era is not only "new" but different, with better science underlaying the promise. Therefore, the lines connecting old eugenics with new human gene therapy are not parallel, and no simple lessons can be drawn.

Indeed, the science underlying the new promise springs from the Human Genome Project, a mammoth, twenty-year, government-funded effort to sequence the entire human genome. The project's goal is to identify what each of our millions of genes do—and they do much. Together, they serve as the blueprint for creating our material bodies and minds. If the role of each gene is known, then we can look for genetic anomalies that set people apart. Almost every week, news reports announce the discovery of more telltale genes. Recently, for example, scientists have reported finding one gene associated with colon cancer, another with "creativity," and yet another with particular forms of mental illness. The Human Genome Project is now well underway, and has identified genes associated with hundreds of different genetic diseases, defects, and characteristics. And the pace of discovery is snowballing.

Physicians have already begun applying this new knowledge to diagnose some diseases. For example, a test is now available to determine if a person has the gene associated with Huntington's disease. It is being used on persons from families plagued by that dread affliction. Family members found not to have the gene now know they are safe; those found to have it now know they will die young. There is no medical cure. Many persons with a family history of Huntington's disease have opted to take the test, others have not, but either way, it has impacted their decisions about having children.

The current tests for individual genes are only a crude beginning, however. By the year 2005, researchers predict that lab technicians will be able to take a single drop of your blood, and quickly analyze it for the complete range of genetic traits. The price will be trivial. The result will be a printout of who you are and what you are likely to become, *materially*. At risk for high cholesterol, cut down on the eggs. Low risk for lung cancer, go ahead with smoking. Susceptible to alcoholism, watch the booze. The response becomes trickier when the trait is depression, or creativity, or criminality, or high IQ— yet scientists project a genetic component for each of these. And since a person's genetic makeup never changes, the analysis can be run at any point after conception. The potential benefits to individuals are legion: reliable information about ourselves and our prospects. This new genetic knowledge and its possible applications raise a host of ethical, moral, and spiritual questions, however.

Everyone, of course, worries about privacy. Who will have access to genetic information about you and me? Can potential employers demand it as part of our job applications? How about schools for tracking potential scholars or the police for identifying possible child molesters? Or insurers for tailoring health or life insurance rates to risk? Of course, most of the genetic information simply reveals increased or decreased probabilities, not certainties. If only one-in-a-thousand people get colon cancer, then an 80 percent increase in likelihood of getting the disease (as is now associated with the so-called colon cancer gene) still leaves a person with a risk rate of less than two in one thousand. Yet that might be enough to influence potential employers and insurers. As worrisome as these privacy issues are, they are not unique to Christians, Jews, or members of any other religious group. They are primarily ethical questions, rather than moral or spiritual ones. Congress and state legislatures have already begun addressing them with protective legislation—and more is sure to come.

At a deeper moral level, there is the specter of eugenics. As discussed above, early in this century, conceptual advances in evolutionary biology and Mendelian genetics led many respected scientists to believe that human heredity could readily be manipulated through selective breeding, or eugenics. As these ideas filtered from the scientific journals into the popular press, many Americans and Europeans changed the way they thought about and treated each other. Massive programs of forced sexual quarantine and sterilization for undesirables were launched by several American states and European countries, culminating with Germany's infamous sterilization and euthanasia program.

Historically, critics (often led by Roman Catholics) typically attacked eugenics on three grounds. First, *the science did not work*. Human heredity was more complex than eugenicists assumed, the critics correctly charged. Selective breeding could never eradicate so-called dysgenic traits for the population. The Human Genome Project now offers surer knowledge of human heredity, however, and raises the prospect of governments' or individuals' actually being able to shape the next generation. At the very least, parents will be able to test the genetic makeup of their unborn children and use it in deciding whether to give birth. This is already happening to a limited extent and is bound to increase.

Second, some religious and secular critics recognized that *the old eugenics programs of forced sterilization infringed on human rights*. At least in America, however, future efforts to discourage dysgenic offspring will probably focus on genetic counseling for prospective parents rather than their forced sterilization. Arguments that the new eugenics infringes on human rights will be countered by claims for a parent's (or woman's) right to choose the genetic makeup of her child. Indeed, parents with a family history of certain genetic diseases have already begun using currently available tests to check their unborn children for those conditions, and some have chosen to terminate pregnancies based on the results. No legal barriers prevent them from doing so. Indeed, many of them see it as their right and, some would add, their responsibility.

With such scientific and liberty arguments weakened, Christians opposed to a new eugenics on spiritual grounds may be forced back to their third and most fundamental objection: *moral concern for the sanctity of all human life*. Neither the unborn or the infirm should be cast aside because of supposed genetic defects. Indeed, Christians who affirm belief in the miraculous power of God to save should not necessarily accept genetic defects as permanent. The Bible records dozens of miraculous healings by Christ and his apostles, some of which may have involved genetic defects (such as the man born blind). And even if our genetic defects are not "healed" in this life, they surely can be in the next one. In any event, Christ loves all, not just the genetic elite.

Yet increased scientific recognition of genetic foundations for human nature will fuel greater popular acceptance of genetic determinism. This has already begun with the rise of sociobiology and the swing from nurture to nature in accounting for a range of human behaviors from homosexuality to criminality. And skeptics have pounced on these developments as a further objection to Christian concepts of free will and individual responsibility. This challenge to spirituality is nothing new. Environmental determinists of the past generation left no room for free will and individual responsibility either. Neither did astrological determinists of the Renaissance nor Stoics of ancient Rome. Christianity survived them all, countering determinism with faith in the sovereign power of God to save individuals and transform lives. In the end, Christians must again rely on the sovereignty of God in responding to the spiritual challenge posed by the new genetics just as they did in responding to eugenics.

## ENDNOTES

1. Richard John Neuhaus, *The Naked Public Square: Religion and Democracy in America* (Grand Rapids: Eerdmans, 1984), vii.
2. Ibid., 36.
3. Stephen L. Carter, *The Culture of Disbelief: How American Law and Politics Trivialize Religious Devotion* (New York: Basic, 1993), 51–52.
4. Ibid., 53.

5.  Ibid., 175.
6.  Third International Exhibit of Eugenics, "What Eugenics Is All About," in *A Decade of Progress in Eugenics: Scientific Papers of the Third International Congress of Eugenics* (Baltimore: Williams, 1934), pl. 3.
7.  For a general discussion of these developments, Daniel J. Kevles, *In the Name of Eugenics: Genetics and the Uses of Human Heredity* (New York: Knopf, 1985); and Phillip Reilly, *The Surgical Solution: A History of Involuntary Sterilization in the United States* (Baltimore: Johns Hopkins University Press, 1991).
8.  For a discussion of the Roman Catholic position on this issue, see Mark A. Haller, *Eugenics: Hereditarian Attitudes in American Thought* (New Brunswick: Rutgers University Press, 1963), 82–83, 131; also, Kevles, *In the Name of Eugenics*, 118–21, 168; and Reilly, *The Surgical Solution*, 118–22.
9.  *Journal of the State of Louisiana* (hereinafter *"La. Senate Journal"*) (1924 Regular Session), 458.
10. *La. Senate Journal* (1924 Regular Session), 75 (calendar). The complete text of the Senate legislation is in "Check on Propagation of Sub-Normal," *New Orleans Post*, 21 June 1924, 3, col. 1.
11. "Check on Propagation," 3, col. 1; and *La. Senate Journal*, 1924 Regular Session, 458.
12. J. W. Shaw, "Eugenical Sterilization Law," *Morning Star* (New Orleans), 28 June 1924, 1, cols. 2–3. For Shaw's background, see Roger Baudier, *The Catholic Clergy in Louisiana* (New Orleans: Louisiana Library, 1972), 527–35.
13. "Sterilization Bill OK'd by This Group," *New Orleans Item*, 2 July 1924, 1, col. 4 and 16, col. 5. In a later retelling of this story about the daughter suffering from the botched abortion, Gordon noted that the woman survived. "Unfortunately," she told a physicians' group, "you doctors cured her and brought her back to the institution" (Jean Gordon, "Discussion," *New Orleans Medical and Surgical Journal* 82 [1929]: 355).
14. "Merely Another Way," *New Orleans Times-Picayune*, 24 June 1924, 8, col. 2; and "Feeble-minded," *Times-Picayune*, 26 June 1924, 8, col. 2.
15. *Journal of the House of Representatives of Louisiana* (hereinafter *"La. House Journal"*) (1924 Regular Session), 830–31; "Asexualization Measure Killed," *Times-Picayune*, 3 July 1924, 1, col. 1; "Dry Bill Smashed," *New Orleans States*, 3 July 1924, 3, cols. 2–3; and "Sterilization Bill Defeated by House Vote," *New Orleans Item*, 3 July 1924, 7, cols. 6–7.
16. "Doctors, Not Lawyers, Due to Stop Crime, Judge Olson Declares, Blaming Heredity," *Times-Picayune*, 29 April 1926, 1, col. 6 and 2, cols. 6–7.
17. John. N. Thomas, "Increasing Insanity in This Country and What Should Be Done to Prevent It," *New Orleans Medical and Surgical Journal* 79 (1926): 334.
18. This summary of the 1926 Senate debate is compiled from "Senate Passes Sterilization in Hot Fight," *The State Times* (Baton Rouge), 15 June, 1926, 5, col. 1; Stanford Jarrell, "Bill to Sterilize Feeble Minded Passes Senate," *New Orleans Item*, 15 June 1926, 8, col. 7; "Sterilization Bill Passed by Senate," *New Orleans State*, 15 June 1926, 6, col. 8; George Vandervoort, "Senate Passes Sterilization Measure 25 to 11," *Times-Picayune*, 15 June 1926, 9, col. 3; and *La. Senate Journal* (1926 Regular Session), 375–76.
19. "Sterile Bill Put to Sleep in House," *New Orleans State*, 30 June 1926, 6, col. 3.
20. This summary of the 1926 House floor debate compiled from ibid.; "House Members Shape Fight Over Sterilization," *The State-Times* (Baton Rouge), 29 June 1926, 5, col. 1; "House Defeats Sterilization Bill 48 to 46," *The State-Times*,

30 June 1926, 6, col. 3; and "Sterilization Bill Is Killed," *Times-Picayune*, 30 June 1926, 6, col. 3. Shaw's letter was reprinted in "His Grace Opposes Proposed Measure on Sterilization," *Morning Star*, 5 June 1926, 4, col. 1.

21. E.g., "Letter from John N. Thomas to the Editor," *Times-Picayune*, 12 June 1926, 8, col. 5.

22. "The Sterilization Bill," *Times-Picayune*, 8 June 1926, 8, col. 1.

23. "Sterile Bill," 6, col. 3; and *La. House Journal* (1926 Regular Session), 1076–77.

24. George Vandervoort, "House Votes Down Tax on Tobacco," *Times-Picayune*, 20 June 1928, 2, col. 3.

25. *La. Senate Journal* (1930 Regular Session), 181; *La. House Journal* (1930 Regular Session), 964–65.

26. Associated Press, "Orleans Women's Leader Is Dead After Operation," 25 February 1931, in Jean Gordon file, Louisiana Collection, Tulane University Libraries.

27. Frank Allen, "Senate Proposal on Sterilization Loses in a Tie Vote," *Times-Picayune*, 16 June 1932, 3, col. 1; *La. Senate Journal* (1932 Regular Session), 422.

28. A second sterilization bill introduced by a physician in the Louisiana Senate during the 1932 session died without action. *La. Senate Journal* (1932 Regular Session), 449, 523.

29. Alabama Code (1923), sec. 1476. Partlow discussed his sterilization policy in "Letter from W. D. Partlow to E. S. Gosney," 9 January 1938, in *Association for Voluntary Sterilization (AVS) Collection*.

30. William D. Partlow, "Pathology of Mental Rehabilitation or Mental Conservation v. Mental Rehabilitation," *Transactions of the Medical Association of the State of Alabama* (hereinafter *"Transactions of MAA"*) (1928): 324. For a particular revealing expression of Partlow's social philosophy, see W. D. Partlow, "The Relation of the Problem of Mental Disease and Mental Deficiency to Society," *Southern Medical Journal* 26 (1933): 1066–68.

31. J. D. S. Davis, "The President's Message," *Transactions of MAA* (1928): 20.

32. See, e.g., W. D. Partlow, "The Relation of the Problem of Mental Disease and Mental Deficiency to Society," *Southern Medical Journal* 26 (1933): 1066–68; and "Social Workers Elect Officers," *Birmingham Age-Herald*, 17 April 1935, 3, col. 1.

33. W. D. Partlow, "Superintendent's Report," Alabama Insane Hospitals, *Trustee's Report* (1934), 85.

34. See Thomas McAdory Owen, *History of Alabama and Dictionary of Alabama Biography*, vol. 4 (Spartenburg, S.C.: Reprint Co., 1978), 1324; *Who Was Who in America*, vol. 5 (Chicago: Marquis Who's Who, Inc., 1973), 556.

35. See "Letter from W. D. Partlow to E. S. Gosney," March 26, 1934, in *Association for Voluntary Sterilization Collection, Social Welfare History Archives*, University of Minnesota, Minneapolis, MN (hereinafter *"AVS Collection"*) (adds "epileptics" to list quoted above).

36. See generally Jacob Henry Landman, *Human Sterilization: The History of the Sexual Sterilization Movement* (New York: Macmillan, 1932). This resource compiled and analyzed the sterilization statutes of every state.

37. J. N. Baker, quoted in "Sterilization in Alabama," *Montgomery Advertiser*, 6 February 1935, 4, col. 3. Partlow claimed credit for drafting the legislation in "Letter from W. D. Partlow to E. S. Gosney," 10 January 1935, in *AVS Collection;* and "Letter from W. D. Partlow to Marian S. Norton Olden," 11 May 1944, in *AVS Collection*.

38. See J. N. Baker, "Medical and Health Legislation in 1935," *Journal of the Medical Association of the State of Alabama* (hereinafter *"Journal of MAA"*) 5 (1935): 157–58; "Report of the Committee on Mental Hygiene," *Journal of MAA* 5 (1935): 27; "Sterilization Progresses," *Montgomery Advertiser*, 11 May 1935, 4, col. 1; William L. Truby, "Today in Both Houses of the Alabama Legislature," *Decatur Daily*, 4 September 1935, 2, col. 4; and "History of the Alabama Division of the American Association of University Women, 1927–1946," in *A. A. U. W.*, *Montgomery Branch Scrapbook, 1941–42*, in *Manuscripts Division, Alabama State Archives*, Montgomery, Alabama (hereinafter *"Alabama State Archives"*).

39. *Journal of the House of Representatives of Alabama* (hereinafter *"Ala. House Journal"*) (1935 Regular Session), 143.

40. 1935 Alabama House bill 87, secs. 1–6, in *Alabama State Archives*.

41. Hugh Sparrow, "Sterilization Bill for State Up to Governor," *Birmingham Age-Herald*, 1 June 1935, 1, col. 3.

42. "Foes 'Run Out' on Measure to Cut Phone Tax," *Montgomery Advertiser*, 5 September 1935, 7, col. 3; Frank Gordy, "House Spotlight Is Taken by Sterilization Measure Passed by Large Majority," *Mobile Register*, 11 May 1935, 1, col. 3; "Sterilization Bill Passes Senate; Up to Governor," *Montgomery Advertiser*, 1 June 1935, 3, col. 5 and 3, col. 1; "Sterilization in Alabama," 4, col. 3; "Sterilization Progresses," *Montgomery Advertiser*, 11 May 1935, 4, col. 1; and William I. Truby, "House Passes Sterilization Bill," *Decatur Daily*, 10 May 1935, 1, col. 8.

43. "Thoughts on Sterilization," *Montgomery Advertiser*, 5 June 1935, 4, col. 2.

44. "Biologist Sees Control of Human Defectives Only Solution of Race," *Montgomery Advertiser*, 30 June 1935, 5, cols. 1–2.

45. *Birmingham News*, quoted in "Thoughts on Sterilization," 4, col. 2.

46. "The House Passes the Sterilization Bill," *Birmingham News*, 11 May 1935, 4, col. 1. The *Montgomery Advertiser* made an almost identical comment in "Sterilization Progresses," 4, col. 1.

47. "Some Aspects of the Sterilization Fight," *Catholic Week* (Birmingham), 26 May 1935, 4, col. 2 (citing *Labor News* of Birmingham). No copies of any May 1935, issues of this union newspaper survive in Alabama public library or archives.

48. "Letter from Lucille Milner to Bibb Graves," 4 June 1935, in *Papers of Governor Bibb Graves* (Second Administration), Alabama State Archives (hereinafter *"Graves's Papers"*).

49. "The Sterilization Bill," *Alabama Baptist*, 4 July 1935, 3, col. 7.

50. "Letter from Hugh DuBose to Bibb Graves," 3 June 1935, in *Graves's Papers*.

51. "Some Aspects of the Sterilization Fight," 4, col. 2.

52. Ralph Hurst, "$2000 Tax-Free Homesteads Is Urged in House," *Birmingham News*, 10 May 1935, 1, col. 6; William F. Obering, "Mobilians Join in State Protest on Dominick Bill," *Mobile Press*, 16 May 1935, in *William F. Obering File*, Spring Hill College Library, Mobile, Alabama; "Solons Hear Opposition to Sterilization," *Catholic Week* (Birmingham), 19 May 1935, 1, col. 4; "Sterilization Bill Is Said to Be Illegal," *Catholic Week* (Birmingham), 1 September 1935, 1, col. 6; and "Letter from A. L. Stabler to Bibb Graves," 26 June 1935 in *Graves's Papers* (Catholic physician denouncing eugenics as pseudoscientific).

53. E.g., William F. Obering, "Authority Says Alabama Sterilization Measure Is Declaration of Slavery," *Catholic Week* (Birmingham), 5 May 1935, 1, cols. 3–5, 6, cols. 4–5, and 7, cols. 2–3; "Social Workers Elect Officers," 1, col. 5; "Father

Obering Attacks Alabama Sterilization Law in Birmingham," *Springhillian*, 29 April 1935, 1, col. 4; Obering's natural-law arguments rested largely on the jurisprudence of Federalist Era U.S. Supreme Court Justice James Wilson, who Obering was then writing about in a book. See William F. Obering, *The Philosophy of Law of James Wilson: A Study in Comparative Jurisprudence* (Washington: Catholic University of America, 1926).

54. Hurst, "$2000 Tax-Free Homesteads Is Urged in House," 1, col. 6 (quotes from resolution).

55. Gordy, "House Spotlight," 1, col. 3; Frank Gordy, "Sterilization Bill Passes, Awaits Governor's Action; Rogers Leads in Opposition," *Mobile Register*, 1 June 1935, 1, col. 3; Sparrow, "Sterilization Bill," 1, col. 3; Truby, "House Passes," 1, col. 8; and William I. Truby, "Sedition Bill Veto Is Under Fire," *Decatur Daily*, 6 August 1935, 1, col. 8.

56. "Sterilization Bill Passes Senate," 1, col. 5 and 3, col. 1.

57. "Sterilization Bill," 3, col. 3 (Baptist); "That Sterilization Bill," *Alabama Christian Advocate*, 23 May 1935, 3, col. 2 (Methodist); and "Totalitarianism," *Alabama Christian Advocate*, 1 August 1935, 2, col. 3.

58. "Sterilization Bill Passes Senate," 1, col. 5 and 3, col. 1. See also Gordy, "Sterilization Bill," 1, col. 3.

59. See, e.g., Obering, "Authority," 6, cols. 4–5 and 7, cols. 2–3 (quote on p. 7, col. 2); "Solon Has Opposition," 2, col. 4; and Letter from W. B. Palmer to Editor, "Objecting to Sterilization Bill," *Montgomery Advertiser*, 15 May 1935, 4, cols. 5–6. The shift in scientific opinion on eugenics is discussed in Haller, *Eugenics*, 179–83; Kevles, *Name of Eugenics*, 166–67; and Kenneth M. Ludmerer, *Genetics and American Society: A Historical Appraisal* (Baltimore: Johns Hopkins University Press, 1972), 121–29.

60. The House passed the bill on a 69–16 vote, *Ala. House Journal* (1935 Regular Session), 640. The vote in the Senate was 17–9, *Journal of the Senate of Alabama* (hereinafter "*Ala. Senate Journal*") (1935 Regular Session), 622–23.

61. "'Sterilization' Bill Gets Veto of Governor Graves," *Mobile Register*, 26 June 1935, 1, col. 3; and "Sterilization Bill Killed by Veto," *Montgomery Advertiser*, 26 June 1935, 1, col. 5.

62. "Dominick's Bill Vetoed by Graves," *Mobile Press*, 25 June 1935, 1, col. 8.

63. William D. Barnard, *Dixiecrats and Democrats: Alabama Politics* (Tuscaloosa: University of Alabama Press, 1974), 17; and John Craig Stewart, *The Governors of Alabama* (Gretna, La.: Pelican, 1975), 174–81 (quote at 176).

64. *In the Opinion of the Justices*, 230 Ala. 543, 547, 162, So. 123, 128, (1935).

65. See *Ala. House Journal* (1935 Regular Session), 1343 (veto message); "Dominick's Bill Vetoed," 1, col. 8; "'Sterilization' Bill Gets Veto," 1, col. 3; and "Letter from J. L. Busby to Hugh B. DuBose," 1 June 1935, in *Graves's Papers*.

66. "'Sterilization' Bill Gets Veto," 1, col. 3; "Under the Capitol Dome," *Alabama Journal* (Montgomery), 25 June 1935, 6, col. 3.

67. "Letter from W. D. Partlow to Bibb Graves," 2 June 1935, in *Graves's Papers*.

68. *Ala. House Journal* (1935 Regular Session), 1342 (veto message).

69. *Ala. House Journal* (1935 Regular Session), 1313–14; see "Senate Approves Decision to Boost Income Tax," *Decatur Daily*, 26 June 1935, 1, col. 2; Hugh Sparrow, "Poll Tax Bill Is Kept Alive," *Birmingham Age-Herald*, 7 August 1935, 4, col. 2.

70. The House vote was 74–21 in favor of the sterilization bill. *Ala. House Journal* (1935 Regular Session), 1994–97. The Senate approved the bill on a 21–8 vote. *Ala. Senate Journal* (1935 Regular Session), 1725–26.

71. *Ala. House Journal* (1935 Regular Session), 2753–54 (veto message).
72. *Ala. House Journal* (1935 Regular Session) 2754 (approving Dominick's motion to table veto override; "Foes 'Run Out,'" 7, col. 3; and Turby, "Today," 2, col. 3.
73. "Letter from 'Citizen of Mobile' to Bibb Graves," 26 June 1935, in *Graves's Papers*. The letters received by Graves on this matter are preserved in *Graves's Papers*.
74. W. D. Partlow, "Discussion," *Transactions of MAA* (1910): 361.
75. "Letter from W. D. Partlow to E. S. Gosney," 9 January 1938, in *AVS Collection*. Later, Partlow privately suggested that "the Catholics . . . persuaded the Governor to veto the bill." Partlow to Olden (1944).
76. "Letter from Bibb Graves to Lucille Milner," 10 September 1935, in *Graves's Papers*.
77. W. D. Partlow, "Superintendent's Report," in Alabama Insane Hospitals, *Trustee's Report* (1935), 89. See also, Partlow to Gosney (1938).
78. *Ala. House Journal* (1939 Regular Session), 1643; and *Ala. House Journal* (1943 Regular Session), 197.
79. "Letter from W. D. Partlow to Marian S. Olden," 10 May 1946, in *AVS Collection*.
80. Kevles, *Name of Eugenics*, 166–67; and Ludmerer, *Genetics*, 121–29.

*An Overview*

The way in which a society applies its technology is inextricably linked to the prevailing philosophy of the time. Today's society combines sociological determinism (something besides human will determines human behavior) with postmodern constructionism (cultural specific truth as opposed to objective universal truth) to create a tenuous philosophical launching pad from which the application of genetic research can be propelled into society. Jim Leffel delineates the ways in which these philosophies view personhood and the implications this view has on the use and misuse of genetic engineering. The Christian perspective can promote and protect human life and value only when it is neither ignorant of nor uninvolved with the philosophical issues of its time. Our belief in God and objective truth compels us to ensure that this is the case.

# Chapter Eight

# GENETICS AND HUMAN RIGHTS IN A POSTMODERN AGE

## Jim Leffel

MEDICAL RESEARCH AND TECHNOLOGY have produced an astounding array of breakthroughs in the last half of this century. Millions of lives have been saved by penicillin, polio immunization, and diagnostic techniques that detect deadly diseases in the early stages. Yet, in recent years, advances in biotechnology have surpassed our ability to anticipate their theological and ethical implications. Nowhere is this more evident than with genetics. As the Human Genome Project nears completion of the effort to map the entire human genetic structure and as scientists become more successful at cloning mammals and primates, a whole new set of dilemmas present themselves. These issues are likely to be at the forefront of human-rights concerns as we enter the next century. As technology continues to advance, human-rights advocates must broaden their scope of concern. Consider just a few technology-driven dilemmas:

1.  With the experimentation on sheep, researchers appear to be bringing us ever closer to having the necessary technology to successfully clone human beings.
2.  A New Jersey family takes their doctor to court for allowing the "wrongful birth" of their Down's syndrome child. Over three hundred similar suits have reached the courts in recent years. Today, as in an earlier time, we hear of "life unworthy of life."
3.  A child is conceived in California for the purpose of serving as a bone-marrow donor for an older sibling. The cells are harvested and her sister lives. Could this be a precedent for the justification of creating human life for "spare parts"?
4.  An embryo conceived in a Louisiana laboratory is protected by state law. But as soon as it is implanted into the mother, it can be aborted by another legally protected freedom.
5.  Researchers at Harvard and Stanford Medical Schools have uncovered over two hundred cases of genetic discrimination. Based on preexisting conditions, insurance companies have denied coverage to people who carry some genetically transmitted disorders even though they currently show no disease symptoms and perhaps never will.

Each of these incidents illustrates the complexities that genetic technology introduces. They involve obvious ethical and legal dilemmas. But a more basic and all too often ignored question must also be explored: What is human personhood? Without an answer to this question, moral and legal debate is almost pointless. How can we speak of protecting human rights without defining what it means to be human?

Citing a lengthy bibliography of current scholarly works on the meaning of personhood, psychologist and social critic Kenneth Gergen observes, "One of the most interesting aspects of this work is that it exists at all, for only under particular cultural conditions would the question be considered worthy of such attention."[1] What are the particular cultural conditions to which Gergen refers? Both in academia and in popular culture, we are experiencing a sweeping ideological shift. It is the decline of Enlightenment assumptions that have guided both Western civilization for the past 250 years and the emergence of a postmodern cultural consensus. This shift in thought has been extensively documented in public opinion[2] and in more scholarly work.[3] However, little critique has been given to the practical implications of postmodernism in regard to the pressing biomedical issues of our day. As postmodern language and concepts become an increasingly significant part of the public discussion about human nature and medical ethics, it is essential that human-rights advocates understand the thinking behind the rhetoric and formulate compelling responses to it.

This chapter attempts to turn the discussion in that direction. We will first examine the meaning of personhood from a postmodernist perspective and then consider its implications for a society entering an age of genetic technology. Finally, we will construct a Christian response that outlines the potential dangers that genetic determinism and postmodern thinking may pose as we enter the twenty-first century.

## FROM THEISTIC TO POSTMODERN ANTHROPOLOGY

### Table 6–1 Comparing Views of Human nature

| THEISM | MODERNISM | POSTMODERNISM |
|---|---|---|
| Rational, but fallen and finite. In need of revelation for true and ultimate knowledge. | Rational and capable of starting from finite human experience and reason to discover ultimate truths. | Reason and truth are not objective. Human thought is limited to and determined by culture. |
| The image of God. Intrinsic human value, even though corrupted by the Fall. | An autonomous, individual "self" exists. | Individuals are the product of cultural determinism. Individuality is an illusion. |

To better understand what's at stake with current issues surrounding genetics, we must first consider how history has defined human personhood from the time of Christ to the present era. Throughout the first millennium and well into the second, biblical theism defined personhood. The onset of modernism at the midpoint of the second millennium defined personhood until the early 1900s when postmodern thinking about personhood surfaced. Consequently, Western culture was built largely on a biblical concept of human nature. Humans were viewed as rational beings but were limited in knowledge by their own finiteness and fallenness. We, as human beings, can reason but, ultimately, the basis for truth (God himself) and the framework of truth is disclosed by divine revelation. Further, humanity is created in the image of God, so even though corrupted by the Fall, we have intrinsic value as individuals. By the late seventeenth century, a new way of conceiving human nature emerged as modernism continued to develop.

French philosopher René Descartes (1596–1650), believing that *humans are rational by nature*, is often considered the father of modern philosophy. Parting company with medieval thought that sought to root reason in the soil of Christian belief,[4] Descartes attempted to discover truth independent of divine revelation. He began inwardly, with his rationalistic deduction, "I think, therefore I am." Descartes' first certainty was that "I exist as a thinking thing." The concept of humanity as rational by nature became the hallmark of Enlightenment thought.

A second modernist assumption suggests that the *self is autonomous*. By autonomous, we mean that the individual self (the "I" that "thinks") transcends, or stands above, environment and biology. Descartes based his theory of an autonomous self on mind-body dualism—the idea that an immaterial mind stands over and apart from nature. Later philosophers rejected this dualism and the theism it presumed, but for more than two hundred years, most maintained the belief in an autonomous self and confidence in the rational objectivity it made possible. The autonomous, rational self became the foundation for Enlightenment humanism and its liberal political theory, free market economics, and radical individualism.[5]

Twentieth-century postmodernism is a direct assault on the entire Enlightenment enterprise. At the heart of it, postmodernists deny the possibility of rational objectivity because they reject the view of the self that modernism presupposes. Rather than seeing humanity as an ocean of autonomous rational selves, as modernists held, postmodernists think of humans as an extension of culture and deny the individual self altogether. Kenneth Gergen notes, "With the spread of postmodern consciousness, we see the demise of personal definition, reason, [and] authority. . . . All intrinsic properties of the human being, along with moral worth and personal commitment, are lost from view."[6] The self stands under "erasure" for postmodernists, meaning they deny all transcendent categories, including essential human personhood, reason, and human value. Postmodern anthropology is based on the idea that humans are "social constructs," or socially determined beings. We have no individual personhood because we are wholly products of culture. There can be no objective access to reality because there is no neutral context from which to think. All thought is "contextual," meaning that the individual can never escape the arbitrary and subjective thought forms and values of the culture from which both personal identity and thought are formed.

Despite much of its "politically correct" rhetoric, postmodernism lifts each culture to a divine status while it devalues the individuals who create and sustain it.[7] There is no universal human essence, no stable personal identity, and consequently, no inherent human value. Humans derive an *illusory* sense of individual identity and value as persons from the arbitrary mores of their culture. So, one's identity, value, and civil rights are accidents of cultural origin rather than some property intrinsic to human nature.

Postmodern concepts of truth and knowledge have attracted the attention of Christians as well. Some argue that postmodernism's notion of "socially constructed truth" provides both a welcome end to modernism's antisupernatural stranglehold on Western culture and a new opportunity for Christians to gain social and intellectual influence.[8] However, the price paid for embracing postmodern constructivism is too high. It is unfaithful to the biblical claim to objective and universal truth,[9] and it negates objective human dignity. Indeed, if all truth is contextual, then truth about human value and rights must also be contextual rather than universal. The unfortunate consequence of postmodern thinking is that it brings an end to any meaningful account of universal human rights. Christian postmodern advocates Middleton and Walsh regrettably conclude that "there simply is no innocent, no intrinsically just narrative, not even the biblical one."[10]

## POSTMODERN IMPLICATIONS IN
## AN AGE OF GENETIC TECHNOLOGY

The insurgence of postmodernism coupled with a growing interest in the genetics industry present two powerful currents that form a potentially menacing riptide against which proponents of human dignity must struggle. We will now focus on some of the possible forces that could influence genetic research and also discuss how postmodern anthropological assumptions increasingly encroach on bioethics and biopolicy.

Generally, scientists are antagonistic to postmodernism because of its assault against reason and the postmodernists' accusation that science is a tool of Western cultural imperialism.[11] Further, the vast majority of scientists properly regard themselves as socially conscious humanitarians, dedicating their professional lives to bettering the human condition. Everyone should be grateful for their dedication and the fruits of their labor. While these humanitarian motivations actually find inspiration in the theistic worldview, some of the ideological assumptions accepted by the general scientific community create a serious concern of no little consequence. Naturalistic materialism, the dominant working presupposition among *secular* scientists, inevitably shares in postmodernism's devaluation of the individual. This creates a dangerous consensus in secular culture today. Consider the unsettling remarks of Robert Haynes, president of the Sixteenth International Congress of Genetics.

> For three thousand years at least, a majority of people have considered that human beings were special, were magic. It's the Judeo-Christian view of man. What the ability to manipulate genes should indicate to people is the very deep extent to which we are biological machines. The traditional view is built on the foundation that life is sacred. . . . *Well, not anymore* (emphasis added). It's no longer possible to live by the idea that there is something special, unique, even sacred about living organisms.[12]

Whether biological machines or cultural constructs, *naturalism and postmodernism strip humanity of all intrinsic value and leave postmodern culture with no meaningful frame of reference to address the pressing bioethical issues of our day.*

An assumption that has been raised in connection with the research of the Human Genome Project portends that human behavior is of genetic origin. Behaviors that in previous times were attributed to environment or moral choice are now thought to be attributed to one's genes. High profile scientists exploiting front-page journalism claim to have discovered the genetic basis for a host of behaviors and characteristics, including alcoholism, homosexuality, promiscuity, I.Q., and violence. Yet, serious scientific doubt about these claims are commonly given little attention, leaving the public with the impression that science is on the verge of solving some of society's greatest concerns. The wide acceptance of genetic explanations for these probing social problems, whether grounded in solid science or not, has contributed to an ideological climate that has serious implications for human dignity.

Beyond these social issues, there are areas of research and technology where families may have a more personal stake. This is where postmodern constructivism is particularly dangerous. For example, as genetic screening becomes more available to potential parents, we can expect to see further erosion in the value of human personhood. Dr. Harvy Lodish of the Whitehead Institute for Biomedical Research in Cambridge, Massachusetts, states, "By using techniques involving in vitro fertilization, it is already possible to remove one cell from the developing embryo and characterize any desired region of DNA. Genetic screening of embryos, before implantation, may soon become routine."[13] As technologies develop, parents will be able to select desirable traits and/or select out undesirable traits for their children. The natural human tendency to compete or be the best will cause those who can afford genetic screening and therapy to attempt to create the "perfect child." The ethical difficulty with this aspect of gene therapy demands that we honestly answer the question: Whose dreams would this therapy help to fulfill, the child's or the parents'? Although gene therapy can serve humanity well as a *healing art*, as a *cosmetic art*, it is too closely linked with unrealistic social pressures and questionable motives! Reproductive consumerism as well as economic and social pressure may turn genetic screening and therapy into a social expectation and, quite possibly, another legal right.

Important market forces are also at work in the genetics research industry. Fortunes will be made through the commercial marketing of genetic material. And scientists have been quick to seize the opportunities. Since 1971, corporations have put on a relentless legal battle to patent genetically altered organisms. After nearly a decade of legal bantering, the United States Supreme Court decided that life forms could be considered "human inventions;" thus patentable by the U.S. Patent and Trademark Office (PTO).[14] Although Christianity is not adverse to people's receiving profit from their work and inventions, financial profit derived from the sale of human tissue or beings is ethically unacceptable.

In 1987, the PTO widened patent rights to include all life-forms on earth, including animals.[15] Human beings, though, were exempt from the ruling, citing the Thirteenth Amendment prohibiting slavery. However, the ruling had significant shortcomings. Attorney Andrew Kimbrell notes, "under the PTO's 1987 ruling, embryos and fetuses, human life-forms not presently covered under Thirteenth Amendment protection, are patentable, as are genetically engineered human tissues, cells, and genes."[16] Corporate America won the right to own, use, and sell all multicellular creatures, including human beings.[17] (For further information on patenting, see chapter 6, "Patenting Life," by C. Ben Mitchell.)

While a storm of pro-life protest resulted in the withdrawal of National Institutes of Health requests for public funding to use human embryos in genetic research, it is still legal. The PTO is now flooded with applications for patents on hundreds of human genes and gene lines. Kimbrell warns, "[a]s patenting continues, the legal distinctions between life and machine, between life and commodity, will begin to vanish."[18] With the potential for human cloning, the picture becomes even less clear. If a researcher clones a human, is the clone a human invention, exempt from civil rights and, therefore, a commodity *or* is it a person with constitutional rights?

Human cloning has been suggested for all kinds of medical applications. Fetal tissue harvested from cloned or genetically engineered fetuses could be used to treat a variety of diseases from Parkinson's disease to leukemia. If human cloning techniques are developed, it will be possible for a person to clone himself to produce the healthy tissue his body lacks. Without stringent ethical guidelines, it's not hard to envision a future in which a clone could be developed solely to provide bone marrow to a patient suffering from leukemia or even organs to patients suffering from other ailments. At present, the idea of cloning humans uncomfortably draws one's mind toward ideas of human slavery, commercialism, and abuse and, therefore, is extremely suspect.

As practical demand for human tissue increases, human value in a postmodern culture experiences a corresponding decline. In today's world of gene mapping and gene therapy, we hear about the "commodification of life," and "the human body shop industry."[19] We are witnessing the depersonalization of human bioscience language: "As body parts and [genetic] materials are sold and patented, manipulated and engineered, we also are seeing an unprecedented change in many of our most basic social and legal definitions. Traditional understandings of life, birth, disease, death, mother, father, and person begin to waver and then fall."[20] In depersonalized language, scientific and legal jargon obscures important moral distinctions. The consequence is that genetic engineering and intervention appear more neutrally scientific than deeply ethical and human. It is imperative that geneticists and policy makers distinguish between what they *can* do and what they *should* do.

At a time when few people can articulate a meaningful defense of human dignity, we are left open to the increasing influence of the postmodern tendency to diminish individuality and, therefore, human value. David Hirsch sets forth an appalling issue: "Purveyors of postmodern ideologies must consider whether it is possible to diminish human beings in theory, without, at the same time, making individual human lives worthless in the real world."[21] There are important indications that Hirsch's fears are being realized. In recent public-opinion surveys, a substantial majority favor genetic screening for a wide range of genetically transmitted disorders.[22] In and of itself, genetic screening does not conflict with the Christian worldview; however, it is not merely serious or fatal diseases that are being singled out. For example, in a recent survey taken in New England, 11 percent of couples polled said they would abort a child genetically predisposed to obesity.[23] In the present climate, abortion as a therapeutic option will nearly always be offered when genetic screening reveals an undesired or unwanted result.[24] This form of eugenics is morally unacceptable.

This popular opinion is also reflected in the medical community. Between 1973 and 1988, the percentage of geneticists who approve of prenatal diagnosis for sex selection rose from 1 percent to 20 percent.[25] In a broader study of gender-selected abortion, 62 percent of American physicians said they would perform genetic screening to identify a fetus' gender or refer patients to a physician who would.[26] Civil-rights activists around the world have rightly condemned abortion based on gender, and we should be equally outraged by the blatant misogyny these studies suggest. The potential for eugenic applications to genetic technology demands a constant vigil to circumvent potential abuse.

## POSTMODERNISM'S FAMILIARITY WITH THE PAST

Postmodernists recognize the potential cost of their antihumanistic denial of objective human value. Kenneth Gergen concedes: "Postmodernism has often been viewed as morally bankrupt because it fails to profess any fundamental values or principles. More forcefully put, postmodernism fails to offer arguments against Nazism or any other forms of cultural tyranny."[27] Gergen's point is grossly understated. There are dangerous historical and conceptual connections between postmodernism's devaluing of the individual and *folkism*, the ideological basis of fascism.[28] In his sobering and timely essay, "Biological Science and the Roots of Nazism,"[29] George Stein states: "German philosophic romanticism was a xenophobic . . . reaction against the idea of 'man' as a species. Rather, 'men' participated in life or had their being through a unique natural and cultural identity. Folkism was established as both a philosophical ideology and as a political movement."[30] For folkism, human value and human rights were associated with cultural identity just as they are for contemporary postmodernism. There simply are no inalienable rights because there is no universal human essence. Individual human value was also illusory for folkism in much the same way it is for contemporary postmodernists. Again citing Stein: "Man is a social species. Individualism is an illusion . . . each individual is subordinate to the social body of which he is a member."[31] Individuals possess value only as they take their place (i.e., their role) in culture. This raises two questions. First, What is culture? Second, What does it mean to have a place in culture? Early fascists found the question of culture easy enough to define: Aryan folkism. And in the post-World War I era when Germany was searching for some way to regroup, folkism provided the rallying point. What it meant to have a place or role in folkish society was another matter. Stein explains: "Without human essentialism, folkish standards came to define normative humanity at the exclusion of other races, and even many within the race. [German social Darwinist Ernst] Hackel and others were thus willing to argue that we must assign a totally different value to their lives."[32] Ideology alone could not accomplish the folkish ideal of the pure German Aryan state. But what if folkish romanticism and Aryan superiority were *scientifically* true? This was the claim of the German social Darwinists and the basis for the Nazi eugenics program. It was a scientific application of what postmodernists today call *social constructivism*. Social undesirables—those who did not fit the folkish ideal—were considered genetically inferior. As such, they had a responsibility to surrender their lives for the good of the state. As Hackel states: "Hundreds of thousands of incurables—lunatics, lepers, people with cancer— are artificially kept alive without the slightest profit to themselves or the general body."[33] This philosophy, which diminishes the value of the "inferior" or disabled, is prominent among proponents of physician-assisted suicide. Not only are the terminally ill presently devalued, one of Kevorkian's most recent victims was a twenty-one year old quadriplegic. We must never come to see ourselves or others as undesirables merely because we are somehow not "physically normal." Human value is inherent in each person as created reflections of God; one's dignity is not determined by appearance or ability.

A growing number of people are expressing concern that the ruthless pragmatism of the past can be cultivated in today's genetics revolution. Arbitrarily assigning value to human life and scientific justification for social engineering is not merely a folkish matter. America has looked to eugenics in the past to address social problems.[34] As economic and social pressures merge with various prejudices, postmodern constructivism provides a compelling basis for manipulating an individual's genes for the betterment of culture. The blond-hair, blue-eyed mentality of a past regime must not be allowed to rear its ugly head anew and corrupt the immense good that genetic engineering can bring to society.

## GENETICS AND HUMAN RIGHTS

Although the lessons of the past should reawaken us to the possible dangers of misusing genetic technology, three other areas where human rights may be compromised by genetic determinism and postmodern constructivism require thoughtful reflection.

### Genetics and Crime

With the prevailing assumption that behavior is reducible to one's genetic code, we should not be surprised that solutions offered to manage social crises will tend to "medicalize" deviant behavior. For example, some have considered proposals to medically treat people who carry the alleged "violence gene," since reform is considered unlikely.[35] Several states are in the process of enacting legislation making it possible to chemically or surgically castrate troublesome sex offenders. But such a proposal is morally unacceptable if the basis of their decision is on the grounds that human behavior is reduced to one's genes. This understanding of human behavior is not proven and, even if it was proven to have some influence on behavior, *there is no justification* for suggesting that psychological and sociological factors do not conjoin with genetic predisposition to define one's character or behavior. Human free will and the reality of a transcendent God makes each human being not just a physical and social person but a spiritual person as well.

The medicalization of criminal behavior is attractive because it provides a scientific solution to the helplessness many feel about violence and the escalating cost of incarceration. It's alluring because it absolves society of accepting culpability or addressing key social, moral, and spiritual failures. Therefore, in a postmodern culture that has no objective basis for social ethics or individual dignity, it is very realistic to expect that society will apply scientific technique to "protect" culture from undesirable behavior. The problem is that only arbitrary social consensus will determine where to draw the line between acceptable and unacceptable behavior.

### Genetics and Racism

Many are disturbed by the popularity of *The Bell Curve*. Written by two prominent academics (one a Harvard researcher, the other a conservative social theorist), the book sparked a heated debate centering on social policy that curbs efforts to educate many poor people based on their presumed limited genetic potential.[36] The book argues that African Americans are less intelligent by nature and, consequently, unworthy recipients of educational and other government programs to help them rise out of poverty. Critics have rightly pointed out the biases and limitations of the study, but there is little question that *The Bell Curve* has fed the undercurrent of racism that plagues our society.[37] The bigoted notion of genetic inferiority and a social policy to reflect it is regrettably and tragically back in the national debate. To point to genetics as a way to diminish the immeasurable value of a human being or race is inconsistent with the Christian position to assist the less fortunate and treat all of humanity without prejudice. Any type of discrimination that is connected to one's genetic endowment represents a gross misuse of scientific research.

## Genetics and Job Discrimination

As correlations are drawn between genetics, potential illness, and behavior, we can expect insurance carriers and employers to consider requiring genetic screening to minimize financial risk. According to a report by the Committee on Government Operations, "[p]ressures to evaluate risk on an individual basis might make genetic assessments a prerequisite to insurance."[38] At a time of enormous health-insurance cost, genetic tests can have the capacity to determine which people will be hired for a job or who receives extended medical coverage. Many public-health experts have expressed substantial concern that the pressures of cost containment and the availability of genetic screening will potentially create a climate of "genetic discrimination" despite passage of the Americans with Disabilities Act.[39]

The issues related to using genetic screening to identify potential illness are complex. Although job discrimination by an employer based on the findings of a genetic test are morally unacceptable, insurance companies do appear to have a real financial interest in knowing the results of a genetic test. However, noninsurability can *never* be an option. It may be that genetic therapy will be viewed by insurers as coverable preventive care. Genetic screening creates many challenges for insurance companies, but fairness and justice can never be sacrificed for financial profit. The plight of human disease is shared by all—it is a community problem. As we presently do, we must all continue to share in the financial risks rather than create a heavier burden on individuals who, for no fault of their own, are inflicted by a genetic abnormality.

## A CHALLENGE TO THE CHURCH

We are entering into a genetic age that will offer a resolution to many human ailments as well as challenge us to be mindful of potential abuses to human rights. Genetic determinism (which leads to a misuse of genetic engineering) and postmodern constructivism (which leads to a misuse of truth and human value) leave little room for the inherent dignity of human life. Only a position that has, as its moral base, a transcendent God who sets absolute standards of righteousness and justice can resist the current momentum toward social constructionism and determinism. Christians must take an informed stand on all the issues that comprise genetic engineering, understanding both the appropriate and inappropriate uses of genetic technology.

## ENDNOTES

1. Kenneth Gergen, *The Saturated Self* (New York: Basic Books, 1991), 272.
2. George Barna, *The Barna Report: What Americans Believe* (Ventura: Regal Books, 1991), 112.

3. See Jim Leffel and Dennis McCallum, "Postmodernism: The Spirit of the Age" *Christian Research Journal*, (fall 1996).
4. Medieval epistemology can be summarized in Anselm's dictum, "I believe so that I may understand."
5. For an excellent discussion of American individualism, see Robert Bellah et al., *Habits of the Heart* (Berkeley: University of California Press, 1985). Bellah does an excellent job of showing the transition from a biblically based concept of human personhood to an Enlightenment or modernist base.
6. Gergen, *The Saturated Self*, 228–29.
7. See David Michael Levin, *The Opening of Vision: Nihilism and the Postmodern Situation* (New York: Routledge, 1988), 405–8.
8. See J. Richard Middleton and Brian J. Walsh, *Truth Is Stranger Than It Used to Be: Biblical Faith in a Postmodern Age* (Downers Grove, Ill.: InterVarsity Press, 1995).
9. For an outstanding critique of Middleton and Walsh, see Peter Payne, "A Review Essay of: *Truth Is Stranger Than It Used To Be*," *Religious and Theological Studies Fellowship Bulletin* 13 (November–December 1996): 16–25.
10. Middleton and Walsh, *Truth Is Stranger Than It Used to Be*, 84.
11. See Jim Leffel, "Postmodernism and the Myth of Progress," in *The Death of Truth*, ed. Dennis McCallum (Minneapolis: Bethany House Publishers, 1996), 45–57.
12. Andrew Kimbrell, *The Human Body Shop: The Engineering and Marketing of Life* (San Francisco: HarperSanFrancisco, 1993), 233–34.
13. Harvey Lodish, "Viewpoint: The Future," *Science*, 267 (March 17, 1995): 1609.
14. *Sidney A. Diamond, Commissioner of Patents and Trademarks, petitioner, v. Ananda M. Charkrabarty et al.*, 65 L 2d ed. 144, 16 June 1980, 144–47.
15. U.S. Patent and Trademark Office, *Animals-Patentability* (Washington, D.C.: U.S. Patent and Trademark Office, 1987), cited in Kimbrell, *The Human Body Shop*, 199.
16. Kimbrell, *The Human Body Shop*, 199.
17. Kimbrell states, "It is important to note that, as described in the last two chapters, current U.S. patent law makes patenting human embryos perfectly legal" (*The Human Body Shop*, 223).
18. Ibid., 212.
19. These terms describe both the rhetoric and the emerging biopolicy surrounding genetic research and technology.
20. Kimbrell, *The Human Body Shop*, 228.
21. David Hirsch, *The Deconstruction of Literature: Criticism After Auschwitz* (Hanover: Brown University Press, 1991), 165.
22. Kimbrell, *The Human Body Shop*, 290.
23. Ibid., 124.
24. "[I]t should be clear that for now and the foreseeable future, a major benefit derived from genetic information by families and individuals is the possibility to prevent the birth of other gene carriers by utilizing selection abortion" (*Designing Genetic Information Policy: The Need for an Independent Policy Review of the Ethical, Legal, and Social Implications of the Human Genome Project* [Washington, D.C.: U.S. Government Printing Office, 1992], 30).
25. Gina Kolata, "Fetal Sex Test Used As Step to Abortion," *New York Times*, 25 December 1988, A1.
26. Kimbrell, *The Human Body Shop*, 123.
27. Gergen, *The Saturated Self*, 231.

28. See Gene Edward Veith, *Today's Fascism* (St. Louis: Concordia Press, 1993).
29. George Stein, "Biological Science and the Roots of Nazism," *American Scientist* 76 (January–February 1988): 50–58.
30. Ibid., 53.
31. Ibid., 56.
32. Ibid., 55.
33. Ibid., 54.
34. For a survey of the development of eugenic policy in the United States, see Kimbrell, *The Human Body Shop*, 250–57.
35. Ibid., 258–59.
36. See Charles Murray and Richard Herrnstein, *The Bell Curve: The Reshaping of American Life by Differences in Intelligence* (New York: Free Press, 1994).
37. For a wide range of responses to Murray and Herrnstein's work, see *The New Republic*, 31 October 1994.
38. Committee on Government Operations, *Designing Genetic Information Policy: The Need of an Independent Policy Review of the Ethical, Legal, and Social Implications of the Human Genome Project*, 16th report (Washington, D.C.: U.S. Government Printing Office, 1992), 17.
39. Ibid., 15–22.

# PART 2

---

# GENETIC ENGINEERING
# AND THE FAMILY

*An Overview*

A general understanding of the technologies associated with assisted reproductivity is necessary for an appropriate and educated Christian response. These technologies are not the topic of brainstorming sessions—they are presently employed around the world to assist couples with infertility issues. Are there any ethical limits placed on them, and are they advancing ahead of serious and thoughtful discussions about the morality and dangers associated with their use? J. Kerby Anderson briefly surveys artificial reproductive technologies that are presently in vogue, as well as those that are on the horizon. Interspersed throughout are statements that reflect a Christian response to the ethical questions many of these technologies raise. This chapter introduces the reader to artificial insemination, artificial sex selection, in vitro fertilization, surrogacy, gene splicing, and cloning. Other chapters in this volume deal with these issues individually and more specifically.

Chapter Nine

# THE ETHICS OF GENETIC ENGINEERING AND ARTIFICIAL REPRODUCTION

J. Kerby Anderson

THE LATTER PART OF THE TWENTIETH century has become the age of genetics. Many believe the genetic revolution may have a more profound impact on society than even the industrial revolution. As knowledge in genetics doubles every few years, ethical considerations frequently lag behind. Although scientists and doctors have the technological capacity to do a multitude of new things, do we have the wisdom and moral capacity to do what is right? The speed of the genetic revolution is breathtaking. Consider the following sample of news items from the last twenty years:

- In 1978, Louise Brown became the first test-tube baby conceived as a result of in vitro fertilization.
- In 1984, a woman in California gives birth to the first baby created from a donor egg. The same year a girl named Zoe is born from a frozen embryo.
- In 1986, surrogate mother Mary Beth Whitehead decides to keep her child, which precipitates a tangled court case.
- In 1994, a postmenopausal woman used donated eggs and her husband's sperm to give birth at the age of sixty-two.
- In 1997, scientists cloned Dolly, the sheep. Also that year, Bobbi McCaughey gave birth to septuplets after taking a fertility drug.
- In 1998, Dr. Richard Seed sets up a clinic in Chicago to clone human beings. Also, scientists announce they have been able to breed headless mice and headless tadpoles; thus opening the way to producing human fetuses without heads that can be used as organ factories.

How powerful a technology is genetic engineering? For the first time in human history it is possible to completely redesign existing organisms, including people, and to direct the genetic and reproductive constitution of every living thing. Physicians can also bypass the normal process of reproduction and, therefore, even further direct the development of these organisms. Humankind has entered a new realm in which the genetics and development of any creature can be artificially manipulated and directed.

## SURVEY OF GENETIC TECHNOLOGIES

The range of technologies available to scientists and physicians at the end of the twentieth century is mind-boggling. Here is a brief list of options already available.

*Artificial insemination* is used as an alternative means of reproduction when male infertility is present. Today there are two types of artificial insemination: using the sperm of the husband (AIH: artificial insemination by the husband) and using sperm of a donor (AID: artificial insemination by a donor; more popularly called DI, i.e., donor insemination). More recently, artificial insemination has also been used for female infertility. Women are impregnated with donor gametes (sperm and egg) so that couples can adopt children born to these surrogate mothers.

*In vitro fertilization* is used for female infertility. Conception takes place outside the womb, which accounts for the popular term *test-tube babies*. The woman is treated with hormones to stimulate the maturation of eggs. The eggs are removed by means of laparoscopy and placed in a dish and fertilized with sperm. After a period of time, the developing embryos are surgically placed in the uterus.

*Artificial sex selection, embryo transfer, and frozen embryos* are other forms of artificial reproduction. Surrogate parenting is possible by using artificial insemination in which the husband's sperm is used to impregnate a donor mother.

*Genetic engineering* is possible through recombinant DNA (rDNA) technology. Scientists cut and paste pieces of DNA to completely redesign existing organisms. In the past, scientists were limited to breeding and cross-pollination. Now these powerful genetic tools allow us to change genetic structure at the microscopic level and bypass the normal processes of reproduction.

*Cloning* allows scientists to make multiple copies of any existing organism or of certain sections of its genetic structure. In the past, this genetic tool has been limited to simpler organisms, but the announcement of the cloning of a sheep suggests the possibility that cloning mammals (including humans) may be possible.

*Genetic surgery and genetic therapy* are developing techniques that will be used to treat and cure genetic diseases. Scientists can already identify genetic sequences that are defective, and soon will be able to replace these defects with properly functioning genes.

## ARTIFICIAL INSEMINATION

Artificial insemination by the husband (AIH) consists of collecting the husband's sperm and injecting it into his wife. Couples often seek this procedure either because the husband is fertile but unable to participate in normal sexual relations or because the husband's sperm count is low.

Periodically collecting sperm can increase the probability of pregnancy.

AIH is much less controversial than artificial insemination by a donor (AID) because it involves the husband. Although the insemination is artificial rather than natural, AIH does not destroy the personal and sexual aspects of the marriage bond and, therefore, is open to less criticism.

Artificial insemination by a donor (AID) is similar to AIH except that sperm from a donor is used instead of sperm from the husband. This singular exception leads to most of the ethical questions surrounding this reproductive procedure.

The major ethical and theological concern with AID is that it introduces a third party or outsider into the pregnancy who is not a part of the sanctioned one-flesh marriage. This is especially true when artificial insemination is used to produce children in the wombs of surrogate mothers. Surrogates are usually arranged through business associations that solicit women through newspaper ads and who then are chosen by couples according to their physical and mental characteristics as well as ethnic and religious backgrounds.

Whether donor sperm or egg is used, both scenarios introduce a third party into the pregnancy. God's ideal for parenthood is for a man and woman to give birth to a child who is genetically related to them. While adoption is an obvious exception to that ideal, the divine ideal should be the standard used to judge AID.

Two Old Testament examples are often cited to support AID. The first is the story of Abraham and Sarah. When Sarah could not bear a child for Abraham, she said to him, "Go, sleep with my maidservant; perhaps I can build a family through her" (Gen. 16:2). The second is the provision of the levirate marriage of the kinsman-redeemer, who was to impregnate his deceased brother's wife if there was no heir (Deut. 25:5–10).

Neither of these examples gives much support for AID. There is no indication of God's approval of the act by Abraham and Sarah. If anything, Sarah's suggestion and Abraham's acquiescence clouded God's lesson for them and unveiled a genuine lack of faith in God. Moreover, the application of either event to today is questionable. Abraham and Sarah's example took place within a polygamous relationship, and the levirate marriage was applicable only to the Old Testament theocracy.

AID cannot be endorsed as a form of artificial reproduction. It violates a biblical view of marriage by introducing a third party or outsider into the pregnancy. Though AID does not involve adultery because sexual relations are not required to present the sperm to the egg, it nonetheless, is morally unacceptable—the married couple is attempting to *produce* a child that is not a product of their marital union. Adoption of a child already born and without a home is acceptable, while intentionally producing children who will require adoption by one or both spouses is quite questionable.

## IN VITRO FERTILIZATION

When Aldous Huxley wrote his famous book, *Brave New World*, in 1932, few thought that what he predicted would take place in their lifetimes. When

Louise Brown was born on July 25, 1978, as the first test-tube baby, many believed a new era had arrived. In some ways, the new reproductive technologies are a fulfillment of that vision; in most ways they are not.

In vitro fertilization (known as IVF) is a procedure that allows an egg to be fertilized outside the womb. The embryo is then injected into the uterus for implantation and maturation. With the future development of an artificial placenta and more advanced incubation technology, an embryo may be able to develop to "birth" having never experienced its mother's womb, or anyone else's womb for that matter.

Since the initial pioneering work on IVF, many other methods have been developed in an effort to treat millions of infertile couples in the United States.[1] These include: gamete intrafallopian transfer (GIFT) in which a physician, using a laparoscope, inserts eggs and sperm directly into a woman's fallopian tube so that fertilization can take place; intrauterine insemination (IUI) in which thawed sperm of the husband, or a donor, is inserted by a catheter into the uterus, bypassing the cervix and upper vagina; zygote intrafallopian transfer (ZIFT), a two-step procedure whereby eggs are fertilized in the laboratory and any resulting zygotes (fertilized eggs) are transferred to a fallopian tube; and intracytoplasmic sperm injection (ICSI) in which a physician, using a microscopic pipette, injects a single sperm into an egg with the resulting zygote then being placed into the uterus.

A number of legal concerns have arisen from these reproductive procedures. The 1981 case of Mario and Elsa Rios demonstrates the legal tangle that can develop. The Rioses wanted children; they decided to travel to a fertility clinic in Australia. Three of Mrs. Rios' eggs were fertilized in vitro with sperm from an anonymous sperm donor. One was implanted and the other two were frozen. Ten days later the implanted embryo spontaneously aborted. But before the clinic could implant the other two, the Rioses were killed in a plane crash in South America.

Two questions surfaced. First, do these frozen embryos have a right to an inheritance and, second, do they have a right to life? Mr. and Mrs. Rios were multimillionaires. Were those embryos potential millionaires? Did they have a right to inherit the Rios' fortune? Did those frozen embryos have a right to life? Are IVF clinics obliged to protect embryos? Should the Australian clinic implant those embryos into a surrogate mother who would carry them to term?

Other questions surfaced as well. For example, who would be the legal father and mother? Here are Mr. Rios, Mrs. Rios, an anonymous sperm donor, a surrogate mother, and possibly, an adoptive father and mother. The child who would be born could have as many as six "potential parents." From a Christian perspective, the two embryos are *living* heirs who should be afforded the opportunity to mature and be born since they should not be discarded as mere human tissue. If either survived implantation and was born, they should be legitimate heirs to some part of the Rios estate. Playing in the genetic playground does not preclude one from the responsibilities that result.

Questions of paternity loom large with surrogate parenting. The most famous case was the battle of custody over "Baby M." William and Elizabeth Stern entered into a contract with Mary Beth Whitehead to carry their child. As her pregnancy progressed, Mrs. Whitehead began to have doubts and developed the inevitable maternal feelings a mother would expect to have for a child she is carrying. She decided to keep the child and forced a judge in New Jersey to resolve this modern-day "Solomon dilemma."

The reverse of the Solomon dilemma also occurred. This was a case in which neither the couple nor the surrogate mother wanted the child. Alexander Malahoff contracted with Judy Stiver to be a surrogate mother. Unfortunately young Christopher was born with an infection and microcephaly. Malahoff disavowed the child and threatened to sue. The issue was uncertain, and the child remained in a foster-care facility. Then, during the airing of the "Phil Donahue Show," blood and tissue tests were brought forward revealing that the child was Judy Stiver's and her husband's. They were required to raise the child.

The various legal issues surrounding IVF and related procedures merely underscore the proliferating nature of the technology. Reproductive endocrinologist Martin Quigley distinguishes "old fashioned IVF" from these newer forms. "The modern way," he notes, "mixes and matches donors and recipients."[2] A woman's egg could be fertilized by a donor's sperm or a donor's egg might be fertilized by the husband's sperm. And any of these matches could then be placed in the wife or in a surrogate mother. The reproductive possibilities are staggering.

The surrogate mother could actually be a surrogate grandmother. In 1988, Pat Anthony, a forty-nine-year-old grandmother in South Africa, was able to give birth to her own grandchildren. She was implanted with her daughter's eggs, which had been fertilized in the laboratory, and subsequently gave birth to triplets.[3]

As this example shows, age may no longer be a limitation for women wanting to become pregnant. Physicians have been able to take an egg from a younger woman and implant it in an older woman (one woman in her sixties gave birth in this way) even if she has been through menopause. Egg donation is also becoming more widely available and accepted as egg brokerage houses match recipients with donors.[4]

Some reproductive technologies open up the possibility of female reproduction without male involvement. Initial research on egg fusion at Vanderbilt University demonstrated the future possibility of taking an egg from one woman and fusing it with the egg of another woman.[5] The procedure has attracted the attention of lesbian groups because the procedure would produce a girl who is genetically related to each of the women who donated an egg. From a Christian perspective, this application of genetic technology seems sexist and is contrary to the biblical view of parenthood, which values the roles of both men and women in the child-rearing process.

A major ethical concern with IVF and other forms of reproductive technology is the status and loss of embryos. The low success rate of some of the procedures and the willingness of some clinics to fertilize many eggs and then choose a likely candidate raises moral questions about the status of the unborn being produced by artificial reproduction. Proponents argue that the loss is not excessive. Opponents argue that the loss is unacceptable or at least call for defining an acceptable level of success.

## ARTIFICIAL SEX SELECTION

Artificial insemination and in vitro fertilization have spawned a separate question: Should parents select the gender of a child? Using new sperm-separation techniques, couples can improve the probability of obtaining a child of the desired sex.

The gender of a child is determined by the sperm of the male. Sperm with Y chromosomes will produce boys, while sperm with X chromosomes will produce girls. Researchers have found at least five methods by which to separate the two types of sperm, using such differences as sperm weight, sperm swimming speed, and electrical charge.

The most commonly used means is the *Ericsson method* developed by reproductive physiologist Ronald Ericsson more than twenty years ago. Because Y sperm tend to swim faster and stronger under certain conditions, physicians can separate them from X sperm by having them swim through a series of viscous layers (layers having a cohesive and sticky fluid consistency). Though not totally foolproof, the method has a published success rate of 75 percent for boys and 69 percent for girls.[6]

While sex selection may be very beneficial in agriculture and animal husbandry, its application to humans is more questionable. Some couples have used the process to prevent a genetic disease that might be sex linked; however, most use it to produce a child of a desired sex.

The social implications are significant. Research has shown that couples would choose the sex of their child if the procedure was relatively simple and inexpensive.[7] Of the couples who expressed a preference, about 90 percent wanted the firstborn to be a boy. If they could only have one child, 72 percent wanted a boy.

The actual impact on society would be difficult to determine. Surveys give only a rough guideline of actual preference. Sex selection may well be influenced by social pressure and personal taste. Thankfully, only a fraction of couples are choosing artificial sex selection, and the technology is not 100 percent effective. However, as more couples choose this procedure and as its effectiveness increases, the impact on society could be significant.

Widespread use of sex selection could dramatically increase the number of boys. And even if the procedure did not increase the number of boys, it could certainly, if the survey mentioned above is accurate, transform society into a nation of older brothers and younger sisters, at least subtly implying that women are second-class citizens.

An important ethical question asks whether parents have the right to determine the sex of a child. A broader question asks whether society at large has a right to decide the sex of children born into it. At a time when more and more rights are being claimed, parents will more likely demand the right to determine the sex of their children. But will that right lead to demands for other rights? Is it not possible that the right of sex selection will eventually lead to the right of genetic specification? Selecting the gender of one's child is considered the most fundamental aspect of that child. Choosing hair and/ or eye color, stature, and other characteristics would logically be the next step.

The Bible teaches that children are a gift from God (Ps. 127:3) and are entrusted to parents for care and nurture. Parents who want control over the gender of their child should evaluate their motives and consider the possible implications of their decision—both to their family and to society. Using genetic engineering to combat disease is one thing; using it to manipulate an otherwise natural selection is quite another.

## CHRISTIAN RESPONSE TO ARTIFICIAL REPRODUCTION

How then should Christians respond to these various reproductive technologies? The first principle is *the sanctity of human life*. Human beings are created in the image of God (Gen. 1:27–28) and therefore have dignity and value. God's special care and protection extend even to unborn children (Ps. 139). Reproductive technologies that threaten the sanctity of human life come under the same criticism as abortion.

The sanctity of life may be threatened in at least three ways. First, there is the potential loss of fetal life. Some reproductive technologies are very inefficient and, therefore, result in an unacceptable loss of life. Second, there is the practice of destroying fertilized ova if they appear abnormal. Third, there is the practice of hyperfertilization in which many eggs are fertilized simultaneously, one is selected for implantation, and the others are thrown away.

This is a concern not only with the clinical use of embryos; it is also a concern for the research use of embryos. In the past, a moratorium was placed on research on embryo and fetal experimentation. The Clinton administration lifted the ban and federal funding has been recommended for research on human embryos up to fourteen days after fertilization.[8] This research also violates the biblical principle of the sanctity of human life.

A second principle is a biblical view of *sexual relations* (Gen. 2:24). Many reproductive technologies separate the unitive from the procreative aspects of human reproduction. To use the vernacular phrases, "making love" and "making babies" were supposed to be associated in the same act. Sexual intimacy, the communication of love, and the desire for children are supposed to be unified within the bounds of matrimony. Artificial reproduction frequently separates these functions and thus poses a potential threat to the completeness God intended for marriage. While some ethicists believe that such an intervention is sufficient to reject all reproductive technologies, most others accept such an intervention as permissible if the gametes that produce the embryo originate from the marital union only.

A third principle is a biblical view of *parenthood* (Gen. 1:28). God ordained marriage as the union of a man and a woman who would give birth to a child genetically related to them. While there may be exceptions to this ideal, this standard should be used to judge reproductive technologies. As stated earlier, procedures such as surrogate parenting and embryo transfer clearly introduce an outsider into the intimate sphere of the marriage union.

Couples considering artificial reproduction should first consider other less ethically questionable options. These include medical options such as reconstructive surgery (tuboplasty) and drug treatments, adoption and foster care, or remaining childless and having more time for a church or community ministry. If these alternatives are unavailable, one may proceed cautiously into the technological reproductive world with a mind-set that will not permit abuses to human life (the embryo) or to the sacredness of the marriage union.

Fundamental to all this should be an attitude of seeking the Lord's will. Abraham and Sarah asked the Lord for a child (Gen. 18). When he did not meet their timetable, they took matters in their own hands with disastrous results. By contrast Hannah (1 Sam. 1) sought the Lord and was patient for his provision. Before a couple seeks medical counsel, they should seek the Lord and then count the costs and consider the ethical issues involved. Remember that there is no actual right to have children; they are a gift from the Lord. Some of us may not be awarded this gift, though numerous other gifts will be awarded as we live out the experience God has planned.

## GENE SPLICING

Recombinant DNA research (rDNA) began in the 1970s with new genetic techniques that allowed scientists to cut small pieces of DNA (known as plasmids) into small segments that could be inserted into host DNA. The new creatures that were designed have been called DNA chimeras because they are conceptually similar to the mythological Chimera (a creature with the head of a lion, the body of a goat, and the tail of a serpent).

Legal concerns also surround this technology. The Supreme Court ruled that genetically engineered organisms as well as the genetic processes that created them can be patented. The original case involved an oil-slick eating microorganism patented by General Electric. Since 1981, the United States Patent and Trademark Office has approved nearly twelve thousand patents for genetic products and processes.[9] Scientists have been concerned that the prospects of profit have decreased the relatively free flow of scientific information. Often scientists-turned-entrepreneurs refuse to share their findings for fear of commercial loss.

Even more significant is the question of whether life should be patented at all. Most religious leaders say no. A 1995 gathering of 187 religious leaders representing virtually every major religious tradition spoke out against the patenting of genetically engineered substances. They argued that life is the creation of God, not of humans, and should not be patented as human inventions.[10] (See chapter 6, "Patenting Life.")

The broader theological question is *whether* genetic engineering should be used and, if permitted, *how* it should be used. The natural reaction for many in society is to reject new forms of technology because they may be dangerous. Christians, however, should take into account God's command to humankind in the cultural mandate (Gen. 1:28). Christians should avoid the reflex reaction that scientists should not tinker with life; instead Christians should consider how this technology should be used responsibly.

One key issue is the worldview behind most scientific research. Modern science rests on an evolutionary assumption. Many scientists assume that life on this planet is the result of millions of years of a chance evolutionary process. Therefore, they conclude that intelligent scientists can do a better job of directing the evolutionary process than nature can do by chance. Even evolutionary scientists warn of this potential danger. Ethan Singer believes that scientists will "verify a few predictions, and then gradually forget that knowing something isn't the same as knowing everything. . . . At each stage we will get a little cockier, a little surer we know all the possibilities."[11]

In essence, rDNA technology gives scientists the tools they have always wanted to drive the evolutionary spiral higher and higher. Julian Huxley looked forward to the day in which scientists could fill the "position of business manager for the cosmic process of evolution."[12] Certainly this technology enables scientists to create new forms of life and alter existing forms in ways that have been impossible until now.

How should Christians respond? They should humbly acknowledge that God is the sovereign Creator and that humans have finite knowledge. Genetic engineering gives scientists the technological ability to be gods, but *they lack the wisdom, knowledge, and moral capacity to act like God.* This fact should never be underestimated, for ignoring the truth of the statement may lead to abuses that match or exceed that of the Holocaust. Even evolutionary scientists who deny the existence of God and believe that all life is the result of an impersonal evolutionary process express concern about the potential dangers of this technology. Erwin Chargaff asked, "Have we the right to counteract, irreversibly, the evolutionary wisdom of millions of years, in order to satisfy the ambition and curiosity of a few scientists?"[13] His answer is no. The Christian's answer should also be no for the simple reason that God is the Creator of life. We do not have the right to "rewrite the fifth day of creation."[14]

What is the place for genetic engineering within a biblical framework? The answer to this question can be found by distinguishing between two types of research. The first is called *genetic repair*. This research attempts to remove genetic defects and develop techniques that will provide treatments for existing diseases. Applications would include various forms of genetic therapy and genetic surgery as well as modifications of existing microorganisms to produce beneficial results.

The Human Genome Project has been able to pinpoint the location and sequence of the approximately one hundred thousand human genes.[15] Further advances in rDNA technology will allow scientists to repair these defective sequences and hopefully remove genetic diseases from our population. Genetic disease is not part of God's plan for the world. It is the result of the Fall (Gen. 3). Christians can apply technology to fight these evils without being accused of fighting against God's will.[16] Genetic engineering can and should be used to treat and cure genetic diseases.

A second type of research is *the creation of new forms of life*. While minor modifications of existing organisms may be permissible, Christians should be concerned about the large-scale production of novel life forms. The potential impact on the environment and on humankind could be considerable. Science is replete with examples of what can happen when an existing organism is introduced into a new environment (e.g., the rabbit into Australia, the rat into Hawaii, or the gypsy moth into the United States). One can only imagine the potential devastation that could occur when a newly created organism is introduced into a new environment.

God created plants and animals as "kinds" (Gen. 1:24). While there is minor variability within these created kinds, there are also built-in barriers between these created kinds. Redesigning creatures of any kind cannot be predicted the same way new elements on the periodic chart can be predicted for properties even before they are discovered. Recombinant DNA technology offers great promise in treating genetic disease, but Christians should also be vigilant. While this technology should be used to repair genetic defects, it should not be used to confer the role of creator on scientists. (See comment by geneticist Francis Collins on page 27.)

## CLONING

In 1970, Paul Ramsey devoted an entire chapter to human cloning in his book *Fabricated Man*.[17] During much of the 1970s ethicists debated the pros and cons of human cloning until scientists were able to convince nearly everyone that cloning a mammal (much less a human being) would be difficult if not impossible.

All that changed when scientists in Scotland announced in 1997 that they had successfully cloned an adult sheep. Commentators were predicting that a "brave new world" was just around the corner, and ethicists began to dust off arguments that had been mothballed in the 1970s. The cloning of the sheep Dolly implied that it might eventually be possible to clone a human being.

A few years earlier in 1993, two scientists from George Washington University announced the first artificial twinning of human embryos. The press erroneously announced that humans had been cloned. Actually this was not the case. What the scientists had done was to begin with seventeen human embryos and multiply them like the Bible's loaves and fishes into forty-eight different embryos. What the scientists in Scotland did was significant because they were able to clone a mammal from cells that were not embryonic.

When an embryo grows, the cells begin to differentiate. Only a certain part of the genetic structure is utilized to form a skin cell, or an eye cell, or a heart cell, and so forth. In a sense, DNA is like a CD album that will only play a single track. The genetic melody for a skin cell is the only track of DNA that is actually played in a skin cell. The scientists found a way to get adult cells to once again play each and every genetic note. They did this by putting them in a state of "quiescence." When the cell became dormant, all the genes once again had the potential of being played.

The scientists took normal mammary cells from an adult ewe and starved them in order to allow the cells to reach a dormant stage, which apparently allowed these cells to be deprogrammed. These were then fused with an egg cell that had its nucleus removed. The cell was then electrically stimulated so that it would begin cell division.

The successful cloning of a lamb raises the question: "Wherever the lamb went, was Mary sure to follow? In other words, how soon will scientists clone humans?"[18] Scientists point out that the procedure used to clone a sheep may not work for other mammals. Human beings use nuclear DNA differently from the way sheep embryos use DNA. And similar experiments, for example, have not worked in mice. Therefore, quite possibly, humans may not be able to be cloned by this procedure. Nevertheless ethicists are once again considering the possibility that humans can be cloned.

While cloning of various organisms may be permissible, cloning a human being raises significant questions beginning with the issue of the sanctity of human life. Human beings are created in the image of God (Gen. 1:27–28) and, therefore, differ from animals. Human cloning would certainly threaten the sanctity of human life at a number of levels. First, cloning is an inefficient process of procreation, as shown in the cloning of a sheep. Second, cloning would no doubt produce genetic accidents. Previous experiments with frogs produced numerous embryos that did not survive, and many of those that did survive developed into grotesque creatures. Third, researchers often clone human embryos for various experiments. Although the National Bioethics Advisory Commission banned the cloning of human beings, it permitted the cloning of human embryos for research. Since these embryos are ultimately destroyed, this research raises the same pro-life concerns that are raised with regard to the abortion issue.

Cloning represents a tampering with the reproductive process at the most basic level. Cloning a human being certainly strays substantially from God's intended procedure of a man and woman who produce children within the bounds of matrimony (Gen. 2:24). All sorts of bizarre scenarios can be envisioned. Some homosexual advocates argue that cloning would be an ideal way for homosexual men to reproduce themselves.

Although cloning would be an alternative form of reproduction, it is reasonable to believe that human clones would still be fully human. For example, some people wonder if a clone would have a soul since a clone would be such a diversion from God's intended process of procreation. A Traducian view of the origin of the soul would imply that a cloned human being would have a soul. In a sense, a clone would be no different from an identical twin.

Human cloning, like other forms of genetic engineering, could be used to usher in a brave new world. James Bonner says "there is nothing to prevent us from taking a thousand [cells]. We could grow any desired number of genetically identical people from individuals who have desirable characteristics."[19] Such a vision conjures up images of Alphas, Betas, Gammas, and Deltas from Aldous Huxley's book *Brave New World* and provides a dismal contrast to God's creation of each individual as unique.

Each person contributes to both the unity and diversity of humanity. This is perhaps best expressed by the Jewish Midrash: "For a man stamps many coins in one mold and they are all alike; but the King who is king over all kings, the Holy One blessed be he, stamped every man in the mold of the first man, yet not one of them resembles his fellow."[20] Christians should reject future research plans to clone a human being and should reject using cloning as an alternative means of reproduction.

## ENDNOTES

1. "Against the Odds: How the Methods Compare," *Newsweek* (4 September 1995): 41.
2. Otto Friedrich, "The New Origins of Life," *Time* (10 September 1984): 46.
3. Stephen Budiansky, "The New Rules of Reproduction," *U.S. News and World Report* (18 April 1988): 67.
4. Traci Watson, "Sister, Can You Spare an Egg?" *U.S. News and World Report* (23 June 1997): 44.
5. Lori Andrews, "Embryo Technology," *Parent* (May 1991): 69.
6. Lisa Busch, "Designer Families, Ethical Knots," *U.S. News and World Report* (31 May 1993): 73.
7. Charles Westoff and Ronald Rindfuss, "Sex Preselection in the United States: Some Implications," *Science* (10 May 1974): 633–36.
8. Thomas Giles, "Test-Tube Wars," *Christianity Today* (9 January 1995): 38.
9. Kenneth Woodward, "Thou Shalt Not Patent!" *Newsweek* (29 May 1995): 68.
10. Ibid.
11. Testimony by Ethan Singer before the Subcommittee on Health and the Environment, House Committee on Interstate and Foreign Commerce, *Hearings* (15 March 1977): 79.
12. Julian Huxley, cited in Joseph Fletcher, *The Ethics of Genetic Control* (Garden City, N.Y.: Anchor, 1974), 8.
13. Erwin Chargaff, cited in George Wald, "The Case Against Genetic Engineering," *The Sciences* (May 1976): 10.
14. Nancy McCann, "The DNA Maelstrom: Science and Industry Rewrite the Fifth Day of Creation," *Sojourners* (May 1977): 23–26.
15. Philip Elmer-Dewitt, "The Genetic Revolution," *Time* (17 January 1994): 49.
16. Skeptics sometimes argue that fighting disease is the same as fighting against God's will. Albert Camus poses this dilemma for Dr. Rieux in *The Plague*. Christians should follow the cultural mandate (Gen. 1:28) and use genetic technology to treat and cure genetic disease.
17. Paul Ramsey, *Fabricated Man* (New Haven, Conn.: Yale University Press, 1970).
18. Sharon Begley, "Little Lamb, Who Made Thee?" *Newsweek* (10 March 1997): 55.
19. James Bonner, quoted in *The Los Angeles Times* (17 May 1971): 1.
20. N. N. Glazer, *Hammer on the Rock: A Short Midrash Reader* (New York: Schocken, 1962), 15.

*An Overview*

For many people, the interest in, and the introduction to, issues of genetics and genetic engineering comes through personal involvement with, or treatment for, infertility. When this occurs, issues that were previously distant and academic suddenly become intensely personal. What are some of the ethical concerns and genetic challenges we face with regard to reproductive technologies and the future? What principles should Christians follow and what latitude, if any, is there in the decision-making process? The rapid advances in science and medicine force us to continually evaluate our ethical principles so that their applications remain current with technology. Physician Bill Cutrer and author Sandra Glahn offer professional and personal perspectives on this timely and crucial issue. The ethical decisions we face individually, as families, and as a society are often intricate and difficult. Christians need to be involved in public discourse on these matters, for the stakes are very high and a biblical perspective is often absent in the public forum.

# Chapter Ten

# DEALING WITH GENETIC REALITY
## *Theological and Clinical Perspectives*

## William Cutrer, M.D. and Sandra Glahn

As a medical doctor who is also an ordained minister, I (Dr. Cutrer) was asked by a Dallas hospital to teach a series on medical ethics to the OB-Gyn residents. One morning as we came together, we began to discuss a recently encountered scenario. A woman had been inseminated by her stepfather's sperm because her mother, having had a hysterectomy, was unable to conceive in her new marriage. They wondered: Is this incestuous? Is it adulterous? Is this right?

As we discussed the case, I found it most interesting that rather than remaining focused on the existing ethical dilemma itself, the conversation kept going back to how this scenario could have been prevented. The focus on prevention seemed significant to me. How interesting that the immediate reaction of medically oriented people was the wish to rewind and change the sequence—to revise the ethical questions and ask how we could keep from having to ask them in the first place. Unfortunately, in the situation described, it was too late. Although this case was not specifically one in which there were questions of genetics and genetic engineering, it is cases such as this that lead some people to ethical discussions in the field of genetics.

Once we're faced with a moral dilemma, we have to act within the set of circumstances we're given; yet preventive ethics is a good way to think, so that we will not be caught off guard when difficult issues arise. That is why we are here thinking through some basic questions—to avoid entering what some might consider unsolvable moral mazes before they come upon us. By making a preemptive ethical strike, we keep from getting ourselves into a moral mess. In our effort to think preemptively, then, we will consider not only current options but also a few that have yet to be realized.

In a very real way, genetics and truth intersect life continuously, and the answers we give to bioethical issues often may be what we think is the best option among difficult choices. Before we consider specific cases, however, we need to take a look at four foundational guidelines for processing these cases.

*First, erect the fence around the evil itself, not around the* potential *for evil.* As Augustine said: "The potential abuse of a thing does not preclude its use."

Yet, often within the Christian community there is a tendency to erect a wider fence around what is acceptable than God himself erects. Rather than opposing the act of immorality itself, Christians sometimes expand the moral limits to include anything that might "lead to sin." Although well meaning, this is detrimental in that it undermines Christian liberty and also can lead to withdrawal from public discourse and limit Christianity's influence on crucial issues.

For example, some argue against drinking because "it can lead to drunkenness." They gloss over verses about Jesus' turning water into wine and Paul's suggestion that Timothy take wine for the sake of his stomach. And consider Proverbs 31:6–7: "Give strong drink to him who is perishing, and wine to him whose life is bitter. Let him drink and forget his poverty, and remember his trouble no more" (NASB). In America this verse may seem surprising, but consider parts of the world where pain killers and anesthetics remain unavailable.

The tendency to broaden the boundary of limitations—to be stricter than God intends—has been around since the beginning. As early as the first few chapters of Genesis, we read, "The LORD God commanded the man, 'You must not eat from the tree of the knowledge of good and evil, for when you eat of it you will surely die.'" (Gen. 2:16–17). Just one short chapter later we see an interesting addition when Eve tells the serpent, "God did say, 'You must not eat fruit from the tree that is in the middle of the garden, *and you must not touch it*, or you will die'" (Gen. 3:2–3, italics ours). According to the record we have, God never said they could not *touch* the fruit; he said they could not *eat* it. As far back as the original first family, we see a drift toward widening the boundary of limitations while at the same time violating the actual limits.

Centuries later, the same expanded boundary problem was still prevalent. The Pharisees considered Jesus to be a lawbreaker because he and his disciples refused to conform to the extra rules they had added to God's commands. In Matthew 12:1–2, we read: "At that time Jesus went through the grainfields on the Sabbath. His disciples were hungry and began to pick some heads of grain and eat them. When the Pharisees saw this, they said to him, 'Look! Your disciples are doing what is unlawful on the Sabbath.'" In the Mishna, the collection of Jewish oral laws compiled ca. A.D. 200, we find a list of thirty-nine acts of labor that Jews prohibited on the Sabbath. Based on the assumption that these same or similar oral laws existed two centuries earlier, we see that the disciples had technically violated four man-made laws. Yet, God's law actually allowed people to pluck grain to satisfy hunger. It was engaging in regular work that he prohibited.[1] The Pharisees had erected a "fence" around the law, which they considered as binding as the law itself.

These biblical illustrations are cited to say that when it comes to medical ethics, we must be careful to avoid doing the same thing. It's easy to be dogmatic in areas where God has not given clear absolutes, and we must continually assess our own opinions on these issues by asking ourselves, "Am I *more sure than right* here?" Emotional certainty and ethical certainty are not always the same and we must not permit emotions to override biblical and ethical principles.

Let's look at some medical examples of actual evil versus *potential* for evil:

> The suction tool used for performing abortions is also used for diagnostic and therapeutic D&Cs and is safer than the old metal curettes. So are we against the tool itself or the wrongful use of it?
>
> The "abortion pill," RU 486, has potential for positive use in that it blocks progesterone production. RU 486 might be helpful for treating some breast cancers. It could also possibly be used to treat ectopic pregnancies, allowing the mother to avoid surgical intervention. Are we opposed to RU 486, or do we oppose its use for elective abortions? True, if it's available for other purposes, some will use it for elective abortions, yet do we outlaw it because of its potential for abuse?
>
> Some people object to genetic screening because insurance companies have used the information to charge enormous premiums for those found to be at risk for future illness. Do we oppose the screening or the wrongful use of this information by insurance companies?

In these cases, the tool, the medication, and the research are amoral. They can be used for ill purposes, but they also have potential beneficial uses. *In the same way, we should not necessarily oppose genetic engineering nor genetic research.* We should oppose that which destroys life and we should oppose the improper application of the knowledge gained. Thus, when we hear the terms *genetic engineering* or the *Human Genome Project*, we must not immediately envision a super race of designer babies nor, at the opposite extreme, a race of people with the I.Q.s of fish who have been designed to do menial tasks. To do so is to seriously misunderstand the realities of genetic research.

*Second, good applications, if they have come via information gained through unethical means, should give us pause.* In the same way that we wouldn't oppose protecting national security even though spies may have killed to get the information that allows the protection, we support the use of good genetic applications, even if embryos were destroyed to gain that information. While we oppose any killing in the process of obtaining the information, we would support the positive use of the knowledge once obtained. Nevertheless, we must hold in reverence the sacrificed lives. We grieve at the loss and must work to support research that seeks alternatives to such destruction.

Take, for example, in vitro fertilization (IVF). In the early stages of the procedure, scientists took enormous risks with embryos, few of which survived. Yet through research and years of practice, IVF is being perfected. While we would have opposed IVF in the late 1970s when Louise Brown was the first baby conceived in a petri dish, today we believe the procedure is generally acceptable as long as the couple allows only those eggs and sperm exposed to each other that they are willing to carry to term. Why? Because the current risk to embryos appears to be greatly reduced, though there is no large scale tracking of the ratio of embryos created to live births.

The same is true of cryopreservation. A decade ago, those holding a high view of life strongly opposed cryopreservation because the thaw survival rates for embryos were so poor. Today, however, the risk to embryos is greatly decreasing, and Christian ethicists are increasingly more comfortable with the practice.

We are reminded of Jesus' parable of the unjust steward. This man's boss charged interest on money he loaned, a practice forbidden when lending to a fellow Jew. When the steward learned he would soon be unemployed, he approached those who owed his boss money and offered them the opportunity to pay off their debts at no interest. Thus, he earned favor in their eyes at a time when he needed connections in the business world. His boss could not go to the Jewish authorities to complain without exposing his own unethical behavior. The steward practiced unethical business, yet he was commended for one thing: He smartly worked the system to ultimately benefit himself. Jesus tells this story and then adds, "the sons of this world are more shrewd in . . . their . . . generation than the sons of light" (Luke 16:8 RSV).

While we must personally commit ourselves to a high standard of medical ethics, we also must be shrewd and wise in recognizing when to use the wrongs of others for good purposes. This is not to say that we secretly support what they are doing. Rather, it says that once the wrong has been done, we look for a way to make good come from it. Some scientific minds approach ethical laboratory dilemmas with a totally different view of life; thus, it is inevitable that research that is ethically problematic for the Christian will take place. This being the case, we must then choose either to reject the information gained or to use it with an appreciation for the cost at which it came and a desire that such costs will not be incurred in the future.

Having established the need to limit our own boundaries to those that we believe God himself has given, we turn to ask: What are those limitations? Below are three presuppositions that we consider foundational for Christians who are considering these issues.

First, we believe that it is wrong to take a life (Exod. 20:13). It is also wrong to impose the sacrifice of one person as a means to benefit others, especially without consent. Because individuals are created in the image of God, human life is to be viewed as a sacred gift. The destruction of life for purposes of scientific or medical research is to be avoided. It is also unbiblical and unethical to require that one individual relinquish his or her life for another. While there are times when an individual voluntarily endangers his or her life for another, one cannot be required to do so.

Second, we assume that life begins when the chromosomes align. We used to say that "life begins at conception." Yet, old medical textbooks define "conception" in the same terms we now use to technically label "implantation." Implantation happens after the living cell mass has found its way down the fallopian tube into the uterus and settles in the uterine wall. Scientific evidence suggests that a unique human life begins before this point.

Thus, in a desire to recognize that life begins before implantation, we began to say, "life begins at fertilization," meaning the point at which the sperm penetrates the egg. Yet, when we became excited about calling fertilization the beginning of life, we became trapped by our own terminology again. For example, in a common test for infertile couples, the hamster egg penetration assay, the husband's sperm are incubated with hamster eggs and watched for signs of penetration. (While penetration of the ova by a sperm is a sign of normal sperm, the reliability and significance of the test is controversial.)

Yet Debra Evans in her book, *Without Moral Limits*, made this faulty assumption: "Food for thought—conception between an animal and a man takes place during this laboratory procedure."[2] This is *very* misleading. When the sperm penetrates the egg, we do not have a *humster* (human-hamster) in embryo form. Why? Because the chromosomes *do not* align. In no sense do the human genes match up and have any relationship with the hamster's. In the same way, if you crack a chicken egg and immerse it in human sperm, you may get egg penetration or fertilization—that is, sperm within the egg— but you do not get a live "chickman" developing cell mass.

Probably the best way to state what we believe about the beginning of life, then, is to say that we believe it begins when the chromosomes align, creating a unique being—generally within the first six to twenty-four hours after the sperm penetrates the egg. How interesting to read Psalm 139:16 in light of what we now know from the laboratory: "Your eyes saw my unformed body. All the days ordained for me were written in your book *before one of them came to be*" (italics ours).

With the possibility of cloning somatic cells on the horizon, we may have to expand our definitions to encompass developments in the future. If it's possible to do in humans what was done in the sheep Dolly—when human chromosomes can align many years before a new individual emerges from them—we face new questions about ensoulment. Perhaps in the next decade, we will speculate that life begins when the chromosomes align and begin to develop *into a new individual* distinct from the donor human whose chromosomes it shares.

*Third, we believe that life, even at the one-celled embryo stage, has full personhood and the full rights of that personhood.* Being made in the image of God is the basis of human dignity. At the point at which life begins, even at the cell-mass stage, humans have individual characteristics based on unique genetics. Thus, it is demeaning or destructive to that life to experiment on or destroy it at this stage. We must uphold a high view of the sanctity of life and seek to be instruments only for good and not for evil.

There is one more question over which theologians, ethicists, and physicians are divided but that has enormous impact on how we view genetics. It is a question that we ask after reading the Genesis 1 account in which God gives the scope of human dominion over creation:

Then God said, "Let Us make man in Our image, according to Our likeness; *and let them rule over the fish of the sea and over the birds of the sky and over the cattle and over all the earth, and over every creeping thing that creeps on the earth.*" And God created man in His own image, in the image of God He created him; male and female He created them. And God blessed them; and God said to them, "Be fruitful and multiply, and fill the earth, and subdue it; *and rule over the fish of the sea and over the birds of the sky, and over every living thing that moves on the earth.*" (Genesis 1:26–28 NASB, italics ours)

Humanity's dominion is a gift—a stewardship—for which we will give account. A question we must ask is this: Does genetic manipulation fall within the scope of humanity's dominion over the earth? If so, how far does that dominion extend? When God says human dominion extends to every living thing, does he include human beings or only the animal kingdom?

How we answer this question has enormous ramifications. For example, it's one thing for a woman to pay to have her own hair color altered every six weeks; but, it's quite another for laboratory technicians to alter her genetic code while she is in embryo form so she will have a certain hair color for life. It's one thing for an athlete to take steroids; it's quite another to genetically manipulate an embryo so that he or she will have an athletic physique. Would such actions overstep the realm of humanity's divinely-sanctioned dominion?

Christians face two options here. We can throw our hands in the air and say, "Don't mess with this stuff! Forget it!" *Or, we can learn the facts and participate in a meaningful way in the dialogue about uses and misuses.* In order to participate, we can introduce a grid for making such ethical decisions in the face of moral uncertainties, recognizing that we need grace to face such complex issues.

## ETHICS AND THE GENETIC FUTURE

Fast forward into the future. Consider a case that genetic therapy might fix. Suppose a pregnant patient presents with a family history of cystic fibrosis. Next, imagine that we have the capability to treat early cell lines in utero. We check the genetic structure early in the pregnancy and determine that the child does, indeed, have cystic fibrosis. We inject the appropriate gene, which corrects the problem totally. If God allows us to do it, should we do it? How would you respond? What would be your counsel, and how would you decide?

In answering this question we might first place it through the grid of three common ethical systems: (1) Teleology: Is this good for the most people? This system generally assumes that the end justifies the means. (2) Virtue-based system: What would a virtuous person do in the situation? (3) Deontology: What does the law say? What are the rules?[3]

We believe that we can use aspects of all three systems for decision making; but as Christians who have the Word of God, we make deontology our foundation. The law is the Bible. If it addresses a situation specifically, we have our answer. Certainly the Bible addresses the sanctity of life. But what about the broader question of manipulating genes?

We then move to the virtue-based system. We have Christ as the ultimate virtuous example. What did he do by way of character and conduct that would apply to the situation? How does compassion, healing the sick, and loving children factor into the decision? What about self-effacement, that willingness for the physician to use his power to take care of the poor and the outcasts? Add self-sacrifice—a willingness to give up our own rights and privileges for others, as did Christ. Certainly it would seem that the compassionate, healing, child-loving option would be to do the therapy.

Finally, we consider teleology. In Christianity we see both an emphasis on one sacrificing for all and the "all" sacrificed for one. Christ died for all; but what about the shepherd who left the ninety-nine sheep to seek the lost one? The "end," from our perspective, then, goes beyond what is best for the most people. It looks at the eternal perspective of what is good for one and all. What would bring the most glory to God? Still, this is difficult to determine. Consider a child with Down's syndrome or any "abnormal" chromosome structure. Let's also assume we have the technology to correct it in utero. We would want to diagnose and treat while organs were still developing. This seems reasonable enough. But we would also have to ask ourselves this: Should we continue further and alter someone's God-given genetic structure to conform them to our view of "perfect"? It is one thing to correct, it is another to perfect.

Beyond the three systems, we continue forward, seeing how the decisions at hand fall within the normal ethical principles as follows:

> Beneficence: Have we succeeded in doing good to the patient? In the case of pregnancy, this principle must apply to both mother and child.

> Nonmaleficence: Have we done no harm in either intent or action?

> Justice: Have we endeavored to do right by the patients—both mother and child? Here we would also have to consider whether the patient has the right to the therapy, and if so, who would pay for it.

> Autonomy: Have we allowed the patient to decide? In the case of embryos, although they have the full rights of personhood, obviously they cannot speak for themselves. So we ask: Would a reasonable person, if he or she had the capacity to decide, choose to be born with cystic fibrosis or Down's syndrome?

In these cases, the future of the unborn is left to scientific research and therapy, the will of God, and the love and compassion of their fellow human beings to assist them.

Further, we must realize that sometimes what is "right" is not always legal. Consider the case of a woman in her fortieth week of pregnancy who came to the hospital bleeding with breech presentation and placenta previa. The initial reaction was to do a C-section. But she refused, and surgery without consent is assault and battery. In this case, the right medical answer (C-section) was wrong and/or unethical, as it would have violated the patient's (mother's) autonomy. Yet her decision jeopardized the baby's rights.

In addition to the three usual ethical considerations in the previous section, there is one more factor that often gets left out of such deliberations. *Fourth, we must leave room for the guidance of the Holy Spirit rather than specifically quantifying how much risk is acceptable in areas where there is Christian liberty*. Life is messy, and as such, we almost always have to take some measure of risk. We take risks when we get into our cars and drive to work. We take risks when we agree to have surgeries that will hopefully improve our health or even save our lives. We seek to minimize the risk, yet we will never fully eliminate it, especially where medicine is concerned. Additionally, there is Christian liberty for individuals to make decisions with regard to areas of medical concern and practice that are not covered in Scripture by a moral command that either commands or prohibits them. Because of this, there must be clear understanding of the ethical and medical principles, problems, and practices in which we engage in order to determine if we are in an area of Christian liberty.[4] (See chapter 11, "The Least That a Parent Can Do," by Brock Eide.)

When considering the risk of conceiving a child with a genetic problem and, in the future, of applying genetic therapy, one couple may feel that a 10 percent risk is acceptable. Another couple may think that one-in-one-hundred odds are unacceptable. We can say in general that taking huge risks is irresponsible. Yet, we must leave room for individual guidance and conviction. The place where a decision falls on the risk spectrum may place it clearly out of bounds for consideration, or it may place it in an area of personal conscience.

## A PERSONAL ILLUSTRATION

As one of my (Sandra's) professors pointed out: "It's amazing how experience makes topics so much more relevant." The difference in perspective from a disinterested person and someone actually in the situation is generally significant. This has certainly been the case in my own life. Before my husband and I experienced infertility, we said we would never consider doing in vitro fertilization. We had always assumed it was (1) not worth taking any risk with embryos, and (2) not worth the high financial cost for such small odds of going home with a child. We saw these as the only significant considerations. Yet, in the situation, we began to see other factors that we had not seen from the outside looking in.

For example, in the face of no clear medical diagnosis at that time, both of us felt driven to discover the cause of our fertility problem. Was it a symptom of a more serious medical condition for one of us? Eventually we concluded that even if IVF did not result in a pregnancy for us, if it would provide some clues to the unexplained cause of my inability to conceive, it seemed worth the risk. Three friends had discovered through IVF that their sperm weren't penetrating the egg. In each case (before the existence of micromanipulation) they were then able to finally shut the door on treatment and move on to adoption. In another case, my surgeon explained that one of his patients had learned through IVF that her eggs were abnormal. Each of these couples was able, through the information gained during a "failed" IVF cycle, to pinpoint the cause of their infertility. Thus, they could find closure and make informed decisions about the future.

Eventually, we learned through careful research that the risk to embryos was not as great as some of the Christian literature had led us to believe. So, despite our initial determination that we would never do IVF, it was medical tests that finally identified the probable cause of our infertility and kept us from going ahead with an IVF cycle. This illustrates some of our earlier comments regarding the need to be informed, engaged, judicious, and prayerful in deciding when and if it is appropriate to use current medical and technological capabilities.

There's more to us—heart, intellect, emotion, spirit, and mystery—than can always be considered when viewing ethical dilemmas from the outside. We must not overlook the psychological and spiritual dimensions of the decisions we face. We are not saying that "outsiders" should refrain from drawing any ethical conclusions. Nor are we suggesting that we should allow our pain to cloud our vision of what is right. And we're not suggesting that couples should "just trust God" and ignore risks altogether. The Scriptures tell us we are not to "test God" by taking enormous risks and then expecting him to have to intervene.[5] We are merely saying that we cannot quantify an acceptable risk that is a standard for everyone, and we are calling for the *involvement* of godly and personally effected people when formulating ethical views to add perspectives that those working in the field may not have considered.

Having said all this, we recognize that an overwhelming ethical consideration in the experimental stages of gene therapy is the human wastage problem. In other words, researchers must take enormous risks with embryos to gain the knowledge needed to reach such a point of treatment. A key consideration, then, is this: How much risk are we allowed to take with a good goal in the experimentation process? Does the end justify the means? We know that we cannot go from cancer to a cure without some experimentation, knowing that some therapies may make it worse. While we allow that some risk is inevitable, and while we concede that we cannot exactly quantify a given percentage, we would still argue that doing experimentation that requires destruction of embryos is unethical.

The more difficult risk to assess is not the clear-cut destruction of human life; it is the possible devastating effects of what appears to be non-life-threatening experimentation. Take for example, the drug thalidomide. It was synthesized in West Germany in 1957 and marketed around the world in approximately forty-six countries under many different brand names from 1958 to 1962. Thalidomide was a sedative found to be effective for morning sickness in pregnant women. It was not realized until it was too late that thalidomide could cross the placental wall and affect the fetus. The drug's side effects were catastrophic. When pregnant women ingested thalidomide during the first trimester of pregnancy—the most critical period—it caused significant birth disabilities and death to babies. Any part of the fetus that was in development at the time of ingestion could be affected. For those babies who survived, birth defects included deafness, blindness, disfigurement, cleft palate, major internal disabilities, and—the most common feature—shortening of or absence of limbs. It has been claimed that between ten and twenty thousand babies were born disabled as a consequence.

Thus, we recognize the very real risk involved in research intended to bring about good, and we must *always* be vigilant to minimize that risk, especially when doing research involving human subjects. Again, while we cannot assign a clear percentage of "what is acceptable," we still issue an urgent request to take every precaution.

## PRESENT REALITIES AND FUTURE HOPES

We will now turn to consider existing means of overcoming genetic difficulties. Consider these couples who must make decisions about genetics before conception:

> Tim and Judy have been wanting to conceive for four years. Judy works for an obstetrician, and for her the birth experience is an essential part of womanhood. But they are both carriers of Tay-Sachs.

> Kevin's family has a history of hemophilia. He and his wife, Katie, don't want to risk having a child with this condition, but they long for a baby. Kevin and Katie married in their late thirties, so most agencies will not approve them as adoptive parents due to their age.

> Cassie and John gave birth to a healthy baby, but his condition soon deteriorated. He was diagnosed with glycogen storage disease (GSD), specifically Pompe's disease, which is invariably fatal by age two. He died at eight months. They desperately want children. Their genetic counselor has explained that they have a 25 percent chance of having another child with GSD. And they know that there is only a one-in-four chance that they will have a noncarrier child. Currently, their options are to use a sperm donor, risk losing another child to the disease, live without children, or try to adopt.

In each of the cases above, the future of genetic engineering and the advances in it provide hope. Genetic engineering may permit them to resolve their medical dilemmas within an acceptable ethical and biblical framework. For couples such as these, genetic research and genetic engineering are not abstract ideas and practices in isolated laboratories, they are issues that are very personal and very real.

## GENETIC RESEARCH AT THE ONE-CELL STAGE

Let's consider some of the ramifications of genetic testing at the one-cell stage. When I (Sandra) served on the board of directors of RESOLVE, a national nonprofit organization for infertility patients and the professionals who treat them, RESOLVE's executive director sat on the Human Embryo Research Panel. This nineteen-member panel was selected to advise the National Institutes of Health about embryo research. NIH in turn recommended to the federal government that tax dollars should be used to fund such research. During that time, the panel issued a statement supporting preimplantation diagnosis, allowing doctors treating couples who carry genes for hereditary diseases to consider genetic tests on embryos so that they could select healthy ones for implantation in the uterus after IVF.[6] When scientists claim they are using this kind of embryo research to cure genetic diseases, what they currently mean by *cure* is really "destroy affected embryos thus preventing the term delivery of children with genetic diseases."

Currently, preimplantation genetic diagnosis is done on embryos after IVF. Three days after the procedure, when each embryo contains four to eight cells, one cell is removed from each embryo and genetically analyzed. During the analysis on the single cell, the embryos remain in culture where they can further divide. Technicians transfer only those embryos with normal genes to the uterus where they can continue to grow.

The projected "gains" in genetic research here are intended to end life earlier rather than improve the quality of life for babies affected. The panel revealed a key presupposition for making these guidelines in their final 102–page report to NIH:

> The preimplantation human embryo warrants respect as a developing form of human life, but it does not have the full legal and moral rights attributed to persons. It does not have the same moral status as infants and children. This is because of the absence of developmental individuation in the preimplantation embryo, the lack of even the possibility of sentience and most other qualities considered relevant to the moral status of persons, and the very high rate of natural mortality at this stage.[7]

They go on to argue that the cells of a preimplantation embryo (i.e., an embryo within the first fourteen days of fertilization) are still "nonspecific." When viewed under a microscope, the cells are undifferentiated: "There are no organs developed and the primitive streak, the precursor of the spinal cord, has not yet appeared. Therefore, no awareness or feeling exists in these cells." Thus, they believe, an embryo within fourteen days of fertilization is, in effect, "fair game" for experimentation and destruction.[8]

In arguing their case, they use careful wording when referring to embryos. They were so good at using these terms that they persuaded some pro-life advocates that this research was acceptable, convincing them that life did not begin until the primitive streak or sometime after that.

The first live birth following preimplantation genetic diagnosis was reported in 1989. Since then, babies have been born after such genetic testing has *ruled out* cystic fibrosis, Tay-Sachs disease, Lesch Nyhan syndrome, Duchenne muscular dystrophy, and diseases carried on the X chromosome. It is possible, in the case of some diseases carried by the mother, to diagnose which eggs (oocytes) have the abnormal gene by using a technique called polar body biopsy. In this technique, only the eggs with the normal gene are fertilized. This technique is only applicable for a limited number of diseases.

And some reports indicate increased technical difficulties with the method. Nevertheless, we favor this option or any like it that puts only eggs at risk and does not lead to the destruction of a living human being.

Our challenge to patients who wish to uphold a high view of life is that they be wary of terms such as *preimplantation embryo, preembryo* (a shortened form of preimplantation embryo, which leaves the impression that it's a before-embryo stage), and *before the primitive streak*. One doctor, who presents himself as pro-life, regularly destroys "excess" embryos in his practice, describing the process as "a natural procedure during which the embryo lives out its normal life span in a petri dish." Some patients hear pro-life and assume that the physician holds their same high regard for the embryo at any stage. We must have a thorough understanding of the terms to navigate the moral maze of embryo research.

For example, in early 1998 the American Society for Reproductive Medicine (ASRM) issued a statement requesting response against several Senate bills that called for bans on some embryo research. The ASRM policy director described one bill saying, "it also poses risks for several promising infertility treatments."[9] A generally well-informed Christian patient forwarded the ASRM warning to us with the following note:

> I am not sure I really understand the medical terms. . . . Is this ban good or bad? I agree with the need to make some moral limits on what can and cannot be done with fertility research (i.e., to protect already fertilized eggs) but is this ban so wide reaching that it limits too many other good things? . . . Can either of you explain in common terms what they are talking about?[10]

The bills did not, in fact, limit ethical research that would benefit infertility patients. Yet, our point at this juncture is not to comment on the bills themselves. It is to demonstrate the difficulty of wading through the carefully constructed terms used by those who believe it is acceptable to experiment on and destroy human embryos. Only if we clearly understand what they are saying can we participate in the discussion and take a stand for the sanctity of life.

On the flip side, we would ask for grace from those who are quick to criticize hurting couples who are persistent in their efforts to have healthy genetic offspring. One scientist who read the ASRM statement expressed disappointment in the profound lack of moral courage on the part of infertile couples, whom he felt should stop pushing for such research.[11] Yet in reality, even the most morally-conscious patients are having difficulty sorting through the rhetoric.

## DILEMMAS OF THE FUTURE

Recently a friend of ours asked about a newspaper drawing of a half-human, half-pig figure accompanying an article on gene therapy. It was reminiscent of H. G. Wells' *Island of Dr. Moreau*, or Dean Koontz's novel, *Fear Nothing*. Someone announces that human genes can be spliced into animal chromosomes with all the possible outcomes, and once again the media sensationalizes the news. This scares people away from gene therapy altogether, which is very unfortunate.

Yet, consider a different future scenario. One of my (Dr. Cutrer's) patients came to me early in her pregnancy. A neonatologist had referred her because her first child, a two-year-old, had a devastating genetic disorder. This child endured multiple seizures, cried incessantly, and could not be comforted. We were uncertain of the exact disease, but we were concerned that it might happen again.

I watched her through an uneventful first trimester. However, we noticed the first sign of trouble when the head failed to grow normally at sixteen to seventeen weeks. I sent her to have a higher resolution sonogram than I could do in my office. While those results demonstrated that the organs were okay, they confirmed that the head was not growing normally. We considered that the father was not a large man, that she might have miscalculated the dates, or that hypertension might be factors here. Before long, however, it became obvious that this child had the same disease as its sibling. The mother gave birth, and eventually both children died. Now I wonder—what if we could develop the technology to alter such children's genes at the embryo stage? Sadly, the cost to get there, in terms of risk to human life, would be far too great at this stage.

Yet, there are cases in which embryos do not have to be sacrificed at the experimentation stage. In these cases, here are some general conclusions: *Saving the life of a child with a genetic illness—Yes.* Take for example, the cystic-fibrosis patient. The possibility of correcting this disease is laudable, and scientists are developing therapies to treat it that do not sacrifice human lives. Or take the case of a mother with AIDS. Certainly it seems appropriate to make alterations in her immune system so that she might better fight the disease and so that her children are protected from contracting it in utero.

*Correcting a serious but not lethal disease—Probably.* Beyond the obvious priority of saving lives, we now consider the treatment of serious disease. What about someone with sickle-cell anemia. How would we view a future gene therapy that can correct this? Sickle cell is problematic, but it's not lethal. In fact, the malaria infection is actually better handled with the sickle-cell trait; thus, the disease has some benefit in parts of the world such as Africa. Nevertheless, quality of life is a good and reasonable matter of concern. Again, a key here would be to look at the risk-benefit ratio involved in research.

*Sex selection and cosmetics—It depends.* With a gender-based disease such as hemophilia, it seems reasonable to select sex before life begins.

In another scenario, we consider that Jesus said we couldn't add a cubit to our life span by worrying, but what about through genetic alteration? It's one thing to treat children with deficiencies of growth hormone. Yet, we would have to limit access to the therapy so that athletic parents don't use it to turn out tall basketball players. It seems clear that there's a vast difference between using the information to treat disease with origins in genetic abnormality versus using it for mere cosmetic improvements.

Since we know that some genetic diseases speed up the aging process, possibly someday scientists will find a way to reverse the process. If found, should we use it? In general, our position is that as long as the intent and action are for diagnosis and treatment of human suffering, within the limits we have outlined, genetic research is a good thing. Again, a key concern is the risk to human life involved in developing those therapies.

*The making of a new individual, whether through twinning or cloning, and any research leading to any of the above positive-outcome scenarios via the destruction of human embryos—No.* When the OB-Gyn residents discussed the ethical dilemma of the woman inseminated by her stepfather, they kept asking: Is it right? In a day when medical technology often runs ahead of its ethical undergirding, we have sought to provide some guidelines for sorting through these complex issues from a Christian perspective. We recognize that "there is a way that seems right to a man, but in the end it leads to death" (Prov. 14:12) in exploring the dominion actually given to us by God whose ways are not our ways. Nevertheless, as a believing community, *we must do the best we can to evaluate, process, debate, and interact on these issues,* always with kindness and graciousness toward not only the researchers involved but also mindful of the hurting families seeking alleviation of their pain.

Developments from genetic research in the next few decades will probably relate to identifying an individual's potential for developing illness and will be aimed at modalities for prevention and treatment. This is a far cry from Michael Crichton's *Jurassic Park.* So, while it's always wise to preemptively consider the potential for extreme abuses before they happen, we must focus most of our energies on issues that currently confront care providers: How do we stop the existing excesses? How can we as leaders in the Christian community constructively provide direction, if not hard-and-fast answers, for those seeking guidance? How do we view the technology? How do we view life? And how can we bring the latter two together for the ultimate glory of our Creator God?

## ENDNOTES

1. See Deuteronomy 23:25 and Exodus 20:10 as well as notes from Matthew 12:2, *Ryrie Study Bible*, 1464.
2. Debra Evans, *Without Moral Limits* (Westchester, Ill.: Crossway Books, 1989), 90.
3. For additional information on each of these systems and their relationship to Christians and the biblical perspective, see, John S. Feinberg and Paul D. Feinberg, *Ethics for a Brave New World* (Wheaton, Ill.: Crossway Books, 1993), 17–45.
4. Ibid., 43–45.
5. Deuteronomy 6:16 and quoted by Christ at the time of his temptation, Matthew 4:7.
6. In part, the statement claimed, "By improving very early diagnostic testing,

couples who carry lethal diseases will be able to ensure that the pregnancy they begin will result in a healthy child. For many it provides a more acceptable option than a later abortion of an affected fetus." See also, John Schwarz, "NIH Panel to Announce Guidelines for Human Embryo Experiments," *Washington Post* (27 September 1994): A3.

7. Executive Summary of the National Institutes of Health Report of the Human Embryo Research Panel, Final Draft (27 September 1994), 2.
8. Ibid. See also, Paul Recer, "Panel Would End Ban on Embryo Research Funds," *Boston Globe* (28 September 1994).
9. Sean Tipton, Letter to Colleagues (4 February 1998).
10. Private correspondence held by the authors.
11. Private correspondence held by the authors.

*An Overview*

How should we respond to the questions raised by the growing availability of genetic and prenatal testing? In this chapter, Dr. Brock Eide draws on personal and professional experiences as well as social and philosophical considerations before formulating a biblical understanding and approach to the issue. Created uniquely and individually bearing the image of God, children are a gift from a sovereign God and are to be welcomed in all of their humanity. The concerns behind the desire for prenatal testing are very real. So also are the embryos being tested, and it is the full affirmation of them as human beings that must be guarded.

Chapter Eleven

# "THE LEAST THAT A PARENT CAN DO"

*Prenatal Genetic Testing and the*
*Welcome of Our Children*

Brock L. Eide, M.D.

RECENTLY I HAD AN EXPERIENCE that brought home to me how extensively prenatal testing has already come to affect the experience of parenthood and how it can exert subtle pressures on the way we view our offspring. My wife and I—both physicians in our midthirties—were expecting our second child. Because of my wife's age, our obstetrician recommended an ultrasound and amniocentesis to screen for the abnormalities for which our child would be at special risk. We declined the amniocentesis because there was nothing it could reveal that would change our decision to carry our child to term or that could lead to beneficial in utero therapy. It also posed a risk to both child and mother. But we decided to consent to the ultrasound because it was harmless and could potentially show something that would affect our actions, such as an obstructed kidney, or hydrocephalus that needed prenatal shunting, or a neural tube defect that would necessitate cesarean section.

On the appointed day, we were shown into the ultrasound suite. Our initial guide was a pleasant young technician who, she told us, had recently had a baby of her own. She seemed bursting with the joy of motherhood and eager to give us our first visual contact with our child. For the next half hour she conducted her ultrasound inspection, flashing the transducer across my wife's abdomen with smooth, efficient strokes and regaling us with shot after shot of our new (and if I may be forgiven a father's pride, extremely lovely) child. She had a real knack for moving the transducer at just the right speed and in just the right line to give a sort of real-time, three-dimensional appearance to the image on the screen. Our baby was twenty-two weeks old, eleven inches long, skull barely two inches in diameter. Everything looked perfect. We watched our baby yawn, rub its eyes, roll over, and stretch. It was an intensely intimate and moving experience. Our child was glory in miniature, and we welcomed it wholeheartedly into our lives. It seemed all too soon when the technician announced she was finished, and we prepared to go only with reluctance. Oh, she said, *you're* not finished, yet. Before you go we need a physician to go over the shots, but don't worry, it's just routine.

We were only too happy to comply, glad, if the truth be told, to get a few extra peeks. Soon the doctor appeared. She was only a little older than the technician, our age, in fact, but she had an air of stale, musty joylessness that sat on her thick as greasy build-up in a bachelor's kitchen. For the next hour she plowed furrows through the transducer goo on my wife's belly with unsmiling intensity. She took shots from every angle imaginable, all the while reminding us that she couldn't guarantee our "fetus" wouldn't have Down's—even though everything looked good; the sensitivity of the ultrasound for that sort of thing was only 50 percent . . . and didn't we want an amnio? Hmm . . . just so we understood that we couldn't really rely on the ultrasound. . . .

By the time she was done, we couldn't wait to get out. Technically, she was a marvelous ultrasonographer, the pictures she took were even better than the technician's. But her view of what we were doing in that suite differed so radically from our own that she grated on our nerves like fingernails on a blackboard. We saw ourselves as the welcome wagon. She viewed herself as quality control.

Unfortunately, this doctor's attitude is far from unique. The view that medicine—and parents in partnership with it—should be in the business of controlling the quality of the offspring delivered has become increasingly prevalent in recent years, fueled by the growing availability of prenatal and genetic testing. As a result, new questions have been raised regarding our proper roles as parents and the nature of our relationships with our children. In addition, as diagnostic advances have surged ahead of comparable advances in treatment, parents have increasingly been faced with difficult and painful decisions regarding their own reproduction and the treatment of their developing children—decisions that have proven especially difficult for those who believe that developing life is sacred, and that the bearing of children is heavily freighted with symbolic, spiritual, and sacramental meanings.

In this chapter, I will examine some of the questions raised by the growing availability of genetic and prenatal testing, and I will seek to determine the implications of the various potential answers both for our understanding of the family and the place of reproduction in human life.

## GENETIC TESTING AND GENETIC ABORTION

Prenatal testing is usually offered in one of several situations: first, when parents are known to be at special risk for carrying a disease gene usually because they are members of an ethnic group known to be at high risk for certain diseases, because they have a previous child or a relative with genetic abnormalities, or because they have had multiple previous miscarriages; second, when maternal age is "advanced"—usually age thirty-five or over; and third, when routine maternal blood screens such as the serum alpha-fetoprotein level yield an abnormal result. Prenatal testing may begin with relatively noninvasive procedures, such as ultrasonography or maternal peripheral blood sampling, but it often progresses to involve the use of more invasive tests, such as amniocentesis or chorionic villus sampling, which require instrumenting the uterus to obtain samples of fetal tissues. Such tests carry risks for the termination of pregnancy of between 0.3 and 4.5 percent.[1]

The information gathered through such procedures may be used in a variety of ways. Several of these uses are widely considered to be morally uncontroversial, even by those categorically opposed to abortion or destruction of embryos. It may be used simply to allay the fears of prospective parents, to prepare them for giving birth to a child with special needs, or to allow for special precautions at the time of delivery. If, for example, a mother were determined early in the second trimester to have an abnormally high alpha-fetoprotein level, an ultrasound could be performed that might reveal the presence of a neural tube defect such as spina bifida or meningomyelocele that would render her fetus susceptible to trauma during normal labor, and an elective cesarean section could be scheduled instead. Such information may also be used to help carriers of disease-causing genes make decisions regarding marriage or reproduction. Evangelical Protestant theologians John and Paul Feinberg have written: "[I]t is hard to argue that early detection of those who will get a [genetic] disease so as to treat it or discovery of carriers of a recessive gene so that they may make informed decisions about marriage and reproduction are immoral uses of genetic screening."[2]

In contrast to such uses, the information gathered from prenatal testing may also be used in ways that generate profound moral controversy, as in decisions to abort genetically abnormal fetuses or to destroy genetically abnormal in vitro fertilized embryos. Indeed, the promise of such uses has frequently been offered as one of the primary justifications for the Human Genome Project, usually under the rubric of "disease prevention." As Evelyn Fox Keller has noted: "[P]revention means preventing the births of individuals diagnosed as genetically aberrant—in a word, it means abortion."[3] Keller supports her contention by citing one scientist who extolled the benefits of the Genome Project as follows: "Pointing to schizophrenia, which he claimed currently accounts for one-half of all hospital beds, Charles Cantor, the former head of the Human Genome Center at the Lawrence Berkeley Laboratory, recently argued in a lecture that the project would more than pay for itself by preventing the occurrence of just this one disease. When asked how such a saving could be effected he could only say: 'by preventing the birth' of schizophrenics."[4] Ruth Schwartz Cowan notes similarly that

> we need to be very clear about what therapy is currently available for most diseases or disabilities that can be diagnosed prenatally: *none*. The only recourse for patients whose fetuses are diagnosed as having Down's syndrome, or spina bifida, or Turner's syndrome, or Tay-Sachs disease, or sickle cell anemia, or one of the thalassemias is abortion, a process that can hardly be described as therapeutic. This means that, for the foreseeable future, the ethical and social implications of the Human Genome Project are going to be inextricable from the ethical and social implications of abortion.[5]

Although the right to obtain an abortion has not been legally prohibited in the United States for over twenty years, abortion is still usually regarded as a moral issue even by those (such as Cowan) who believe the procedure justifiable. This is particularly true in the case of abortions that are obtained for genetic reasons, which for ease of usage will be referred to as "genetic abortions." Indeed, it is rare to find anyone, either in the professional literature or in a public-policy forum, who denies that there are serious moral considerations attending to this issue. While a variety of justifications have been offered for the practice of genetic abortion, I will focus on three that are most frequently given.

## FIRST JUSTIFICATION: FETAL BENEFIT

The first and most common means of justifying genetic abortion is by pointing to the benefit it provides the fetus. According to this line of thinking, since fetuses with severe genetic disorders are destined to have lives of poor quality, the most merciful thing one can do for them is prevent their birth. In his recent book, *The Lives to Come*,[6] philosopher Philip Kitcher provides a typical discussion of one who holds such views and of the ways in which the lives of those suffering from severe genetic defects may be viewed as being of poor quality.

According to Kitcher, an individual's quality of life can be measured along three axes.[7] The first of these axes reflects the individual's ability to form a sense of what is valuable and important to him- or herself as a person. According to Kitcher, an individual must be able to form such a sense of values to attain the status of "personhood" that is required for membership in the human moral community. In employing this criterion, Kitcher follows a line of thought that has its beginnings with Immanuel Kant. According to Kant, human dignity is a product of the human capacity for autonomy or moral self-legislation, a capacity belonging solely to rational creatures. By virtue of this capacity, rational beings are creatures "of infinite worth" and "deserving of respect." For Kant this meant that a rational being must be regarded only as "an end in itself" and never simply as a "means." Kant referred to rational beings as "persons," while he called nonrational beings "things."[8] Only the former were considered "objects of respect" and hence deserving of protection from "arbitrary use." Kitcher uses similar arguments in setting standards that he believes any human life must meet to be considered even minimally valuable. For Kitcher, any individual who, as a result of genetic disease, is destined never to attain this state of personhood may justifiably be aborted. Kitcher gives the example of Tay-Sachs: "Doctors, parents, even many religious leaders agree on the permissibility of terminating pregnancies when the fetus is diagnosed as positive for Tay-Sachs, not because the baby will suffer pain, that can relatively easily be avoided, but because neuro-degeneration will start before the distinctive life of an individual person can begin."[9]

The second of Kitcher's quality-of-life axes reflects the extent to which an individual's autonomously chosen values and desires are satisfied. According to Kitcher, there are certain genetic disabilities that, though they may not affect an individual's ability to form a system of values, inevitably prevent their realization of goals that are typically regarded as of central importance to most human lives. As such, quality of life is diminished, often to the point where that life may be considered not worthwhile. In this regard, Kitcher cites as paradigmatic any disorders that result in severe immobilization and dependence, though he also implies that disorders resulting in infertility or shortened life span may similarly deprive life of worth.

Kitcher's third quality-of-life axis reflects the balance of pleasure and pain that are expected to occur in an individual's life. His typical examples include Tay-Sachs disease, which results in an early onset of painful neurological degeneration, and Lesch-Nyhan syndrome, which results in painful, compulsive self-mutilation.

According to Kitcher, when faced with a developing fetus that is known to have a genetic defect that we believe will cause it to have a life of poor quality, it is morally permissible, and in fact even morally commendable, to abort that fetus. Most contemporary bioethicists agree. Others go even farther, calling such abortions morally obligatory. One philosopher, Margery Shaw,[10] has even charged that parents who knowingly give birth to a seriously impaired child are guilty of negligent child abuse and has urged that courts and legislatures develop standards by which parents should be held accountable for the genetic health of their children.[11]

Although the near consensus among secular thinkers that quality-of-life considerations are sufficient justification for genetic abortion is not entirely unexpected, what *is* perhaps surprising is the apparent acquiescence to this view among a number of religious groups that have traditionally been strongly opposed to abortion. Such groups include the Greek Orthodox and Roman Catholic churches in Cyprus and Sardinia, where beta-thalassemia is rampant, and certain Orthodox Jewish communities afflicted with a high incidence of Tay-Sachs disease. While we might expect the leaders of such communities to agree with secular thinkers that children affected by severe genetic disabilities are destined to a quality of life that we would not willingly *choose* for them, we might expect them to oppose the premise that we are therefore justified in taking their lives through genetic abortion.

Even if we set aside our concerns about abortion in general, we should still be troubled by the fact that the quality-of-life criteria that Kitcher adduces could equally well be used to justify the killing of severely handicapped infants and mentally impaired children and adults. Such criteria could also be used to justify abortion for sex selection, a practice almost universally condemned by Western bioethicists, especially in countries such as India and China where there are clear differences in expected quality of life for male and female children and where females can be highly restricted in forming and fulfilling their own sets of values. Indeed, such subjective third-party assessments of quality of life are unavoidably elastic, capable of stretching to accommodate whatever concerns or biases the assessor might have. Such considerations should give us pause, and lead us to wonder whether Leon Kass was perhaps right in claiming that the principle, "Defectives' should not be born," is a principle without limits.[12]

There are other reasons to question both the validity and wisdom of this first type of justification; but as they apply equally to the two justifications we have yet to consider, they will be considered below.

## SECOND JUSTIFICATION: SOCIETAL BENEFIT

The second kind of justification commonly offered for genetic abortion is that it increases the well-being of the society as a whole and of future generations in particular. Those with genetic diseases, it is argued, consume a large quantity of limited societal resources that yield only a limited benefit to themselves and no benefit whatsoever to the rest of society. These resources, it is claimed, could better be used to fund immunizations, disease prevention, or biomedical research that could ultimately benefit millions. Philip Kitcher provides a characteristic argument along these lines: "To the extent that funds for social programs are tightly limited, support for [children born with severe disabilities] diverts money that could be used to improve the quality of the lives of many others."[13] What should be the proper response to this fact on behalf of parents? Kitcher writes: "[B]ecause reproductive decisions do not occur in social vacua, responsible reflections must recognize that new lives impose demands: If everybody acted as we are inclined to, what would be the effect on the well-being of other children and adults in our society?"[14]

Kitcher's arguments are predicated on a number of claims, the validity of which he seems to assume but that others may be inclined to doubt. First, his claim that genetically handicapped children will deprive others of scarce and costly medical resources is predicated on the premise that the total amount of money available for the care of the ill is somehow gravely limited—a claim that, however often repeated, is lacking in factual support. The actual quantity of money that will be available for such purposes—especially in the affluent societies of the West—will be a function of the value that the citizens of those societies place on such uses. As such, a better response to a shortage of funds would be to explain both the inherent value and the neediness of our handicapped citizens and to appeal to the public at large for their support. Arguing as Kitcher has done will only increase societal prejudice against handicapped persons, implying as it does that their births were somehow the result of selfish or even antisocial acts. Such prejudice can only decrease the public's willingness to assist the handicapped.

Kitcher's arguments are also predicated on the claim that genetically disabled persons can confidently be known to consume more societal resources than their nondisabled counterparts. While this claim seems to have greater relevance for some disorders than others, it would be hard to demonstrate its accuracy for any known disorder. As Leon Kass has pointed out,

> many questions can be raised about [such an] approach. First, how accurate are the calculations? Not all the costs have been reckoned. The aborted "defective" child will in most cases be "replaced" by a "normal" child. In keeping the ledger, the costs to society of his care and maintenance cannot be ignored—costs of educating him, or removing his wastes and pollution,

not to mention the costs in nonreplacable natural resources that he consumes. Who is a greater drain on society's precious resources, the average inmate of a home for the retarded or the average graduate of Berkeley? I doubt that we know or can even find out.[15]

There is additionally the hidden cost to society that the "normal replacement" child has if he or she is a carrier for a recessive genetic disease and passes that disease gene on to subsequent generations—something that the handicapped person himself or herself will most often be unable to do. Indeed, there is actual empirical data to suggest that for certain kinds of disorders, genetic testing as it is currently practiced actually has the "dysgenic" effect of raising the frequency of disease alleles that are passed on to subsequent generations. Marc Lappe has written that

> the process of aborting a fetus with a deleterious recessive disease and then compensating for the loss of the expected child by trying to have more children ultimately results in a subtle increase in frequency of the recessive gene over many generations. This is true because with reproductive compensation, two-thirds of all of the live children will be carriers of the recessive gene at issue, instead of the one-half normally expected without prenatal diagnosis.[16]

A similar effect can be expected with X-linked disorders as well.

Perhaps the strongest objection to such societal good arguments is that we have powerful reasons for doubting the claim that our society's good is to be found in the intentional killing of any of its members. Even without appealing to divine standards of justice, we should remember that our society has been founded on the notion that all human beings possess an "unalienable right" to life, and that all of us have been created equal; not equal in every respect of course—not equal in talents or capacities or intellectual abilities—but equal in the politically important sense that we possess an "unalienable right" to life, simply by virtue of our membership in the human community.[17] Once this membership ceases to be awarded to each and every individual simply on the basis of his or her descent from human parents—in other words, it is awarded only to those possessing certain abilities or capacities—the guarantee of unalienable rights that has been the backbone of our society will be formally meaningless, and human rights will belong only to those who are beloved by the powerful. It is for this reason more than any other that all people in our society—whether believers in the divinely ordained value of human life or not—should be highly suspicious of any purported societal good that requires the abandonment of our society's belief in the moral equality of all human beings.

## THIRD JUSTIFICATION: FAMILIAL BENEFIT

The third justification for genetic abortion is that it benefits the family into which the defective child would otherwise be born. Severely defective infants, it is argued, place such great demands on a family that they significantly reduce the quality of the lives of the other family members. Philip Kitcher again provides a typical example of such an argument when he urges that we take account of such facts when we think about genetic abortion. He bases his argument on the oft-recited contemporary claim that human beings, until they attain the status of autonomous persons, are devoid of any intrinsic value, and as such, any value that they possess as nonpersons must be conferred on them by others. When an essentially worthless prenatal life poses a great threat to the quality of already existing lives, it is only reasonable to abort it. Kitcher expresses this view in the form of a paraphrase of Ronald Dworkin:

> Liberals about abortion take the value of human lives to arise as the result of human investment in lives. In consequence, they view the continuation of some pregnancies as greatly diminishing the value of lives, the lives of parents, children already born, others who are affected, in which there has already been substantial human investment, and see this diminution of value as a far greater loss than the cessation of a human life that has not yet "begun in earnest."[18]

Even if we ignore the question of whether a fetus has any intrinsic value, we may still question the apparent confidence of Kitcher and Dworkin that they can know in advance what sorts of events would or would not be good for "families" as such. While many families have no doubt experienced considerable grief and disruption after the birth of a handicapped child, many others have found the experience deeply enriching. Author Pearl Buck, for example, has written movingly of the experience of having a daughter gravely retarded from PKU:

> A retarded child, a handicapped person, brings its own gift to life, even to the life of normal human beings. That gift is comprehended in the lessons of patience, understanding, and mercy, lessons which we all need to receive and to practice with one another, whatever we are. My feelings can be summed up, perhaps, by saying that in this world, where cruelty prevails in so many aspects of our life, I would not add the weight of choice to kill rather than to let live.[19]

Another Nobel Prize-winning novelist, Kenzaburo Oe of Japan, has written extensively of his and his family's enriching experience of raising a mentally handicapped child. In his recent memoir, *A Healing Family*, he writes:

> Twenty-five years ago, my first son was born with brain damage. This was a blow, to say the least; and yet, as a writer, I must acknowledge the fact that the central theme of my work, throughout much of my career, has been the way my family has managed to live with this handicapped child. Indeed, I would have to admit that the very ideas that I hold about this society and

the world at large—my thoughts, even, about whatever there might be that transcends our limited reality—are based on and learned through living with him.[20]

This birth was for Oe "a case of 'perfect timing,' an immensely important event that occurred at a vital moment in my life,"[21] and he can say of it now that

> my greatest source of pride these days is the fact that my brain-damaged son is a decent, tolerant, trustworthy human being who also happens to have a good sense of humor. And his strength of character has had no small influence on our family. In the course of living with him, I have come to know many disabled people, their families, and those who help with their rehabilitation, and I have seen how each shoulders his or her own burden. The signs of this suffering are clearly visible on the faces of the handicapped, even when they have reached the stage of acceptance; and those around them are no doubt similarly marked. But I believe there is another sign that all these people share: their common decency.[22]

Leon Kass captures well the difficulties of the view that familial hardship is inevitably harmful:

> It is not entirely clear [in any family] what would be good for the other children. In a strong family, the experience with a suffering and dying child might help the healthy siblings learn to face and cope with adversity. Some have even speculated that the lack of experience with death and serious illness in our affluent young people is responsible for their immaturity and lack of gravity, and their inability to respond patiently and steadily to the serious problems they encounter in private or community life. Doubtless many American parents have unwittingly fostered childishness by their well-meaning efforts to spare their children any confrontation with harsh reality.[23]

Christians, especially, would seem to have reason to question this unquestioning desire to avoid suffering, even at the cost of another's life, and the low value that contemporaries ascribe to the sacrificial care of the helpless. This is not to make light of the very real sufferings that those who give birth to handicapped children experience, but it is an attempt to do justice to the very real value that suffering may sometimes have in human life, and to question those who pretend to know in which direction the good for a family inevitably lies.

Each of the three putative justifications for genetic abortion that I have discussed contain additional difficulties in their thinking about the family, the most fundamental of which involve misunderstandings of the ultimate purposes of parenthood and of the relationship between parents and children. It is to an examination of these misunderstandings that I will now turn, and since we are seeking the sources of misunderstandings in predominantly secular thought, I will begin by examining the ideas that are most characteristic of contemporary secular views of the family.

## SECULAR VIEWS OF THE FAMILY

Aristotle was perhaps the first secular philosopher to address seriously one of the most fundamental questions regarding the nature of the family: why parents desire to have children. In *De Anima* he wrote:

> For this the most natural function of living creatures . . . namely to make another thing like themselves . . . so that in the way that they can they may partake in the eternal and the divine. . . . Now the living creature cannot have a share in the eternal and the divine by continuity, since none of the mortal things admits of persistence as numerically one and the same, but in the way that each creature can participate in this, in that way it does have a share in it . . . and persists not as itself but as something like itself.[24]

For Aristotle, then, the desire to procreate is tied up with the deepest desires of the soul: the desires for immortality and transcendence. In his *Nicomachean Ethics*, Aristotle says further of the relationship between generations that parents love their children as "a part of themselves"—an offshoot, as it were—"for one's offspring is a sort of other self in virtue of a separate existence."[25]

Contemporary philosopher David Heyd expands further on the topic of parental desires, revealing both its positive and its negative aspects:

> It is a universal cultural fact that human beings desire to have children and that they raise them more or less "in their own image." Empirical research enumerates a wide variety of motives for having children: economic need (children as work force), security (for old age), status, power, psychological stimulation, expression of primary group ties (love), companionship, self-realization, the preservation of lineage, the continuation, multiplication, or expansion of the self, a religious or moral duty (to God or society), even simple fun. This long list indirectly supports a generocentric view of procreation, as the list conspicuously does not consist of "altruistic" motives, that is, those concerned with the good of the future child. The decision to have children is one of the most selfish of human choices, and parentocentric motives guide not only the positive choices (to create another happy child), but also the negative (refraining from begetting a handicapped child). For as a matter of psychological fact, we rarely face a case in which the parents wish to have a (handicapped) child but decide to assign an overriding weight to the "interests of the child" not to be born. It is the parents who do not want a suffering child. . . . We want to have children for our own satisfaction; we want them, therefore, to be of a particular nature (identity), that is, sufficiently similar to us; and we want them to be of a certain number, such that we can maintain that kind of quality of life (for us and for them) that would secure that satisfaction.[26]

Thus, in the contemporary view of the parent-child relation, the children are not only *from* the parents but also *for* the parents, and their existence is to be valued only insofar as it furthers parental aims or pleasures. This view is behind the following claim of H. Tristram Engelhardt that prerational children are a form of parental possession:

> One also owns what one produces. One might think here of both animals and young children. Insofar as they are the products of the ingenuity or energies of persons, they can be possessions. There are, however, special obligations to animals by virtue of the morality of beneficence that do not exist with regard to things. Such considerations, as well as the fact that young children will become persons, limit the extent to which parents have ownership rights over their young children. However, these limits will be very weak, at least insofar as they can be made out in general secular terms, with regard to ownership rights in human zygotes, embryos, and fetuses that will not be allowed to develop into persons, or with regard to lower vertebrates, where there is very little sentience.[27]

The view that parents possess absolute rights over their offspring is not, of course, new. Historically it was embodied in the Roman law of *patria potestas*, which gave absolute power over the life and death of children to their father, and with only slight modification this has been the controlling principle in parent-child relations in most cultures throughout most of history. Such views, however, began to be questioned in the West beginning in about the seventeenth century. At that time, the rights of parents over their children came to be viewed as being analogous to the rights of kings over their subjects—rights that at that time were beginning to come under heavy fire.

Nowhere was this subject more keenly debated than in England. Thomas Hobbes and his contemporary Robert Filmer were the most powerful defenders of the old order. Hobbes argued in his book, *Leviathan*, that based on their relations in the state of nature, parents have no fundamental obligations to their children. Their primary duty rather is to protect themselves, which entitles them to keep their children in a state of submission by threat or, if need be, by violence. For Hobbes, the war of all against all extended even into the family. Filmer echoed Hobbes in claiming that parents—or rather fathers—possess absolute authority over their children. For Filmer, this power is given by God: divine in origin, and in authority.[28] Through procreation, the father becomes owner of his children. He made them, and they are his property to do with as he will. His authority is absolute and unlimited, extending to the right of life or death over his children.

Later in that same century, John Locke argued that such views are fundamentally unsound. Locke based his argument on the fact that such views are incompatible with the Bible's teaching that each individual is fundamentally equal in the eyes of God, and that parents are given power over their children by God solely for the children's benefit. According to Locke, "The power . . . that parents have over their children arises from the duty which is incumbent on them to take care of their off-spring during the imperfect state of childhood."[29] Because God is the maker of children, children are not man's property; rather, they belong to God. For Locke, the child does not exist to serve the wishes of the family, but the family to serve the child. Jacob Joshua Ross has summarized Locke's views by saying that "this Lockean conception demotes parents from their status as absolute monarchs and turns them into trustees whose children are temporary wards and whose actions are subject to constant . . . divine scrutiny."[30]

Locke's view has been extremely influential in subsequent Western thought, and in many ways it still forms the theoretical basis for many of our laws governing the relations of parents and postnatal children. However, as the divine command on which Locke's argument was based has lost its authority in our increasingly secular culture, the child-centered view of human procreation that it embodies has become increasingly rare. Indeed, we have now reached the point where prenatal fetuses and "defective" infants are viewed as having no intrinsic value but only such value as is conferred on them by their parents—a value that is usually assessed according to the extent to which the child is seen as furthering parental goals and desires. In consequence, it is now largely among religious communities that views of the human family such as Locke's can be found. Indeed, the views that these communities espouse are frequently even richer than the largely fiduciary image of trusteeship presented by Locke, for they incorporate additional teachings from the Bible regarding the nature of the human family. It is to such teachings that I will now briefly turn to see what guidance they can offer for our understanding of the family and our attitudes toward the new genetic technologies.

## BIBLICAL VIEWS OF THE FAMILY

The Bible clearly teaches, both in Old and New Testaments, that there is tremendous spiritual significance to the fact that God has chosen to give each of us physical life through a particular pair of human parents—situating us in a particular family, and giving us a particular genetic, cultural, and spiritual heritage.[31] He has created both parents and children with the capacity to love each other—a capacity that is of equal or even greater importance than the sense of obligation cited by Locke in forming the basis of their relationship. The Bible also teaches that the relationship between human parent and child has been ordered by God to represent his relationship to his earthly children. As such, our care for our children is intended to be both an imitation of and a thanksgiving for God's gracious care for us. The Bible explicitly endorses the notion that parents have duties to their children that include, among other things, nurture and kindness,[32] love,[33] and the provision of basic necessities.[34]

This biblically inspired view of the family and the parent-child relationship in particular stands in marked contrast to those contemporary secular understandings that view parental rights as superseding absolutely those of the prenatal, or even prerational, child. Put quite simply, the biblical understanding of the family, which incorporates a fundamental obligation to the sacrificial service of the needy child, could not be more at odds with the new and starkly utilitarian visions of the family that would justify the sacrifice of the needy child for the happiness of the powerful parent.

## CONCLUSION

How, then, should those who are persuaded of the relevance of this biblical view of the family respond to the availability of the new genetic technologies that I have been considering? Should they avoid the use of such technologies as unpardonable incursions into areas of divine prerogative? Should they seek testing before marriage, like many Orthodox Jewish communities, and abstain from marriage to those with whom they would be at high risk of giving birth to a child with a severe genetic disability? Should they marry but refrain from reproduction? Or should they make use of prenatal testing and pursue an abortion when a severe genetic defect is detected?

Responding first to the last of these questions, for those religious communities that hold that all human life is sacred—even prenatal human life—the practice of genetic abortion has usually been regarded as an unwarranted usurpation of a divine prerogative. Even within those communities, however, certain voices have been calling for a loosening of such prohibitions in the case of certain genetic disorders that carry particularly grim prognoses. Religious ethicist Allen Verhey, for example, said recently:

> There are, I think, genetic conditions which justify abortion. There are conditions like Tay-Sachs which consign a child not only to an abbreviated life, but to a life subjectively indistinguishable from torture; and there are conditions like trisomy 18 which are inconsistent not only with life but with the minimal conditions for human communication. Prenatal diagnosis and abortion, I think, can be used responsibly.[35]

Certainly those who are committed to a biblical view of the family will be sympathetic to Verhey's desire to minimize the suffering of infants born with such conditions (even if, like Philip Kitcher, we are not so pessimistic about the possibility of relieving the conscious suffering of those afflicted with disorders such as Tay-Sachs). Such persons, however, must also notice the extent of Verhey's departure from traditional Christian belief regarding the impermissibility of intentionally taking innocent human life. It is important to note in considering Verhey's recommendations that his arguments must either entail an acceptance of other life-taking practices such as infanticide or euthanasia or the devaluation of prenatal human life. If intense suffering and the inability to communicate are regarded as sufficient justifications for taking human life, then voluntary euthanasia of the intensely suffering and involuntary euthanasia of the comatose, vegetative, or severely retarded would seem to be countenanced. Indeed, if termination of life under such circumstances is regarded as beneficial and appropriate for the unborn, it would only seem cruel to deny termination of life to those already born. Take, for instance, the case of Tay-Sachs: If we feel justified in aborting a fetus diagnosed with Tay-Sachs, should we not equally feel justified in euthanizing a year-old infant who is just beginning to develop symptoms? or even a day-old newborn who can expect several months of presymptomatic existence—a time that will most likely only increase its parents' eventual suffering? If we do not feel justified in aborting these postnatal infants, it must only be because we believe that prenatal life is somehow inherently less valuable than postnatal life. There is simply no way around the fact that if we believe we are justified in taking a particular human life, we must either reject outright the belief that innocent human lives *as such* must not be taken, or we must believe that the particular life in question is of insufficient worth to merit protection under the general prohibition. Either way, such a view would carry tremendous implications both for our understanding of the inherent worth of human life and for our treatment of the unborn and the infirm. Surely we must think carefully about such implications before adopting Verhey's recommendations; otherwise it is not only possible but highly likely that we will be led into evil by our desire to do good.[36]

How else might we respond to Verhey's quite legitimate desire to minimize the suffering caused by genetic disorders without resorting to genetic abortion? One way is by preventing the conception of children with severe genetic diseases through a program of adult genetic screening and counseling in which couples who are found to be at high risk of giving birth to children with severe genetic defects could be given the option of foregoing reproduction. Would such a program be consistent with the kind of biblical view of the family presented above? While this point is not beyond dispute, I believe that it would. Such a practice seems consistent with many Protestant understandings of our mandate as beings created in the divine image to use our creative powers to introduce back into a fallen creation God's own standards of compassion for the suffering. Such a practice will, of course, require sustained reflection on the part of each couple involved as to precisely which genetic diseases are severe enough to warrant such action; Lesch-Nyhan syndrome, with its tendency to produce painful and disfiguring self-mutilation in addition to mental retardation, would seem a likely candidate, as would Tay-Sachs disease, Fragile X-chromosome syndrome, and a variety of syndromes resulting from stable genetic translocations that lead to shortened life span and the early onset of severe mental disabilities. But what about cystic fibrosis? Sickle-cell anemia? Huntington's disease? Familial Alzheimer's disease? Hemophilia? All of these disorders are now compatible with years of potentially enjoyable life. Are the health problems faced by those with these disorders severe enough to warrant avoidance of reproduction by their parents? Such questions are extremely difficult to answer and are probably best left to the individual consciences of those involved. Given, however, the growing availability of prenatal testing, such questions will inevitably have to be addressed, and we would do well to address them in advance of any attempt on the part of the government to form any national-policy guidelines on such issues.

I would like to address two potential objections to this policy. The first is that any attempt to prevent the birth of genetically handicapped children—no matter how effected and irrespective of motives—will inevitably lead to discrimination against other handicapped persons. Such efforts, it is claimed, inevitably carry the message that we view such lives as not worth living and that we wish such persons had never been born. These arguments are admittedly powerful when directed against efforts to prevent the birth of severely handicapped children because such children are a strain on their families and society. Such arguments would appear especially powerful against efforts that employ abortion to take lives that have already begun. Such arguments, however, would appear to be less powerful when directed against efforts that are motivated by a concern for the plight of the potential persons who could be affected by handicaps, especially when such efforts embody a respect for the inviolability of such lives once they have begun and a willingness on the part of parents to forego the pleasures of reproduction for the benefit of others. Indeed, in a community where persons would be freely willing to forego their opportunities to reproduce—and possibly even their unconstrained choice of marital partners—for the sake of their potential offspring, an other-centered attitude would be fostered that would create a view of human relationships that placed a high value on caring for the needs of others. Such an attitude would only increase the community's concern for the needs of the handicapped. It would also lead to a new and truer understanding of quality of life as measured not according to the possible quality attainable to some mythical normal child but as the best quality available to each really existing individual child.

The second objection is that a growing acceptance of such practices will usher in an increasingly mechanistic and production-oriented view of human reproduction—that procreation will be undertaken with a specific end or kind of product in mind and that such a practice is invariably dehumanizing. As with the previous objection, such a complaint seems apt when directed against the kind of practice in which decisions to abort or refrain from reproduction are based mostly on parental desires to give birth to a particular type of offspring; but it seems less apt against those efforts that are motivated by a sincere interest to avoid causing harm to another individual. In the latter case, procreative decisions are motivated by parental love for their potential offspring, which would seem to affirm rather than deny the humanity of the procreative process.

How then should we respond to the growing availability of prenatal genetic testing? And, what implications will such testing have for the relations between parents and their children? Several options are available. Certain of these options are predicated on the belief that not every human conceptus should be carried to term but only those that meet certain standards: freedom from genetic defects; ability to fulfill parental desires or expectations; capacity to develop rational thought and personhood; and likelihood of living free of significant suffering. To those who meet such standards, family membership is given; to those who fall short, it is denied. Parental choice is absolute, at least until late in gestation: they made it, they own it, they may do with it what they will.

Another option is based on the notion that each human conceptus is a unique and valuable individual and is, as such, fully invested with the rights and liberties belonging to human beings. Though these individuals are of us, by us, and from us, they are not ours in the sense of property to do with as we will. Rather, they are members with us of one great family whose children we are and whose father is God. He is our maker, and he alone holds the rights of ownership over all humankind; and though Scripture teaches that he has invested us with extensive powers of stewardship over all creation, it has never taught that those powers extend to our deciding which innocent human beings may be deprived by us of his sovereign gift of life.

Our responsibility as parents and stewards to the life God has given through us is, while more limited, no less divine. Ironically, this responsibility has perhaps never been stated more eloquently than by that great modern herald of human isolation, Franz Kafka, who wrote in his *Letter to His Father:* "The least that a parent can do for a child is to welcome it when it arrives."[37] May we all give our children such welcomes.

## ENDNOTES

1. Because of the limited space available in this chapter, I will not address directly the prenatal screening of *in vitro* fertilized embryos.
2. John S. Feinberg and Paul D. Feinberg, *Ethics for a Brave New World* (Wheaton, Ill.: Crossway Books, 1993), 265.
3. Evelyn Fox Keller, "Nature, Nurture, and the Human Genome Project" in *The Code of Codes: Scientific and Social Issues in the Human Genome Project,* ed. Daniel J. Kevles and LeRoy Hood (Cambridge: Harvard University Press, 1992), 296.
4. Ibid.
5. Ruth Schwartz Cowan, "Genetic Technology and Reproductive Choice: An Ethics for Autonomy," in *The Code of Codes,* 246.
6. Philip Kitcher, *The Lives to Come: The Genetic Revolution and Human Possibilities* (New York: Simon & Schuster, 1996).
7. Ibid., 289.
8. Immanuel Kant, *Grounding for the Metaphysics of Morals,* trans. James W. Ellington (Indianapolis: Hackett, 1983), see esp. 35–36 (*Akademie* 428).
9. Kitcher, *The Lives to Come,* 288.
10. Margery W. Shaw, "The Potential Plaintiff: Preconception and Prenatal Torts," in *Genetics and the Law II,* ed. Aubrey Milunsky and George J. Annas (New York: Plenum, 1980), 225–32.
11. This proposal bears many resemblances to the German "Law for the Prevention of Genetically Diseased Offspring," enacted in July 1933.
12. Leon R. Kass, *Toward a More Natural Science: Biology and Human Affairs* (New York: The Free Press, 1985), 89.
13. Kitcher, *The Lives to Come,* 298.
14. Ibid.
15. Kass, *Toward a More Natural Science,* 92.
16. Marc Lappe, "Eugenics: Ethical Issues" in *The Encyclopedia of Bioethics,* ed. Warren T. Reich (New York: Macmillan, 1995), 773.
17. See Kass, *Toward a More Natural Science,* 84.

18. Kitcher, *The Lives to Come*, 229.
19. Pearl Buck, foreword to *The Terrible Choice: The Abortion Dilemma*, ed. Robert E. Cooke (New York: Bantam Books, 1968), as quoted in Kass, *Toward a More Natural Science*, 93.
20. Kenzaburo Oe, *A Healing Family* (New York: Kodansha International, 1996), 44.
21. Ibid., 28.
22. Ibid., 52.
23. Kass, *Toward a More Natural Science*, 95.
24. Aristotle, *De Anima* (London: Penguin Classics, 1986) II:4, 165.
25. Aristotle, *Nichomachean Ethics* (London: Penguin Classics, 1976), 279.
26. David Heyd, *Genethics* (Berkeley and Los Angeles: University of California Press, 1992), 199–200.
27. H. Tristram Engelhardt Jr., *The Foundations of Bioethics*, 2d ed. (Oxford: Oxford University Press, 1996), 156.
28. It was Filmer, in fact, who coined the well-known phrase "the divine right of kings."
29. John Locke, *Second Treatise of Government* (Indianapolis: Hackett, 1980), 32.
30. Jacob Joshua Ross, *The Virtues of the Family* (New York: Free Press, 1995), 140.
31. A particularly helpful discussion of the biblical teachings on the human family (as interpreted by the Family Life Committee of the Lutheran Church, Missouri Synod) can be found in Oscar E. Feucht, ed., *Family Relationships and the Church: A Sociological, Historical, and Theological Study of Family Structures, Roles, and Relationships* (St. Louis: Concordia, 1970).
32. See, e.g., Ephesians 6:4, Colossians 3:21.
33. See, e.g., Titus 2:4.
34. See, e.g., 2 Corinthians 12:14.
35. Allen Verhey, transcript of an oral presentation given at The Christian Stake in Genetics Conference, July 1996, at Trinity International University, Deerfield, Ill., conducted by the Center for Bioethics and Human Dignity, Bannockburn, Ill.
36. See, e.g., the apostle Paul's discussion of performing an action evil in itself with the aim of producing the greatest of all goods—i.e., the glorification of God—in Romans 3:8.
37. Franz Kafka, *Letter to His Father. Brief an den Vater* (New York: Schocken Books, 1966).

*An Overview*

Because of the many advances in medical technology, life-and-death decisions have become more complex and often require the assistance of a third party to gather insight for making the best possible decisions. Genetic counselors are quickly becoming an essential channel through which patients must pass before deciding on a medical or genetic therapy. Rebecca D. Pentz offers insightful information regarding the pros and cons of genetic testing and the importance of applying the biblical principles of stewardship and call in determining the potential value of genetic therapy.

# Chapter Twelve

# GENETIC COUNSELING

*Guidance for Chilling Choices*

Rebecca D. Pentz

DURING THE SUMMER OF 1997, my family had the opportunity to backpack in the southwestern corner of Yosemite National Park. As I was walking through one of God's most magnificent natural creations, I couldn't help feeling like a flesh flake (a small insignificant piece of the whole) in the universe nor marveling that God should care for such flakes as humanity. What is more amazing, God not only cares for humans, he gives us incredible responsibilities over this creation. While gazing at the massive stability and power of the granite that surrounded me, it crossed my mind that humanity is developing genetic technologies that may irretrievably change the natural order that God has given us dominion over, and most crucially, change the not-so-insignificant flesh flakes he loves so dearly. How are people of faith, and specifically Christians, to respond to the possibilities that genetics offer us? I intend to propose a few tentative "rules of thumb" that Christians may find helpful as they face challenges posed by new genetic technologies. I particularly hope these may be helpful to genetic counselors who provide guidance for difficult choices.[1]

First, let me describe some of the challenges. A couple from our church called late one afternoon. They had had a routine amniocentesis, and there was a worrisome result. They were to meet with a genetic counselor the following day at 9:00 A.M. Would I accompany them? They wanted an ethicist, who was also a Christian, to hear the news with them and help them sort through the options. The couple had three healthy children at home, ages eight, five, and three. This child was to be the completion of the family, the last arrow in the quiver. The couple was blessed with adequate resources to raise four children, and they had chosen to have what, by today's standards, is a large family. The wife was thirty-six—the obstetrician had recommended amniocentesis. Without a thought they had accepted. Now they might be facing a choice they had not anticipated.

One of the most difficult aspects of today's technological expansion is that knowledge brings choices that humans previously didn't have to make. A generation ago none of these technologies existed and couples went through pregnancy in blissful ignorance. Should we avoid the technologies? Not necessarily, but we must recognize that they create options and choices we may not want to face. My husband and I chose against amniocentesis when I was thirty-six and pregnant. We did, however, meet with a genetic counselor *before* we attempted pregnancy to see what our odds at my age would be—three hundred to one in favor of having a normal child. That seemed good enough for us. This couple made the opposite, though I don't mean to imply wrong, decision.

The couple and I sat in the genetic counselor's waiting room and tried to make small talk; instead we made ourselves more anxious by avoiding discussion about our unexpressed fears. Finally, the counselor was ready and with clear diagrams and measured words, she explained how the preliminary tests showed an abnormality on one of the chromosomes consistent with a syndrome called cri du chat, so named because those afflicted are mentally handicapped and cry incessantly in a high-pitched sound resembling the cry of a cat in distress. More tests would have to be run to confirm the tentative diagnosis, but the counselor wanted us to know that there were choices available if the diagnosis was confirmed. We all knew that the words were coming that none of us had wanted to hear: The pregnancy could safely be terminated. We were all opposed to "therapeutic" abortion, but would this child be doomed to a short life of unrelieved suffering for no point at all? As we left each other that morning, I promised to find out everything I could about cri du chat and, more importantly, to pray for my friends. We all were tearful—what had been a joyful hope for a complete family was now a disheartening nightmare.

Two days later I received another call. The further tests showed nothing. The first test was most likely a testing artifact. No choices had to be made, just sleepless nights to catch up on. Months later a healthy baby boy joined the family. To test or not to test is no longer restricted to the prenatal period. I work in a tertiary cancer center and help design the testing protocols for cancer genes such as BRCA1. Although most cancers are not caused by inherited genes, there are inherited gene alterations that drive one's risk for cancer sky high. Women who carry the BRCA1 mutation have an 80 to 85 percent lifetime risk of breast cancer. A woman who has no inherited mutation faces a lifetime risk of 10 percent. The catch-22 for genetic breast cancer screening is that we are unsure what to recommend to women who test positive. Certainly there should be increased surveillance, but all women should be vigilant in their surveillance. As of yet, we do not know if there are preventive strategies; the tamoxifen prevention trial is not complete. We do not know if the radical prophylactic mastectomy and oophorectomy (surgical removal of the ovary) are truly beneficial, though some women only feel comfortable when they take radical steps. So, once again, there are more choices but no good data to make them informed.

Nor do the choices end there. We now have a few options for experimental genetic therapies. For ovarian cancer, rather than replacing a gene, we are experimenting with inserting a multidrug-resistant gene type into bone marrow cells to protect them against destruction by high-dose taxol. We, therefore, hope to give the patient a high enough dose of taxol to destroy her ovarian cancer, while protecting her bone marrow from destruction. In brain cancer, the opposite approach is being studied. Research is progressing on inserting a gene into the brain tumor that attracts the antitumor drugs. In lung cancer we just began injecting a retrovirus with the tumor suppresser gene p53 into the lung tumor. Our hope is that the p53 gene will stop the tumor's growth. All of these projects are in beginning stages; we must be realistic about gene therapy. *We currently are in no position to cure anyone's breast cancer by inserting nonaltered BRCA1 genes or wipe out colon cancer with a new improved hMSH2 or hMLH1 gene.* But genetic therapies are the future, and we need to be ready for them.

What are the ethical issues involved in using genetic tests or genetic therapies? For testing, the most important question to ask is: Will the information I may possibly get from this test (sometimes the tests do not provide new information) change anything I will do? If there is nothing to be done with the information, no preventive steps to take, is the information useful? Perhaps the information will change how you feel, but caution must be exercised. Even people with negative test results who do not have an identified dangerous mutation may become depressed or experience so-called survivor's guilt.

## CONSIDER POTENTIAL RISKS IN GENETIC TESTING

Undergoing genetic testing does carry risks; until all states have satisfactory genetic discrimination laws, there is the possibility that insurance, both health and life insurance, may be dropped or rates increased. Instances of discrimination in employment have already occurred. There is also the risk that family members may react negatively to another in the family undergoing testing that could possibly uncover a problem with the family's genes. A genetic counselor told me of a patient whose estranged father refused to give her the names of her aunts and forbade her half sisters from talking to her when he learned that she was contemplating genetic testing. The father's side of the family was riddled with cancer and all were at high risk. One of the unique aspects of genetic information is that it is inescapably familial and members of families differ in their desire to have such information.

Genetic therapy, on the other hand, raises the same ethical questions as does any so-called heroic therapy. Many physicians rely on the benefit-burden test to determine whether to recommend a therapy. Do the potential benefits of the therapy outweigh the burdens? This test requires that the physician be able to correctly determine what would count as a benefit for any particular patient. Usually this is not too difficult: improved health is a benefit. But in the case of heroic therapies, what a patient considers a benefit may not be what the physician judges to be a benefit. A particular patient may value quality of life at home above longevity, or just the reverse. These are individual decisions.

## DECISION-MAKING PRINCIPLES

In making decisions about heroic therapies, I counsel Christians to consider two Judeo-Christian principles: *stewardship* and *call.* God has charged us to be good stewards of the resources he has given us. Is using this particular medical technology good stewardship? Cost is not the only or even the most important factor in stewardship. We are charged to care for that which is entrusted to us, including our own bodies. That care sometimes involves great expense. But when the therapy proposed has little chance of being effective and is invasive and expensive, stewardship dictates that it be foregone. God has also placed us here for a purpose: Each Christian has a call. Before refusing a life-prolonging therapy, we must consider whether or not the therapy will give us a chance to proceed with God's purposes for our lives. Please do not underestimate God's many and varied purposes—one being prayer for oneself and others, which does not require great physical ability.

Two cases illustrate how stewardship and call impact decisions. A thirty-six-year-old woman, married with two small children, was diagnosed with ovarian cancer. Her oncologist gave her a 60 percent chance of long-term remission if she underwent aggressive therapy. She refused. The oncologist, a Christian, stormed into my office and asked how we could force her to take the therapy. Of course, we can't force her in any way, but from a Christian perspective, it surely seemed that she had made an unfortunate decision. At least one part of her call was not complete—she had a young family to raise—nor was the stewardship equation dismal. Certainly the treatment is more than unpleasant—at times, it would be totally debilitating; however, it offered her years of quality time with her husband and young children. We should not judge her, but if I could counsel her, I would urge her to proceed with therapy.

Another woman came to us with terminal lung cancer that had not responded to the best standard therapies. She wrote a note in her own medical chart stating that she wanted full resuscitation and intensive care on a ventilator should she go into respiratory arrest. Short of a miracle, such a resuscitation had a zero chance of curing her and close to a zero chance of restoring her life to the level of quality before the arrest. In fact, after the resuscitation that she demanded, she spent four weeks in an intensive care unit unconscious before she died. I cannot see how the resuscitation was either good stewardship or a furthering of God's call.

Stewardship and call also assist decisions about genetic therapies. Geneticists have informally adopted two ground rules over the last few decades that govern their research. The first ground rule states that somatic therapy, changing an individual's genes, is acceptable but germ-line therapy, therapy on the sperm and the egg or on the early fertilized egg that would result in a positive change that benefits future generations, is strictly forbidden. And yet, if I carry the BRCA1 mutation, which creates an 80 percent likelihood of developing breast or ovarian cancer in my lifetime, what would be wrong with changing that gene in my ovaries so future generations of Pentzes would not need to face the horror of knowing they may carry that mutation? I think it could be argued that stewardship actually indicates that we should do germ-line therapy in this case. A single intervention would provide healing not only to me but to my future children.

The Great Physician would be pleased with an intervention that brought healing to generations.

Clearly we must be particularly cautious in germ-line therapy—we are not omniscient and can never know all the long-term consequences of our actions. Presently, we do not understand enough about mutations or the possible benefits germ-line therapy may yield simultaneously with its detriments. Maybe BRCA1 protects against some other dreaded disease. But this present lack of knowledge does not preclude future advancements in our understanding that might allow us to reasonably weigh the risks and benefits of deleting a gene mutation from our own genetic line. I think that the early ground rule against germ-line therapy is losing its force.

## GENE TESTING AND EUGENICS

An important rule of thumb has been that curing diseases is ethical but enhancement of humans (eugenics) is not. Yet, every mother strives mightily to enhance her children. We sing to them in the womb, read to them as babes, challenge them with wide-ranging experiences, hand pick their schools or teach them at home, join churches with strong youth programs that promote Christian values and are led by adults who love Jesus. Parenting is, at least, an eighteen-year-long endeavor to enhance our children. What if in the future—it certainly is not possible today—there were a certain series of genetic changes that would give children a keener problem-solving sense so that they could be better stewards in this increasingly complex world God has given us to superintend? What value would such a change jeopardize? Perhaps such enhancements may never be possible. Perhaps any that are possible will have negative side effects, e.g., increasing problem-solving ability decreases creative ability. Clearly there are dangers in such technology. Parents who choose enhancement may be calculative, overbearing, shortsighted, and hasty. Enhancement may lead to devaluing the "unenhanced." Parents unable to afford the costs associated with this type of procedure will suffer the agony of seeing their children become unnaturally disadvantaged and underprivileged. Enhancement may only reflect fads and not true enhancements. *The list of dangers is impressive; so impressive that the no-enhancement rule is well justified today*. Enhancement now is reckless. It may not be reckless for our grandchildren, who may discover that the ability to trust God has a physiological component that is, in part, genetically determined. Perhaps individuals with a certain balance of chemicals in their brains find it easier to be trusting, just as individuals with the proper amount of serotonin do not as easily get depressed. These physiological characteristics are not determinative—God made humans much too complex for that—*but they do create tendencies*. If our grandchildren find such a chemically produced tendency that is in part triggered genetically, would they be wrong to offer genetic therapy to the biologically susceptible? Wouldn't good stewards take advantage of this enhancement? These issues are complex and provocative; I am glad we do not have to decide today. But I do not think we should hastily write off every enhancement therapy.[2]

## CONCLUSION: FOUR DECISION-MAKING RULES OF THUMB

Besides the general principles of stewardship and call, there are additional Christian rules of thumb that are particularly helpful in making decisions about genetic testing or therapy.

*First, God does not abandon us in our times of weakness.* He chose not to remove Paul's thorn in the flesh, and he does not always choose to remove adversity from us but instead may choose to use adversity to "mature us." What he does promise is to be with us, to guide us, to comfort us, and to strengthen us no matter what the circumstance. Be confident that deleterious genetic mutations will not separate us from the love of God.

*Second, people with disabilities reflect the image of God.* Christians, perhaps more than others who do not understand the theological reason why all humans are sacred, must resist any form of discrimination against those who have "thorns in the flesh." A person with Alzheimer's (chromosome 1), colon cancer[3] (chromosome 2), lung cancer (chromosome 3), Huntington's (chromosome 4), diastrophic dysplasia (chromosome 5), spino-cerebelaratrophy (chromosome 6), cystic fibrosis (chromosome 7), Werner's syndrome (chromosome 8), malignant skin cancer (chromosome 9), endocrine tumors (chromosome 10), Long-QT syndrome (chromosome 11), phenylketonuria (chromosome 12), breast cancer (chromosome 13), Alzheimer's (chromosome 14), marfan syndrome (chromosome 15), polycystic kidneys (chromosome 16), breast-ovarian cancer (chromosome 17), pancreatic cancer (chromosome 18), myotonic dystrophy (chromosome 19), severe immune system disorder (chromosome 20), Lou Gehrig's disease (chromosome 21), neurofibromatosis (chromosome 22) or Fragile X syndrome (chromosome x) is a creature created in the image of God and, therefore, must be treated with respect and dignity. An individual's worth must not be determined by physical disabilities or conditions but rather by natural connection with the divine.

*Third, remember why we are here.* We are not here for self-aggrandizement, nor for freeing the "god" within us, nor for creating a superhuman race. We are here to glorify God and enjoy fellowship with him and his creation. Any genetic test or therapy must meet a threefold test: (1) Does it further the goal of glorifying God? (2) Does it better equip our children to be faithful servants of God and stewards of his world? (3) Does it respect humans as bearers not just of genes but of the image of God?

*Fourth, never decide on a genetic test or therapy in isolation.* Pray about the decision, asking God to clarify your motives and to give understanding about the potential benefits and burdens. Seek counsel from your pastor or another in your local church whom you trust as a confidant. We are all too sinful to make such decisions without prayer and Christian consultation. Know the God of Scripture! God has given us the special gifts of himself and his community when we are faced with "impossible" choices. Use these gifts consistently and wisely.

We have no reason to fear the advances offered by science. I view science as a tool that God gives us to better understand his creation and make us better stewards of it. As long as genetics remains a tool to these ends, it is to be celebrated and embraced, not feared.

## ENDNOTES

1. My own view is that genetic counselors should jettison nondirective counseling and state explicitly the values they hold. Nondirective counseling, though well intentioned, usually masks the values that pervade the discussion. It is more helpful for the clients if the values are stated explicitly.
2. See both Nils Holtug and Glenn McGee, "Parenting in an Era of Genetics," *Hastings Center Report* 27, no. 2 (1997): 16–22, for other statements regarding gene-enhancement therapy.
3. Most cancers, as far as we know, are not a result of inherited gene mutations.

*An Overview*

Although we may look to genetic research for future potential assistance in the prevention of complex chromosomal abnormalities, presently we also must care for infants with those same conditions in a wise and compassionate manner as provided through perinatal hospice for example. It is in difficult circumstances such as these that our beliefs, values, and actions are put to the greatest test and require our greatest commitment. The termination of late-term pregnancies when fetal anomalies have been detected, while performed under the guise of reducing suffering, threatens the best interests of both the mother and the infant. An alternative to such procedures as partial-birth abortion is perinatal hospice which recognizes the value of bringing these infants to term by treating them as human beings conceived with a tangible future. Perinatal hospice affirms the biblical teaching of the dignity and worth of each fetus, supports parents through their grief when their infant dies, and maximizes the opportunity for authentic mourning.

Chapter Thirteen

# PERINATAL HOSPICE
*A Response to Early Termination for*
*Severe Congenital Anomalies*

## James S. Reitman, M.D., Byron C. Calhoun, M.D., and Nathan J. Hoeldtke, M.D.

THE PUBLIC DEBATE OVER PARTIAL-BIRTH abortion—or dilatation and extraction, as termed by its proponents—has received much press.[1] Proponents have maintained that most of these abortions were performed only for congenital defects or to save the life of the mother.[2] A well-known abortion activist and others finally admitted "that the vast majority of these abortions are performed . . . on healthy fetuses and healthy mothers."[3] However, even if public opinion eventually prevails and the procedure is banned for "healthy" pregnancies,[4] roughly 0.5 to 1 percent of all live-born infants are still afflicted by severe genetic defects.[5]

Many infants with congenital defects die in utero, and most with complex chromosomal abnormalities who do survive to birth will die shortly thereafter.[6] Partial-birth abortion—like intrauterine lethal injection—is intended to ensure that those who survive to late pregnancy will not be born alive,[7] thus avoiding the prospect of even greater anguish after birth when the infant "becomes" a person.[8] While this approach appears to have the benefit of reducing human suffering, it actually threatens the best interests of both mother and infant. The following case will illustrate the hidden dangers of early termination when fetal anomalies are detected late in pregnancy.

A 25 year old woman, Gravida 3, Para 1, Ab 1, presented at 22 weeks of gestation with the question of how to manage the remainder of her pregnancy after sonography revealed findings highly suggestive of trisomy 13. Because hospital policy allowed for termination of pregnancy only if "pregnancy would endanger a woman's life," her obstetrician sought assistance from the hospital Ethics Committee, which met ad hoc to recommend whether to approve or disapprove termination of the pregnancy. The patient was not present at the meeting. While there was no evidence of any impending danger to the mother's life, the obstetrician asserted that a decision *not* to terminate the pregnancy would be detrimental to her mental state. Further discussion unmasked concern that this would be further aggravated if the parents were forced to bear the expense of the procedure at a different institution where health-care costs would not be "covered." The obstetrician did not know the circumstances of the patient's previous abortion at four weeks of gestation. Notwithstanding the vigorously stated moral and legal concerns of the hospital chaplain and attorney, the committee voted 7 to 2 in favor of administrative approval to terminate the pregnancy.

How much can an obstetrician in such cases "read into" parents' preferences? Would the committee have been justified in seeking more information regarding the previous pregnancies and the parents' feelings about termination? Were the potential adverse consequences of pregnancy termination openly discussed? Did the committee consider all the relevant options? We argue that the committee in this case reached premature closure in the decision and failed to pursue the best interests of either the parents or the fetus.

Care providers involved in prenatal and perinatal care should evaluate the basis for their own approach to decision making when fetal anomalies are detected and be prepared to challenge potentially flawed reasoning behind early termination. On the one hand, the unexplained suffering in such cases raises key questions of meaning that all too often remain unexplored when attempts to mitigate that suffering are based on categorical, unreflective advocacy for the right of self-determination. On the other hand, these issues are openly addressed by Old Testament wisdom, which provides the basis for our argument.[9]

The serious pitfalls associated with early termination of pregnancy for fetal anomalies argue for a radically different approach to decision making that offers parents in their anguish an opportunity for meaning not afforded by early termination. Perinatal hospice emphasizes the value of bearing infants afflicted with severe congenital anomalies by treating them as beings with a tangible future, even though they will die soon. This approach allows for the resources and time needed to enjoy that future by supporting the family through the added ambivalence and anguish entailed in bringing the pregnancy to term.

## THE FLAWED JUSTIFICATION FOR EARLY TERMINATION

### The "Right" of Self-Determination

The most prevalent rationale used to justify abortion in general is that of preserving the presumed "right" of self-determination or autonomous choice, despite the recognized dangers of acceding too readily to external preferences in similarly ambiguous and uncertain end of life decisions.[10] So pervasive is this presumption in reproductive decisions that it usually goes unchallenged in discussions such as that held by the ethics committee in our case presentation. The right of self-determination in reproductive decisions has been enshrined in American jurisprudence through the recent acceptance of a preeminent right to "privacy" and an irreducible social and philosophical "pluralism."

*Privacy and the Problem of Informed Consent.* While *Roe* found that a pregnant woman's decision to terminate her pregnancy was protected by a right to privacy, this right was not found to be absolute—it was qualified by "the state interests as to protection of health, medical standards, and prenatal life."[11] Although reaffirmed by *Casey*,[12] the argument had to be modified because of the rapid development of the doctrine of informed consent, which has been deemed necessary to guarantee true liberty in medical decisions, including abortion.[13] It was soon recognized that rigid adherence to a presumed right of privacy would jeopardize a truly informed decision.[14]

Unfortunately, a similar level of attention has not been focused on what specific information a woman bearing a congenitally defective fetus needs to know in order to be truly "informed." For example, studies assessing the predictors of disordered mourning following perinatal loss are fraught with significant methodological weaknesses that limit conclusions about the psychological sequelae in these cases, whether from stillbirth[15] or abortion for fetal anomalies.[16]

While a recent review of studies of psychological complications within two years of therapeutic abortion revealed a frequency of adverse sequelae averaging only about 10 percent, a disproportionate number of these were related to therapeutic abortion for fetal abnormalities.[17] A recent case-control study evaluating the grief responses of women who terminated their pregnancies for fetal anomalies concluded that "[w]omen who terminate pregnancies for fetal anomalies experience grief as intense as those who experience spontaneous perinatal loss, and they may require similar clinical management. Diagnosis of a fetal anomaly and subsequent termination may be associated with psychological morbidity."[18] Psychological stress three months after delivery for fetal anomalies has been found to be significantly greater for women whose pregnancies were terminated between twenty-four and thirty-four weeks of gestation than those who delivered after thirty-four weeks.[19] When disordered mourning is studied beyond the early postpartum period, it "seems to be related to lack of or problematic social support and significant life stresses in pregnancy. . . . The marital relationship may be especially important."[20]

These data should be quite arresting to those who "might . . . assume that if a woman is aborting because of a suspected fetal anomaly, her post-abortion adjustment would be easier because she could rationalize the medical necessity of the procedure."[21] They suggest that in the case we presented earlier, the obstetrician—not to mention the committee that voted for termination—either was unaware of this information or rationalized away the need to discuss this data in order to satisfy the requisites of fully informed consent.

It is possible that primary care physicians face important structural barriers to the full utilization of opportunities in the consultation to assist the process of considered, autonomous decision-making. For example, time considerations may exert pressure on clinicians to focus more or less exclusively on the presenting problem and its quick solution rather than deliberately broadening the consultation to explore relevant psychological aspects of decisions. Because the procedure is so common, some clinicians may regard termination as fairly routine and thus underestimate its impact for some women.[22]

Despite the necessity to satisfy certain criteria before a pregnancy is legally terminated, some patients, families, and physicians may consider that primary care physicians' efforts at providing a structure within which the pregnant woman can explore ambivalence and alternatives constitute meddling in the exercise of a personal right. Patients can bypass their primary care physician, however, and go directly to an abortion provider without the primary care physician's knowledge.[23]

All this suggests that the problem of inadequate consent regarding the psychological sequelae of elective termination is seriously underestimated by most providers and alone warrants serious consideration of other alternatives. There is, however, another significant barrier to such consideration.

*Pluralism and the Problem of Conscience.* Notwithstanding *Casey's* recognition of the importance of informed consent, the Court subtly redefined the notion of liberty in a way that bore witness to an increasingly unquestioned societal presumption. "At the heart of liberty is the right to define one's own concept of existence, of meaning, of the universe, and of the mystery of human life."[24] The hidden premise of this definition is that our society is characterized by irreducible pluralism, and this presumption has increasingly insinuated itself into discussions of ethical decision making, including decisions concerning abortion.[25]

At the core of the presumption is a denial that certain elements of moral awareness are common to all humans.[26] Without a common moral ground on which to base such decisions, it is argued, on the one hand, that mutual tolerance is the only feasible way to maintain a "peaceable" society.[27] On the other hand, wisdom teaches that each of us possesses a conscience that confers some level of awareness of transcendent purpose in life.[28] Moreover, we remain accountable for this awareness, even in decisions concerning the appropriate timing of life and death.

> [A] wise man's heart discerns both time and judgment,
>      Because for every matter there is time and judgment,
> Though the misery of man increases greatly.
>      For he does not know what will happen;
> So who can tell him when it will occur?
>      No one has power over the spirit to retain the spirit,
> And no one has power in the day of death.
>                         —Ecclesiastes 8:5b–8a[29]

Humans are aware of some transcendent order and design to human destiny even though they cannot discern the content of the future. They know that even amid severe affliction they do not retain the prerogative to determine the timing of life and death, yet they all too commonly presume to exercise that prerogative, as evidenced in decisions to electively terminate pregnancy. A simple yet extraordinary secular argument accords fully with this wisdom.

> When I am killed, I am deprived both of what I now value which would have been part of my future personal life, but also what I would come to value. Therefore, when I die, I am deprived of all of the value of my future. Inflicting this loss on me is ultimately what makes killing me wrong. This being the case, it would seem that what makes killing *any* adult human being prima facie seriously wrong is the loss of his or her future.[30]
>
> The claim that the primary wrong-making feature of a killing is the loss to the victim of the value of its future accounts for the wrongness of killing young children and infants directly. . . . [I]t meshes with a *central intuition concerning what makes killing wrong.*
>
> [This] claim . . . has obvious consequences for the ethics of abortion. The future of a standard fetus includes a set of experiences, projects, activities, and such which are identical with the futures of adult human beings and are identical with the futures of young children. Since the reason that is sufficient to explain why it is wrong to kill human beings after the time of birth is a reason that also applies to fetuses, it follows that abortion is . . . seriously morally wrong.[31]

The higher frequency of grief reactions observed among women who terminate their pregnancies for fetal anomalies[32] may well be explained by the operation of such "intuition" in these decisions. The mother who chooses to terminate her pregnancy when she finds that her fetus is defective can expect to struggle between two powerful but conflicting emotional drives: the compulsion to relieve the anguish of a pregnancy that projects the sense of personal failure and the dread that follows active participation in the early termination of the infant's "future,"[33] however brief and bittersweet that future might have been.

The strong influence of conscience among these women is attested by the experience of clinicians whom they have consulted for help in resolving the psychological sequelae of such termination. One such clinician relates that

> attaching to the fetus as a real child clearly complicated the meanings and feelings behind the decision to terminate. Simply and bluntly put, many women described their action as murder, justifiable and excusable to be sure, but murder no less. This helps to explain the usually profound guilt that follows this loss, exceeding, at least in my clinical experience, that resulting from spontaneous perinatal loss. . . . Many of the women I worked with demonstrated the importance of *recognizing their child's existence* and the guilt over feeling they had *denied them just that* by the decision to terminate.[34]

The wisdom perspective would suggest that they are rooted in normally operating conscience. Leon's description of specific manifestations of such guilt in his patients[35] is remarkably similar to that of post-abortion counselors confronted with cases of women who have self-referred—often years later—after having aborted normal pregnancies.[36] The guilt reactions that come to clinical attention may represent only a small proportion of those that remain for the most part "successfully" repressed for years.[37]

## Relief of Suffering—the Real Agenda Behind "Liberty"

The operation of conscience among these women would suggest that a more compelling need than preserving the right of self-determination must be driving most decisions to abort. The arguments of *Roe* and *Casey* can both be demonstrated to hinge at least in part on the conviction that any suffering deemed unpalatable by patient (or care provider) must be eliminated.[38] This result merely reflects the natural emotional response to unjust suffering that makes abortion seem reasonable for both mother and infant:

> I saw the tears of the oppressed—
>    and they have no comforter;
> power was on the side of their oppressors—
>    and they have no comforter.
> And I declared that the dead,
>    who had already died,
> are happier than the living,
>    who are still alive.
> But better than both
>    is he who has not yet been,
> who has not seen the evil
>    that is done under the sun.
> —Ecclesiastes 4:1b–3

By expressing the sentiment that some suffering is worse than death, the passage reflects the all too prevalent justification for ending the life of a preborn infant overwhelmed by the "oppression" of congenital anomalies[39] and shortening the anguish faced by the family before death finally ensues.[40]

This rationale may also underlie the more subtle "professional judgment" of the genetics consultant or obstetrician who recommends abortion in the "best interests" of mother and fetus,[41] as in the case presented earlier. By subtly insinuating that the infant will suffer less if it is destroyed, prenatal counseling—even that which is purportedly nondirective—may thus reinforce a societal expectation to terminate the pregnancy and move on.[42] Such logic follows naturally from the perspective of suffering avoidance portrayed above. But how can anyone determine before the fact that a given life will be "too painful to live" or that death should be accelerated because the infant will "eventually die anyway"? On the contrary, the largely inscrutable future of the fetus and its suffering supports an entirely different approach to decisions.

## A BETTER STANDARD FOR DECISION MAKING:
## THE WISDOM PERSPECTIVE

### "Personhood" and Distinctive Human Life

Debates over the "personhood" of the fetus have shed little light on the morality of decisions that touch on the value and welfare of the fetus. While proponents on either side of the debate attempt to justify drawing the line of personhood at various stages of gestation, these arguments beg the question of what value we may assign to the human life that exists at any point along this continuum of development.[43] Apart from such considerations of personhood, the assertion that human life begins at conception is strongly attested by wisdom:

> My frame was not hidden from you
>     when I was made in the secret place.
> When I was woven together in the depths of the earth,
>     your eyes saw my unformed body.
> All the days ordained for me
>     were written in your book
> before one of them came to be.
>     —Psalm 139:15–16

However, does this justify deferring the inevitable demise of infants afflicted with severe congenital anomalies, thereby only prolonging parental anguish?

### The Image of God, Transcendent Purpose, and the Limits of Life

Biblical wisdom establishes the image of God as the basis for human dignity and worth.[44] Since it is evident that preborn human life is equally imbued with God's image, great worth also attaches to the humanity of each fetus.[45] Moreover, it is a logical fallacy to assume that there exists some threshold of congenital defectiveness beyond which the birth of such an infant has no conceivable value. Exodus 4:11 says, "Who gave man his mouth? Who makes him deaf or mute? Who gives him sight or makes him blind? Is it not I, the LORD?"[46]

If every infant is created with value, it follows that each is also created with a distinctive purpose—regardless of physical characteristics or chromosomal complement—even if we cannot discern that purpose beforehand:

> As you do not know the path of the wind,
>     or how a body is formed in a mother's womb,
> so you cannot understand the work of God,
>     the Maker of all things.
>     —Ecclesiastes 11:5

Realizing how little is known about divine prerogative in fetal development should enjoin those in the moral community of the fetus to give due consideration to its created nature and inscrutable purpose—in a word, its *future*.[47]

The vicarious suffering of parents and physicians does not justify an assault on the fetus, for there is no way to predict before birth what good may come of a child's life, however brief.[48] The real problem with early termination is that it is based on the false presumption that parents have the capacity and full authority to determine which infants shall live, how long, and with what "quality of life." It is not their place to dictate the parameters of continued existence and preempt purposes that cannot be known ahead of time. Consequently, we remain accountable for wise stewardship over such life and should not presume to destroy it as long as a future for that infant can still be realized.[49]

## The "Opportunity" of Mourning

Further wisdom supports parents' choosing, in spite of suffering, not to destroy their unborn children who have even severe anomalies.[50] We all share an essential kinship with each of these infants. Each of us carries the elements of physical imperfection that ultimately dictate the common, inescapable legacy of humankind—death (Eccl. 3:19–21; 9:2–3; cf. also 1 Cor. 15:48; Rom. 5:12–21). While each of us is allotted a particular period of time to live,[51] we cannot determine in advance how long it will be (Eccl. 9:11–12). Perinatal death presents an occasion to acknowledge and mourn our collective mortality and to contemplate the potential value and purpose of all life.

Even though this purpose—the "work of God"—cannot be fully appreciated ahead of time (Eccl. 8:16–17; cf. 3:10–11; 11:5), the wisdom perspective provides ample grounds for the hope of realizing such meaning. Despair over the prospect of suffering and death often leads to the discovery of new meaning in life, even when it is deformed and all too brief:

> It is better to go to a house of mourning
> than to go to a house of feasting,
> for death is the destiny of every man;
> the living should take this to heart.
> —Ecclesiastes 7:2

Such authentic mourning[52] can transform one's initial response to overwhelming suffering (Eccl. 4:1–3) into the conviction that "Anyone who is among the living has hope—even a live dog is better off than a dead lion!" (Eccl. 9:4). The testimony of those who have persevered through such a pregnancy and birth illustrates, on the one hand, the advantage of responding to the discovery of fetal anomalies by "taking to heart" the implications of mortality on meaning in life.[53]

On the other hand, valid concerns over artificially prolonging the biological existence of infants born with truly marginal conditions like anencephaly warrant exercising reasonable judgment over the boundaries of supportive care for these terminally ill infants.[54] Such decisions are still taken with care and respect for the image of God and the lost future represented in that infant. As the trajectory of the dying child's life emerges over time, parents ultimately gain the wisdom to discern when it is "time to die."[55] The evolving standard of care for families facing perinatal loss reflects flexibility and sensitivity to the variable needs of individual family members during the dying process.[56] These priorities are best supported in a given health-care program through the implementation of some form of perinatal hospice.

## THE ADVANTAGE OF PERINATAL HOSPICE

Those obstetrics-gynecology and neonatology programs in which the funding of abortions is restricted (to situations when the life of the mother is truly at risk) provide an opportunity to evaluate parental responses to the limitation of the option of early termination for problem pregnancies. Approval for an abortion in U.S. military treatment facilities, even under circumstances such as ectopic pregnancy or maternal pulmonary hypertension, generally requires agreement among at least three obstetricians that the pregnancy poses a genuine threat to maternal life. When this condition is not met, many military parents expecting infants with congenital anomalies choose not to procure an abortion outside the system.[57] Under these circumstances parents are given the opportunity to seriously consider the alternative of perinatal hospice.

Perinatal hospice coordinates the combined efforts of obstetricians, Maternal Fetal Medicine (MFM) staff, neonatologists, anesthesia services, labor and delivery nursing, neonatal intensive care nursing, chaplains/pastors, and social services. Patients are given the fetal diagnosis and expected prognosis during extensive discussion with MFM subspecialists, who participate in ultrasound evaluation, amniocentesis (if desired), birth planning, and ongoing medical management in the antepartum, intrapartum, and postpartum periods. However, it is the patience, sensitivity, and sense of interdependence of nurses at the bedside—as well as their willingness to facilitate the mourning process—that most ensures the ultimate success of perinatal hospice.[58]

The main burden of effort for physicians consists in antepartum counseling and preparation. Patients need to see the baby on ultrasound and be allowed to begin grieving. Most birth defects are not nearly as grotesque at birth as parents may imagine.[59] Extensive support is provided in labor through encouragement by the nursing staff and pain relief administered by the anesthesia service. Fetuses with conditions not expected to be lethal, such as Down's or Turner's syndromes, are managed with fetal heart rate monitoring in the same way as other labors.

Immediately after delivery the infant is handed to the parents to share the baby's remaining life. Many of these infants are stillborn, but some may live for minutes to days. The parents are allowed to stay in the delivery suite with the child as long as they wish.[60] We encourage dressing and naming the baby, taking pictures of the baby, and, if desired, holding of the baby by all family members, including children.[61] Nonanomalous features of the baby are emphasized to the parents such as cute hands and feet or soft skin. Comfort measures are emphasized to the family. The infant is kept warm and cuddled, and some may even be able to feed. Neonatologists provide comfort for the baby as needed. If the parents are feeling overwhelmed, those infants who survive for longer periods may be kept comfortable in the nursery during the postpartum period.

This supportive environment has been offered on our antenatal service since 1989. Contrary to the expectations of those who favor early termination, the response has been overwhelmingly positive.[62] We are convinced that most parents instinctively recognize that their infant has a "future like ours," however brief that future may be. When parents permit God to determine their paths and allow life to run its course, they are much more content; they can more freely experience and mourn the bittersweet birth and the all-too-soon departure of their awaited child. Grief lessens as time passes, and they can rest secure in the knowledge that they did not dismember or destroy their baby.

## CONCLUSION

Physicians and nurses committed to authentic care can provide a genuine alternative to the horrific destruction wrought by partial-birth abortion. They may refer to physicians who advise their patients of the life-affirming choice to bear and comfort their terminally ill fetuses. Since this choice is undoubtedly facilitated when such care is fully "covered," we assert that even in nonmilitary settings financial concerns should not preclude offering this option. Physicians and hospitals can foster the establishment of perinatal hospice by being willing to waive or adjust fees, or by helping to set up payment plans.

Perinatal hospice and the wisdom perspective provide a "better way" than merely hastening death. When given the opportunity and support of perinatal hospice, most parents will choose to bring their infants with congenital anomalies to term. Parents are given the opportunity to genuinely mourn our common fallibility and mortality and acknowledge the sovereign prerogative of God as Creator over each individual life. While they mourn the premature loss of that life, they come to rejoice in the confidence that God delights in cultivating joy out of the sorrow that characterizes so much of our present existence.[63]

## ENDNOTES

1. Diane M. Gianelli, "Shock-Tactic Ads Target Late-Term Abortion Procedure," *Am. Med. News* ( July 1993), 3, 21–22; and "Outlawing Abortion Method," *Am. Med. News* (November 1995), 3, 27.
2. Diane M. Gianelli, "Medicine Adds to Debate on Late Term Abortion: Abortion Rights Leader Urges End to 'Half truths,'" *Am. Med. News* (March 1997), 3, 28.
3. Ibid., 28.

4.  Ibid., 3, 28–29. See also Diane M. Gianelli, "ACOG Draws Fire for Saying Procedure 'May' Be Best Option for Some," *Am. Med. News* (March 1997), 3, 27–28, documenting opposition to the procedure from a group of obstetricians within the American College of Obstetrics and Gynecology.

5.  N. P. Kuleshov, "Chromosome Anomalies of Infants Dying During the Perinatal Period and the Premature Newborn," *Human Genetics* 31 (1976): 151; and Rhona Bauld, Grant R. Sutherland, and A. Douglas Bain, "Chromosome Studies in Investigation of Stillbirths and Neonatal Deaths," *Archives Diseases Childhood* 49 (1974): 782.

6.  Bonnie J. Baty et al., "Natural History of Trisomy 18 and Trisomy 13: I. Growth, Physical Assessment, Medical Histories, Survival, and Recurrence Risk. II. Psychomotor Development," *Am. J. Med. Genetics* 49 (1994): 175–88, 189–94; and Jonathan P. Wyllie et al., "Natural History of Trisomy 13," *Archives Diseases Childhood* 71 (1994): 343.

7.  Joan Callahan, "Ensuring a Stillborn: The Ethics of Fetal Lethal Injection in Late Abortion," *J. Clinical Ethics* 6 (1995): 254.

8.  Bethany Spielman, "Certainty and Agnosticism About Lethal Injection in Late Abortion," *J. Clinical Ethics* 6 (1995): 270.

9.  See James S. Reitman, "The Structure and Unity of Ecclesiastes," *Bibliotheca Sacra* 154 ( July–September 1997): 281–303.

10. See James S. Reitman, "The Debate on Assisted Suicide—Redefining Morally Appropriate Care for People with Intractable Suffering," *Issues in Law and Med.* 11 (1995): 299–329; "The Dilemma of Medical Futility: A 'Wisdom Model' for Decisionmaking," *Issues in Law and Med.* 12 (1997): 231–64; "A 'Wisdom' Perspective on Advocacy for the Suicidal," in *Suicide: A Christian Response*, ed. Timothy J. Demy and Gary P. Stewart (Grand Rapids: Kregel, 1998).

11. *Roe v. Wade*, 410 U.S. 113.

12. *Planned Parenthood v. Casey*, 505 U.S. 833 (1992).

13. See, e.g., Jay Katz, *The Silent World of Doctor and Patient* (New York: Free Press, 1984).

14. This important correction to abortion jurisprudence was developed in a line of cases beginning with *Danforth*, 428 U.S. 52 (1976) and continuing with *Akron*, 462 U.S. 416 (1983); *Ashcraft*, 462 U.S. 476 (1983); *Webster*, 492 U.S. 490 (1989); and, ultimately, *Casey*. See Bo Schambelan, "Postscript," in *Roe v. Wade: The Complete Text of the Official U.S. Supreme Court Decision* 101–16 (1992).

15. Charles H. Zeanah, "Adaptation Following Perinatal Loss: A Critical Review," *J. Am. Acad. Child Adolescent Psychiatry* 28 (1989): 467, 476; and Charles H. Zeanah et al., "Initial Adaptation in Mothers and Fathers Following Perinatal Loss," *Infant Mental Health J.* 16 (1995): 80.

16. Charles H. Zeanah et al., "Do Women Grieve After Terminating Pregnancies Because of Fetal Anomalies? A Controlled Investigation," *Obstetrics and Gynecology* 82 (1993): 270.

17. G. Zolese and C. V. R. Blacker, "The Psychological Complications of Therapeutic Abortion," *British J. Psychiatry* 160 (1992): 742, 747.

18. Zeanah, "Do Women Grieve?" Up to 77 percent of such women may experience an acute grief reaction and 46 percent may remain symptomatic six months after termination. See J. Lloyd and K. M. Laurence, "Sequelae and Support after Termination of Pregnancy for Fetal Malformation," *British Med. J.* 290 (1985): 907.

19. J. A. M. Hunfeld et al., "Emotional Reactions in Women in Late Pregnancy

(twenty-four weeks or longer) Following the Ultrasound Diagnosis of a Severe or Lethal Fetal Malformation," *Prenatal Diagnosis* 13 (1993): 603, 609.

20. Zeanah, "A Critical Review," 476 (citations omitted).

21. Teri Reisser, "Personal Characteristics as Predictors of Post-Abortion Emotional Distress," unpublished thesis for Master of Science Degree in Counseling (December 1994), 24.

22. Chris Butler, "Late Psychological Sequelae of Abortion: Questions from a Primary Care Perspective," *J. Family Practice* 43 (1996): 396, 398 (citations omitted).

23. Ibid., 399.

24. *Casey* at 851.

25. See e.g., H. Tristram Engelhardt, *The Foundation of Bioethics*, 2d ed. (New York: Oxford University Press, 1996), 239–87.

26. Ibid., 42–45.

27. Ibid., 239–87. This argument is, however, seriously flawed. See Stanley Hauerwas, "Not All Peace Is Peace: Why Christians Cannot Make Peace with Engelhardt's Peace," in *Reading Engelhardt*, ed. Professor Minoque (Kluwer, 1997), 17; and D. A. Carson, *The Gagging of God: Christianity Confronts Pluralism* (Grand Rapids: Zondervan, 1996).

28. "I have seen the burden God has laid on men. He has made everything beautiful in its time. He has also set eternity in the hearts of men; yet they cannot fathom what God has done from beginning to end" (Eccl. 3:10–11). Scripture citations are from the *New International Version*, unless otherwise indicated.

29. *New King James Version* (NKJV).

30. Don Marquis, "Why Abortion Is Immoral," *J. Philosophy* 86 (1989): 183, 189–90.

31. Ibid., 192 (emphasis added).

32. Zeanah, "Do Women Grieve?" 270.

33. The powerful influence of existential dread that can be associated with the loss of such a perceived future is explored by Reitman, "Dilemma of Medical Futility," 243–46.

34. Irving G. Leon, "Pregnancy Termination Due to Fetal Anomaly: Clinical Considerations," *Infant Mental Health J.* 16 (1995): 112, 119 (emphasis added).

35. Ibid.

36. See Teri Reisser and Paul Reisser, *Help for the Post-Abortion Woman* (Toronto: Life Cycle Books, 1994), 35–45.

37. Ibid.

38. Byron C. Calhoun, James S. Reitman, and Nathan J. Hoeldtke, "Perinatal Hospice: A Response to Partial Birth Abortion for Infants with Congenital Defects," *Issues in Law and Medicine* 13 (1997).

39. Hauerwas' perception of the societal unease that attends the prospect of a mentally handicapped child applies as well to the prenatal detection of any congenital anomaly:

> I suspect that at least part of the reason it seems so obvious that we ought to prevent retardation is the conviction that we ought to prevent suffering. No one should will that an animal should suffer gratuitously. No one should will that a child should endure an illness. No one should will that another person should suffer from hunger. No one should will that a child should be born retarded. That suffering should be avoided is a belief as deep as any we have. That

someone born retarded suffers is obvious. Therefore if we believe we ought to prevent suffering, it seems we ought to prevent retardation.

Stanley Hauerwas, "Suffering the Retarded: Should We Prevent Retardation?," in *Suffering Presence: Theological Reflections on Medicine, the Mentally Handicapped, and the Church* (Notre Dame, Ind.: University of Notre Dame Press, 1986), 164. See also Martin S. Pernick, *The Black Stork: Eugenics and the Death of "Defective" Babies in American Medicine and Motion Pictures Since 1915* (New York: Oxford University Press, 1996).

40. Stanley Hauerwas, "The Retarded, Society, and the Family: The Dilemma of Care," in *Suffering Presence*, 189–210; and James Bopp and Richard E. Coleson, "A Critique of Family Members as Proxy Decisionmakers Without Legal Limits," *Issues in Law and Med.* 12 (1996): 133, 140–56.

41. See e.g., Callahan, "Ensuring a Stillborn," 254.

42. Stanley Hauerwas, "Community and Diversity: The Tyranny of Normality," in *Suffering Presence*, 211–17; and Bopp and Coleson, "Proxy Decisionmakers Without Legal Limits"; Spielman, "Certainty and Agnosticism," 270.

43. See, e.g., "Respect for Persons and Their Agency," in *On Moral Medicine*, ed. Stephen E. Lammers and Allen Verhey, (1987) 273–304; and Engelhardt, *The Foundation of Bioethics*, 135–54.

44. See Genesis 4:9; 9:5–6; James 3:9.

45. Evidence supporting this conclusion can be adduced from Psalm 139; Jeremiah 1:5; Genesis 1:26–27, and the recorded reactions of the fetus to events in the outside world (cf. Luke 1:39–44, citing the in utero reaction of John the Baptist to the voice of Mary, the mother of the preborn Christ).

46. Indeed, specific instances of such divine purpose are revealed elsewhere in Scripture to answer natural questions of attribution for congenital anomalies, such as the case of a man who was born blind "so that the work of God might be displayed in his life" (John 9:3).

47. See Marquis, "Why Abortion Is Immoral."

48. "For who knows what is good for a man in life, during the few and meaningless days he passes through like a shadow? Who can tell him what will happen?" (Eccl. 6:12).

49. This assertion is the moral foundation of Exodus 21:22–25. While scholars have tried to prove that the "life for life" provision specified in this passage applies only to the mother and not the fetus (see, e.g., Robert N. Congdon, "Exodus 21:22–25 and the Abortion Debate," 146 *Bibliotheca Sacra* 132 [1989]), the most cogent and exegetically consistent understanding is that the death in view is of either the mother or the fetus. See John S. Feinberg and Paul D. Feinberg, *Ethics for a Brave New World* (Wheaton, Ill.: Crossway Books, 1993), 63–65.

50. Victoria A. Vincent et al., "Pregnancy Termination Because of Chromosomal Abnormalities: A Study of 26,950 Amniocenteses in the Southeast," *Southern Med. J.* 84 (1991): 1210; Marlon S. Verp et al., "Parental Decision Following Prenatal Diagnosis of Fetal Chromosome Abnormality," *Am. J. Med. Genetics* 29 (1988): 613; and Arie Drugan et al., "Determinants of Parental Decisions to Abort for Chromosome Abnormalities," *Prenatal Diagnosis* 10 (1990): 483.

51. "There is a time for everything, and a season for every activity under heaven: a time to be born and a time to die" (Eccl. 3:1–2a).

52. The sense intended for "mourning" in Ecclesiastes is reviewed by Reitman, "Unity of Ecclesiastes," 290–91. Zeanah gives a clinically useful description of the relationships among grief, mourning, and bereavement.

> [G]rief refers to all of the painful affects associated with loss of an infant, such as sadness, anger, guilt, shame, and anxiety. . . . [M]ourning . . . refers to a complex interplay of all the psychological processes that are triggered by the loss. This includes biological reactions, behavioral reactions, and cognitive and defensive operations related to the loss. Therefore, . . . mourning is the total psychological experience of the bereaved individual with respect to the loss. Mourning is considered to be the process by which an individual resolves a loss, that is, accepts the reality of a change in the external world and reorganizes and reorients his or her . . . world accordingly. . . . Bereavement refers to the period of time during which mourning is largely unresolved (Zeanah, "A Critical Review," 467–68).

53. See e.g., James H. Pence, "A Road Not Chosen," *Dallas Theological Seminary's Kindred Spirit* 20 (August 1996): 4–7.
54. While supporters of the sanctity-of-life principle have historically denied any significant role for quality-of-life criteria, cases such as "Baby K" raise legitimate questions about what should be considered "futile therapy" (Reitman, "Dilemma of Medical Futility," 231–55). To blindly apply any and all possible life prolonging therapy when it becomes obvious that it is time to let go is also to risk presuming on divine prerogative (cf. Eccl. 8:5–8; 11:5). See further Jerome R. Wernow, "Saying the Unsaid: Quality of Life Criteria in a Sanctity of Life Position," in *Bioethics and the Future of Medicine: A Christian Appraisal*, ed. John F. Kilner et al. (Grand Rapids: Eerdmans, 1995), 93–111.
55. Ecclesiastes 3:1–2a; cf. Reitman, "Dilemma of Medical Futility," 256–64.
56. Zeanah, "A Critical Review"; Irving G. Leon, "Perinatal Loss: Choreographing Grief on the Obstetric Unit," *Am. J. Orthopsychiatry* 62 (1992): 7–8; and Irving G. Leon, "Perinatal Loss: A Critique of Current Hospital Practices," *Clinical Pediatrics* 31 (1992): 366–74.
57. While this choice may involve financial considerations—a second or third trimester abortion may be costly, often requiring prior payment—it should nevertheless raise substantial concerns about the embarrassing ease with which abortions can otherwise be procured under *Roe* and/or *Casey* for the "health" of the mother.
58. The rich dynamics of perinatal hospice from the nursing perspective is described in detail in a wonderful collection of narratives from Vanderbilt University Medical Center. See Andrew Todd, *Journey of the Heart: Stories of Grief As Told by Nurses in the NICU*, vol. 1, 2d ed. (Nashville: Vanderbilt University Press, 1995), 59.
59. Ibid., 238.
60. Ingela Rådestad et al., "Psychological Complications after Stillbirth—Influence of Memories and Immediate Management: Population Based Study," *British Med. J.* 312 (1996): 1505.
61. Todd, "Journey of the Heart," Appendix B.
62. Out of more than twenty cases of fatal anomalies detected in our experience at Madigan Army Medical Center, only one family opted to pursue early termination.

63. Ecclesiastes 11:7–12:1. See Reitman, "Dilemma of Medial Futility," 255–56, for an exposition of the implications of this passage for wise and joyful stewardship under similar circumstances of so-called medical futility.

*An Overview*

This chapter is a reprint of an article that appeared in the September 1993 issue of *Clinical Obstetrics and Gynecology*. Its publication identified a serious misuse of a genetic screening test called, at that time, triple screen for Down's syndrome. It is included in this volume as an example of the potential misuse that can accompany advanced technologies and to underscore the importance of publicly addressing misuses so that corrections can be achieved. As a result of this article and the work of others who identified this misuse, the name of the genetic screening test has been changed to simply, triple screen, and a population of people (those with a mutation of chromosome 21, also known as trisomy 21) once heavily demeaned is now receiving better recognition for the contribution they can make to society.

Thomas Elkins and Douglas Brown discuss the unavoidable discrimination that is inherent in an ethic that determines the significance of a person by cost effectiveness or by weighing burdens against benefits. Genetic screening is an important advancement in the struggle against human suffering; however, it should not be used with the intent to seek out and eliminate society's undesirable fetuses (persons). The ability to identify genetic disorders in adults, children, infants, and the unborn will help make decision making easier, especially as genetic therapies are developed and improved. Consider the patient who is a carrier of Tay-Sachs disease. Once the disorder is identified in the patient, the easier choice is to determine who to court and marry. Should this carrier fall in love and marry another carrier, the decision to adopt is much less risky than the couple's choosing to conceive their own child (one in four chance of producing a child with Tay-Sachs). The most difficult decision of what to do about a fetus who has the disease could become obsolete if people are willing to take the information they gather through genetic screening and use it responsibly. In the world of disease, we are not all equal and, therefore, our opportunities differ from one another. As cures become more available, opportunities widen; however, it is always our responsibility to honor all human life in all situations.

# Chapter Fourteen

# THE COST OF CHOICE

## A Price Too High in the
## Triple Screen for Down's Syndrome

### Thomas E. Elkins, M.D. and Douglas Brown

MUCH HAS BEEN WRITTEN THAT emphasizes the dramatic increase in diagnostic and decisional choices that genetic advances are making possible in obstetrics. In this chapter, the question: At what cost? is raised.

The premium assigned to "choice" remains a rarely critiqued assumption in an enlightened, technologically advanced, wealthy society, such as that in the United States. We still have the cultural myth, "You can be whatever you want to be," recited in America. This enlightened worldview challenged and eventually replaced the theologic fatalism of medieval times and promoted choice as the cornerstone of societal revision. Technologic advances, accordingly, have been pursued and introduced as having inherent value because choices are increased. Choices allow us to exercise more control over destiny. The story of reproductive medicine, especially in light of the expanding impact of genetic technology in obstetrics, should be seen within this larger cultural context.

It should be noted that the perception of human beings as being capable of and accountable for choice has been understood variously. Some claim that choice is really only an illusion because we are so shaped by genetics and social conditioning. Others have contended that the issue is not whether human beings are free to choose, but how responsible their decisions are and how willing they are to accept limitations to unrestricted freedom of choice. The pretext of genetic prenatal counseling is that every effort should be made to provide adequate information to a pregnant woman so that she may have a full range of available choices about fetal outcome.

At two national medical society meetings in 1992, researchers from a major university medical school presented their data on a triple screen of maternal serum tests for the detection of fetal Down's syndrome.[1] Low maternal serum levels of estriol and alpha-fetoprotein, along with a high level of human chorionic gonadotropin can predict pregnancies at risk for trisomy 21 or Down's syndrome.[2] Through further studies with ultrasound and amniocentesis, the fetal presence of Down's syndrome may be determined. The authors of these presentations argued that a statistical analysis of these three serum tests is as successful as the maternal age risk factor in predicting the presence of Down's syndrome in utero. The 1 in 270 risk at age thirty-five is similar to the 1 in 197 risk identified by the serum tests.[3] These presentations were hailed as significant progress in prenatal genetics, but are they really? At both meetings, the presenters were questioned openly about the cost effectiveness of such testing. Both from the speaker's platform, and now in print, these researchers have presented a cost analysis that is tied directly and solely to the termination of pregnancies with fetal Down's syndrome. For years, geneticists have claimed that prenatal testing was cost effective because of the choices provided to pregnant women—not necessarily the "cost" of the potential future person being identified. The triple screen for Down's syndrome represents a significant event in prenatal genetics because the cost analysis, now appearing in medical literature, no longer discusses the concern for a woman's choice but seeks to demean and to estimate harshly the value of a significant population group in our society. A thorough evaluation of the researchers' own cost analysis for the triple screen is necessary to understand the extent of the problem that this thinking represents. As stated in *Obstetrics and Gynecology* in September 1992, the cost analysis of the triple screen includes several concerns.

In their cost-impact analysis, the authors claimed that a person with Down's syndrome costs approximately $196,000. This included health, education, and "residential" costs. The total cost was claimed as higher because of the "loss of productivity of parents, counseling and social work services, increased divorce rates, and problems with siblings." This gave a "favorable benefit-cost ratio" for the triple screen that costs only about $100,000 per fetus found with Down's syndrome.[4] The contemporary accuracy of such statements and the entire methodology of such an analysis must be challenged.

## SIMPLE ECONOMIC COSTS

A look at simple economic costs brings many questions to mind immediately. The first national presentation focused on the screening of teenage pregnancies for trisomy 21.[5] According to the authors, the serum tests cost $40, and these were used in 2,067 pregnancies ($82,080 total cost). This first step identified 150 women at "high risk" for carrying a fetus with Down's syndrome. For these, an ultrasound evaluation followed, costing a study price of $100 per test ($15,000 total cost). For ninety-seven of these patients, ultrasound revealed reasons other than fetal Down's syndrome for the serum test results. The remaining fifty-three patients were offered amniocentesis, and only thirty-one patients agreed to this test, at a study cost of $175 per test ($9,300 total cost). Thus, the cost, at the reduced study rates, for screening 2,067 pregnant teenagers with the triple serum tests was approximately $106,480. (By contacting three other centers, it was found that the usual costs of these evaluations are two- to threefold greater than the study costs presented by the researchers. In fact, at the second national presentation, the researchers admitted that the simple economic cost would rise significantly after the study period was concluded.) In the initial study, one fetus with

Down's syndrome was found, and as the presenter stated, the pregnancy was terminated. The medical scientists, therefore, called the screening "cost effective" and recommended the triple screening for all pregnant adolescents. This was surprising to many because the cost of triple screening the one million pregnant teenagers each year in America would be staggering, perhaps as much as $100 to $300 million would be spent to find fewer than one thousand fetuses with Down's syndrome. By what standard is this screening cost effective to find what even the investigators described as a rare event in adolescent pregnancies?

The second national presentation by the same researchers reported the results of screening 8,431 patients who were younger than age thirty-five and pregnant (including the 2,067 women younger than age nineteen, presented previously).[6] This has now been published, and the simple costs of the tests remain similar to those already discussed. The authors claim that the simple economic costs to the patients remain at approximately $100,000 per fetus found with Down's syndrome.[7] Again, the $450,000 spent in the pilot study would translate to more than $1 million in other institutions contacted. For that total cost, four fetuses with Down's syndrome were identified. Three other fetuses with Down's syndrome were missed by the tests because of the low accuracy of the triple screen. On the basis of the cost analysis presented by the authors in print, they claimed that the triple screen was cost effective and should be recommended to all women at all ages for detection of Down's syndrome in utero. Simply describing the vast costs envisioned by these researchers makes the practice of using such a screen questionable, at best.

The cost analysis presented by prenatal geneticists encouraging use of the triple screen for Down's syndrome demands much more analysis than the brief economic concerns presented. Both the accuracy of such an analysis and the validity of using such a dehumanizing approach toward a population group also must be questioned.

## THE PROBLEM OF FALSE ASSUMPTIONS ABOUT PERSONS WITH DOWN'S SYNDROME

The litany of negative comments about persons with Down's syndrome included in the published cost analysis of the triple screen seems terribly unbalanced and must be questioned. Some recent studies show no increase in divorce rates for families that include persons with Down's syndrome.[8] In fact, a review of the information regarding marital problems and divorce in families with handicapped children in general is at best "sparse and contradictory."[9]

There is no evidence to support the authors' assumption of reduced productivity for parents of persons with Down's syndrome, or the presumption that persons with Down's syndrome have a negative effect on families. One group found that parents of severely retarded children reported the greatest amount of negative impact on family adjustment.[10] Because persons with Down's syndrome generally are found to have mild to moderate mental retardation, it is likely that such a negative impact would be less common.[11] Reviews of the literature show clearly that children and youths with disabilities often make positive contributions to their families.[12] Several reviewers have argued that the negative effects have been overstated and the positive effects ignored.[13]

The comment of one group, concerning the high cost of residential facilities, also seems noncontemporary.[14] The move away from institutionalization, especially for persons as highly functioning as those with Down's syndrome, and the impact of supported employment efforts nationwide have created a new financial setting for adults with Down's syndrome.

The negative effect of persons with Down's syndrome on siblings is certainly not supported universally in medical and mental retardation literature. One report noted that as many siblings showed benefits as those who showed harm from having a sibling with a developmental disability.[15] In a 1971 review of 104 brothers and sisters of persons with Down's syndrome, no specific behavioral disturbances were noted.[16] In fact, it was noted that the siblings of persons with disabilities showed greater tolerance, compassion, awareness of prejudice and its consequences, and a more focused personality than did others who had no contact with persons with disabilities.

The negative assumptions listed by the authors are simply not supported by contemporary literature and clinical observations about persons with Down's syndrome.

## COMPLEX COSTS: MATTERS OF INTEGRITY, KNOWLEDGE, MOTIVATION, AND COMPASSION

Triple screening threatens the integrity of the medical profession. Genetics counselors pride themselves in promoting nonbiased, fully nondirective informed consent, but the cost analysis description of Down's syndrome under review is anything but accurate or nondirective. Some within the genetics community consider nondirective counseling to be impossible because of the inherent setting of the counseling.[17] This is especially true when testing is conducted in such a way that one anomaly is singled out above all others for detection. The negative bias of the triple screen toward persons with Down's syndrome is inherent in the marketing of the test. The triple screen has been shown to identify a high risk for a number of genetic disorders, including trisomy 13, trisomy 18, and anencephaly,[18] but, as one marketing person explained, "we use Down's syndrome because people know it—it sells." Four industrial exhibits marketed the test for Down's syndrome at the 1992 annual American College of Obstetricians and Gynecologists meeting. Whenever any group is singled out for prenatal identification (and elimination), the data and reasons for such actions will be questioned.

After a pregnant woman has been offered a test for Down's syndrome, the inherent negative bias is there that tells her that this is an individual whom we who are learned and who care for human welfare think is so negative that we need to seek them and find them before birth—in an effort to prevent birth defects. However, the biases are not this subtle in many other ways.

One group of geneticists lists Down's syndrome among the "serious anomalies" that can be found in utero.[19] In their list, Down's syndrome stands with such lethal or near-lethal anomalies as trisomies 13 and 18, triploidy, and other aneuploidies. The term *Down's syndrome* identifies persons with hope and a future in today's world, but it is described within the context of this list as having a "severe prognosis."

These same professionals claim to offer nondirective counseling. A recent study questioned this negative bias among genetic counselors concerning Down's syndrome and why it exists.[20] A routine film describing Down's syndrome was shown to a group of parents and to a group of medical professionals. Eighty-nine percent of the parents thought the film accurately represented persons with Down's syndrome. However, only 14 percent of the genetic counselors agreed with the parents; the majority thought the film was too positive.

Even when facts are known, counseling that emphasizes the "wide variation" in physical and mental disabilities associated with Down's syndrome—including such potential physical problems as heart defects, leukemia, and future Alzheimer's dementia—can easily be conducted in such a way that prospective parents are reluctant to carry such a pregnancy to term. Certainly, if the counseling is as misleading as the "factual" cost analysis included by the genetics experts in the article cited,[21] its validity must be questioned. Physician counseling about Down's syndrome should become more balanced because persons with Down's syndrome continue to progress beyond their previously expected physical and social limitations. For example, the majority of persons with Down's syndrome are in the mild-to-moderate mental retardation range (consistent with a third- to ninth-grade reading level). Less than 1 percent have leukemia. In the 5 to 20 percent who need cardiac surgery, it is usually successful. Less than 3 percent have inoperable cardiac disease. As life beyond age fifty-five becomes the norm, Alzheimer's dementia among those with Down's is not as common clinically as it was once thought. Attitude, bias, and motivation make a large difference in the way "facts" are presented, even if they are accurate (and not the negative presumptions offered by some in defining the burdens of cost).[22]

Perhaps one of the most disturbing aspects of the published negative cost analysis was the isolated use of a dollar figure for a person with Down's syndrome ($196,000), which was presented without reference to anything else.[23] What is the cost to a family and society for a normal person who becomes a physician or who pursues doctoral level education? What is the cost for anyone who spends even a brief number of years in a prison? Or consider the cost for someone who becomes the object of court-room hearings for even a few days. How much do we spend today to rear a normal child who eats an American fast food diet and enjoys television and movies? To state a contrived dollar figure for a person with Down's syndrome without a reference to other similar costs is misleading and demeaning.

The reasons for the negative counseling shown by obstetricians and genetics counselors have not been defined clearly by any studies. Disability advocates and pro-life critics claim that a conflict of interest exists for the physician who counsels patients about genetic problems—performs the blood tests, ultrasound, amniocentesis, chorionic villus sampling, and pregnancy termination—and then is reimbursed financially for all the services connected with such counseling. This seems especially upsetting if the same physicians or counselors do not participate in the remainder of the prenatal care or the delivery of the patients for whom they provide genetic services. Even some in the international community of genetics professionals have voiced concerns about the exclusive focus on prenatal genetics by those who have no contact later in life with the persons who have genetic disorders.[24] The International Society for Genetics professes a dedication to working for and with those patients with genetic disorders, but seldom is this dedication found among those who do prenatal counseling.[25]

Many geneticists in obstetrics and gynecology are victimized by these criticisms. In a large survey recently done to assess the availability of health care for adults with mental retardation, gynecologic care was the one area of medicine noted to be minimally available for persons in New England.[26] Few obstetricians and gynecologists belong to the American Association for Mental Retardation. The reading material for obstetricians and gynecologists does not include professional journals concerning persons with mental retardation. Obstetricians (including those with an emphasis on genetics) usually see very little of the person with a genetic disorder after the neonatal period—when the shock and grief of parents are at a peak, and no "positive" aspects of Down's syndrome can be imagined. The progress made by persons with Down's syndrome over the past twenty-five years has gone largely unnoticed by prenatal genetics counselors. It is not surprising that the information provided in prenatal counseling does not concur with that understood by parents and professionals who work with persons with Down's syndrome over a lifetime.[27]

Another cost that is difficult to measure includes the value placed on the maternal, paternal, and familial anxiety caused by genetic screening tests. In the case of the triple screen, a patient is told that she may be at high risk for fetal Down's syndrome. This high risk is only a risk, in reality, of 1 in 197 births. Furthermore, the test that identifies even that high risk carries at least a 55 percent false-positive rate.

The overall process of screening may take days and even weeks to complete. During that time, extreme anxiety may escalate, resulting in a loss of productivity and even signs of physical illness or despair. As the tests, initial and ultimate, become more involved, the time between counseling and diagnosis lengthens—as does the mental anguish for those tested.

## COMPLEX COSTS: THE PARADOXIC LOSS OF CHOICE TO JUSTIFY A PRICE TOO HIGH

As chairman of the professional Advisory Board for the National Down's Syndrome Congress, the first author of this chapter became accustomed to receiving complaints from persons who felt coerced into genetic counseling.

One memorable complaint came from a fellow in a genetics program who became angry at the behavior of the staff geneticist who was unreceptive to the choice a couple was making. When the couple informed the staff physician that they would prefer to carry the pregnancy to term, even knowing that the fetus had Down's syndrome, the geneticist claimed that he could not understand such a choice, argued with the decision, and pointedly refused to see the patient again. Often, this attitude is more subtle but still coercive. "The serum tests are just like any blood test. Let's at least do that much." "Ultrasound is painless, and it will tell us a great number of facts, besides genetic problems."

Is the preservation of maternal choice actually being accomplished in the triple screen for Down's syndrome? Such reasoning reminds many of us of the ethical issues of the Infant Doe arguments in the 1980s. Rival groups championed different levels of normative principles. The American College of Obstetricians and Gynecologists professed a preference for a "burdens versus benefits" view of ethical decision making for handicapped newborns and their families.[28] The corollary to this was the underscoring of parental autonomy or choice in the newborn nursery setting. Many of the same reasons for the unacceptableness of that reasoning in the newborn nursery also exist for the management of the handicapped fetus in utero. The true prognosis for a fetus with Down's syndrome is not known, but the vast majority will do well medically (with routine, equivalent care), will be highly functional mentally, and will be integrated socially in today's society. They will become the center of controversy in the triple screen program, as they were for the Infant Doe discussions of the 1980s. Most importantly, such articles as the one cited at the outset of this chapter[29] will emphasize again the problem with using a burdens versus benefits method of assessment for persons with disabilities. We in America seem very skilled at assessing the financial burdens that we cause each other, *but we seem unable to discuss the benefits, especially in the presence of a handicapping disability.* Without this aspect of the discussion, no real choice is ever provided to women who undergo prenatal counseling.

Many of us who parent children with Down's syndrome acknowledge readily that we have been given an additional burden of education—for ourselves. This translates into one of life's great benefits. Having and caring for a child with Down's syndrome teaches us about our limitations and shared disabilities. It teaches us to value persons for reasons other than performance. It teaches us the importance of developing a community of caring rather than a community of competition. It teaches us about the philosophic ideal of unconditional love, the theologic concept of grace. It teaches us to experience joy in the most mundane and menial tasks accomplished. It teaches us to devalue physique, to see a disability as only a small part of a person's life, to be adaptive in setting lifetime goals. Until geneticists begin to understand the positive side of Down's syndrome and it becomes part of their cost effectiveness analysis, they are failing to offer a true choice in genetics counseling. One of the greatest costs of the triple screen for Down's syndrome, as it is now being discussed, is the loss of choice that occurs.

Barbara Katz Rothman[30] discusses prenatal diagnosis and choice in a similar framework. The dilemmas inherent in genetic counseling are those imposed on women by the technologies of prenatal diagnosis, which most women feel compelled to accept.

> The technologies of prenatal diagnosis are offered to people in terms of expanding choices. However, it is always true that although new technology opens up some choices, it closes down others . . . prenatal diagnoses serves as a technology of quality control, based on a given society's ideas about what constitutes "quality" in children. The ability to control the "quality" of our children may ultimately cost the choice of not controlling that quality.[31]

Rothman claims that prenatal diagnosis, because of its inherent pressures, gives an illusion of choice in an ever narrowing structure. Issues of basic values, beliefs, and the larger moral questions will be lost in this narrowing of choices as decisions become pragmatic, often clinical, and always individual.[32] As stated by Zola:

> Bombarded on all sides by realistic concerns (the escalation of costs) and objective evidence (genetics) and techniques (genetic counseling), the basic value issues at stake will be obfuscated. The freedom to choose will be illusory. Someone will already have set the limits of choice (cuts in medical care and social benefits . . .), the dimensions of choice (if you do this then you will have an x probability of a defective child) and the outcomes of choice (you will have to endure the following social, political, legal and economic costs). . . . The "choice" being presented is effectively lost.[33]

## COMPLEX COSTS: SOCIETAL CONCERNS

Others suggest that our social character is measured by our capacity to welcome the disabled into our midst.[34] Triple screening is not finally about good medicine or economics. Triple screening for Down's syndrome is about our social character. The effort to prevent (or eliminate) Down's syndrome with triple screening builds from a view of what it means to be a man or woman who cannot seriously consider an affirmation of persons with Down's syndrome. It is a view that can judge the allocation of $100,000 to $300,000 per Down's syndrome fetus found and eliminated as money well spent.

Are we a society that would choose to pay that amount (or more) rather than make the necessary changes inherent in welcoming such a responsive and expressive group of people as those with Down's syndrome into our moral community? How far are we willing to go as a society to deny persons with Down's syndrome a life with us in this land of freedom? How much are we willing to spend to try vainly to eradicate a group for whom many have become so grateful? What is the ultimate cost of such efforts?

## CONCLUSION

In this chapter, we have argued against attaching a price tag to persons with Down's syndrome. Determining cost effectiveness is fraught with difficulties, even when more defensible subjects are considered, because it often emphasizes economics at the expense of clinical or social outcome. Serious consideration must be given to using other methods of determining cost effectiveness when dealing with procedures that affect humanity and society so directly.

One method would be to look more directly at medical features and clearly identifiable prognoses. Some fetal anomalies clearly bring greatly diminished life expectancy if brought to term gestation (e.g., anencephaly and trisomy 13 or 18). Other fetal conditions, such as Tay-Sachs disease or acquired immune deficiency syndrome predictably lead to extreme infant suffering. These are vastly different from Down's syndrome and would make any form of genetic screening seem more reasonable. Alternatively, the discovery of genetic traits, rather than disorders, would not be seen as important enough to warrant such extensive screening.

Some would recommend the use of "value analysis," which is based on an integration of decisional theory and evaluation science. The goal of value analysis is to establish a range of outcomes that might be viewed as important from various perspectives (e.g., patients, families, medical staff, providers, payers, and society as a whole). This would allow the incorporation of a wide range of viewpoints and would encourage regionalization and committee or consensus opinions about what prenatal genetic counseling should include at different institutions. However, individual cases would remain problematic.

Many methods of health care rationing await the American medical system. A large number of factors must be considered before any system of limiting costs and choices is selected in a pluralistic society. Accepting the fact that *limitations to choice must occur* is the first step toward future reasonableness in genetic counseling.

## ENDNOTES

1. O. P. Phillips et al., "Maternal Serum Screening for Fetal Down's Syndrome Using AFP, HCG, and UE3 in Women Less Than Twenty Years of Age" (paper presented at the Annual Meeting of the North American Society for Pediatric and Adolescent Gynecology, Nashville, Tenn., 4 April 1992); also, O. P. Phillips et al., "Maternal Serum Screening for Fetal Down's Syndrome in Women Less Than Thirty-five Years: AFP, HCG, AND UE3" (paper presented at the Annual Clinic Meeting of the American College of Obstetricians and Gynecologists, Las Vegas, Nev., 25 April 1992).

2. O. P. Phillips et al., "Maternal Serum Screening for Fetal Down—Fetoprotein, HCG, and Unconjugated Estriol: A Prospective Two-Year Study," *Obstet Gynecol* 80 (1992): 353–58; and J. E. Haddow et al., "Prenatal Screening for Down's Syndrome with Use of Maternal Serum Makers," *N Engl J Med* 327 (1992): 588–93.

3. N. G. Wald et al., "Maternal Serum Testing for Down's Syndrome in Early Pregnancy," *BMJ* 297 (1988): 883–85; and M. L. MacDonald and R. N. Slotnick,

"Sensitivity and Specificity of Screening for Down's Syndrome with AFP, HCG, Unconjugated Estriol, and Maternal Age," *Obstet Gynecol* 77 (1991): 964–70.

4. Phillips et al., "Maternal Serum Screening for Fetal Down—Fetoprotein, HCG, and Unconjugated Estriol: A Prospective Two-Year Study."

5. Phillips et al., "Maternal Serum Screening for Fetal Down's Syndrome Using AFP, HCG, and UE3 in Women Less Than Twenty Years of Age."

6. Phillips et al., "Maternal Serum Screening for Fetal Down's Syndrome in Women Less Than Thirty-five Years: AFP, HCG, and UE3."

7. Phillips et al., "Maternal Serum Screening for Fetal Down—Fetoprotein, HCG, and Unconjugated Estriol: A Prospective Two-Year Study."

8. S. E. Waisbren, "Parents Reactions After the Birth of a Developmentally Disabled Child," *Am J Ment Retard* 84 (1980): 345–51.

9. K. A. Ornie, W. N. Friedrich, and M. T. Greenberg, "Adaptation of Families with Mentally Retarded Children: A Model of Stress, Coping, and Family Ecology," *Am J Ment Retard* 88 (1983): 125–38.

10. J. Blacher, K. Nihira, and C. E. Meyers, "Characteristics of Home Environments of Families with Mentally Retarded Children: Comparison Across Levels of Retardation," *Am J Ment Retard* 91 (1987): 313–20.

11. S. Pueschel et al., *Down Syndrome: Growing and Learning* (New York: Andrews, McMeel, and Parker, 1986), 73–75.

12. A. P. Turnbull and H. R. Turnbull, "Developing Independence in Adolescents with Disabilities," *J Adolesc Health Care* 6, no. 2 (1985): 108–19.

13. Ibid.; R. A. Humphrey and R. B. Jacobson, "Families in Crisis: Research in Theory in Child Retardation," *Soc Casework* 60 (1979): 597–601; and M. A. Murphy, "The Family with a Handicapped Child: A Review of the Literature," *J Dev Behav Pediatr* 3 (1982): 73–82.

14. S. M. Pueschel et al., *New Perspectives on Down Syndrome* (Baltimore: Brookers, 1987), 335–77.

15. F. K. Grossman, *Brothers and Sisters of Retarded Children* (Syracuse, N.Y.: Syracuse University Press, 1972), 84.

16. A. Gath, "The School-Age Siblings of Mongol Children," *Br J Psych* 123 (1978): 161–67.

17. A. Clarke, "Is Nondirective Genetic Counseling Possible?" *Lancet* 338 (1991): 989–90.

18. J. A. Canick and G. J. Knight, "Multiple-Marker Screening for Fetal Down's Syndrome," *Contemporary Obstetrics and Gynecology Technology Symposium* (1992): 25–42.

19. A. Drugan et al., "Determinants of Parental Decisions to Abort for Chromosomal Abnormalities," *Prenat Diagn* 10 (1990): 483–90.

20. W. C. Cooley et al., "Reactions of Mothers and Medical Professionals to a Film About Down's Syndrome," *Am J Dis Child* 144 (1990): 1112.

21. Phillips et al., "Maternal Serum Screening for Fetal Down—Fetoprotein, HEG, and Unconjugated Estriol: A Prospective Two-Year Study."

22. T. E. Elkins et al., "Baby Doe: Is There Really a Problem?" *Obstet Gynecol* 65 (1985): 492–95.

23. Phillips et al., "Maternal Serum Screening for Fetal Down—Fetoprotein, HEG, and Unconjugated Estriol: A Prospective Two-Year Study."

24. A. Clarke, "Genetic, Ethics, and Audit," *Lancet* 335 (1990): 1145–47.

25. A. Lippman, "Prenatal Genetic Testing and Screening: Constructing Needs and Reinforcing Inequities," *Am J Law Med* 17 (1991): 15–50.

26. P. M. Minihan and D. H. Dean, "Meeting the Needs for Health Services of Persons with Mental Retardation Living in the Community," *Am J Public Health* 80 (1990): 1043–48.

27. W. C. Cooley et al., "Reactions of Mothers and Medical Professionals to a Film About Down's Syndrome," 1112.

28. Committee on Bioethics, *Statement on Withdrawing and Withholding Treatment* (Washington, D.C.: American College of Obstetricians and Gynecologists, 1985), 1–5.

29. Phillips et al., "Maternal Serum Screening for Fetal Down—Fetoprotein, HCG, and Unconjugated Estriol: A Prospective Two-Year Study."

30. B. K. Rothman, "Prenatal Diagnosis" in *Bioethics and the Fetus: Medical, Moral, and Legal Issues*, ed. J. M. Humber and R. F. Almoder (Totowa, N.J.: Humana Press, 1991), 173–75.

31. Ibid.

32. Ibid.

33. I. K. Zola, *Socio-Medical Inquiries: Recollections, Reflections, and Reconsiderations* (Philadelphia: Temple University Press, 1983), 296.

34. S. Hauerwas, *Responsibility for Devalued Persons: Ethical Interactions Between Society, the Family, and the Retarded* (Springfield, Mo.: Charles C. Thomas, 1982), 57–65.

# PART 3

## GENETIC ENGINEERING AND THE INDIVIDUAL

*An Overview*

As we consider and utilize the findings of the scientists, physicians, and researchers involved with the Human Genome Project and other genetic investigations regarding the physiological and scientific dimensions of what it means to be human, we should not neglect the biblical record that provides the unique and foundational perspective of what it means to be human. The biblical view of creation and Old Testament anthropology clearly separates humanity from the remainder of the created order. Humanity was created as the image of God, and there is a uniqueness and responsibility in humanity that is not to be found in any other living entity. Biblical and scientific understanding of humanity need not be antithetical, and, when properly understood and combined, they can provide valuable and necessary boundaries for scientific investigation and experimentation.

Chapter Fifteen

# "WHAT IS MAN?"
## *A Study of Old Testament Anthropology*

### Eugene H. Merrill

## INTRODUCTION

At the dawn of the third millennium, when genetics research has not only yielded many of the biological secrets of human life but has also begun to experiment with ways of radically altering it, one might well ask what possible good can come from a study of Old Testament anthropology. How can a collection of sacred texts written more than twenty-five hundred years ago by and for a culturally encapsulated people with a prescientific worldview have any relevance to cutting-edge theoretical and practical science?

The answer to that question will, of course, depend on one's view of the Old Testament. Those who see it as Hebrew texts that reflect only the thinking of its ancient composers and compilers will, quite correctly, devalue its significance in defining the nature and implications of modern genetics. One could as well ask what the Bible has to say about rocket propulsion. Albeit, those committed to the timelessness of the Old Testament record, its ongoing relevance as a function of its divine revelation and authority, will and must inquire of it to determine if it has anything at all to say to the existential crisis that dogs modern genetic science.

Genetics is different from rocket science not least because genetics has to do with who and what we are, whereas rocket science is an example of what we can do. The one pertains to ontology, the other to function. If the Old Testament has any central anthropological concern at all, it is precisely to address questions of human essentiality, the same concerns as those of social and even biological science.[1] The purpose here is to examine the Hebrew Scriptures to discover what (if anything) they have to say about human existence in general and modern genetics research in particular.

## GENETICS AND GENETICS RESEARCH

The technical, scientific aspects of genetics research and its applications are dealt with elsewhere in this volume. In this section, it is sufficient to survey very briefly the moral, ethical, and theological issues attendant to the scientific enterprise with a view to discovering if and how the Bible speaks to the debate.

First, the point must be made that genetics research is not inherently evil. If God created all things in the universe—from the atoms to the galaxies—he did so, among other reasons, to display his wisdom, power, and glory. If one can gaze at the heavens and marvel at the illimitability of God as displayed in the vastness of the universe (Ps. 19:1–6), then surely one can study the microscopic nature of the human genetics system and see in it the infinite design and care of the Creator. Reverent scientific research and interpretation can do nothing other than draw one to the God of truth.

Second, biological and medical breakthroughs have made possible such lifesaving measures as organ transplantation. Even with its attendant questionable or clearly evil excesses—such as interspecific organ exchanges or organ "harvesting" of fetuses and the like—it is undeniable that much good has come from a sober application of genetic principles.[2] Skin auto-transplants, organ donation from the deceased to the living, and kidney transplants among related persons can hardly be condemned on biblical moral and theological grounds.

The issues of cloning and mutation are of a different kind, however.[3] The latter, of course, has proven to be an effective tool in producing hybrids in plants and animals, enhancing their growth rates and productivity to humankind's advantage. Even cloning as a theoretical principle seems to be amoral at worst. As with all scientific principles, it is the application for good or ill that determines its morality and biblical justification. Nazi experiments in cloning research that were designed to produce the "super race" is an extreme but instructive example of where misguided genetics can take its practitioners. Few scientists engaged in such research today would harbor these evil designs, but frequently unexpected and unintended deleterious consequences issue from processes uncontrolled or undisciplined by well-thought-out systems of ethical and theological belief. To the evangelical, that system of belief is one rooted and grounded in biblical revelation. The discussion at this point, then, turns to the witness of the Old Testament, particularly to those texts that speak most directly to the idea of biblical anthropology.

## "WHAT IS MAN?" AN EXEGESIS OF PSALM 8

A central question in genetics research must surely be, "What is humankind?" Is it only a fortuitous result of a random evolutionary process? Or is humankind the most sublime evidence of all that there exists an intelligent Creator who has made man and woman in his own image? Basic philosophical and theological premises will of necessity determine the answer to that question. It is not a new question posed only in response to modern scientific investigation. David raised the same query three thousand years ago in his inimitable treatise on the nature and function of humankind—Psalm 8. Of YHWH God the psalmist asked, "What is man that you are mindful of him, the son of man that you care for him?" (v. 4). This psalm, one of the texts most quoted by the New Testament,[4] is a proper point of departure.

The psalm begins with a praise of God (vv. 1–2), named here "LORD, our Lord" (v. 1a).[5] LORD translates as the Hebrew word *YHWH*, the name by which God expresses his immanence, especially his covenant relationship with his chosen people. The word *Lord* translates Adonai, a term suggesting dominion. David is confessing that the God of covenant is the God of lordship to whom he and his fellow Israelites are accountable.

The lordship theme continues in verse 1b with its assertion of the majesty of God's name, a majesty universally applicable even if not recognized. *Majesty* (*'addîr*) connotes loftiness or transcendence,[6] and *name* is figurative for YHWH himself. He is "our Lord" (near) but also "majestic" (afar). In the second half of verse 1, David locates God (represented by his glory) not just in heaven but "above the heavens." The purpose of such lofty praise is to elevate God to another realm, one impervious to human access or even apprehension. This makes the contrast in verse 2 all the more astounding. The utterly transcendent God can be praised by human beings and by infants at that! Such praise is not weak and feeble, however, but powerful. When it is uttered, all of God's enemies must be shamed into silence. If the sophisticated and scientific among us cannot see God or recognize his work, tiny children can do so because they have the spiritual naïveté to see.

David next speaks of God's priorities (vv. 3–5) by the surprising juxtaposition of the apparently contradictory ideas of God's exaltation and humankind's lowliness. Having studied the limitless and awesome expanse of the heavens, David wonders how God could possibly even notice his earthbound creation, let alone oversee his every move ("care for him," v. 4b; *paqad*). Verse 3 underscores divine eminence and verse 4 human insignificance, but verse 5 provides a bridge of reconciliation—humankind is "a little lower than the heavenly beings" (v. 5a) whom God has crowned "with glory and honor" (v. 5b).

The theological deduction is this: God, the altogether sovereign One, has taken humankind, though comparatively of no worth or dignity, and has elevated him to a position of preeminence in the created order. The more full exposition of this idea follows in verses 6–8 and, as we shall show, in the creation accounts of Genesis 1 and 2.

The New Testament book of Hebrews makes use of this psalm to describe the humiliation and then the exaltation of Jesus Christ (Heb. 2:5–10). Having been made man ("son of man"; Heb. 2:6) in the Incarnation (cf. Phil. 2:7), Christ was elevated to unlimited sovereignty by his resurrection and ascension (Heb. 2:7–9; cf. Phil. 2:8–11). This interpretation and use of the psalm by the author of Hebrews does not negate its Old Testament contextual meaning, however. In fact, Jesus' exaltation was in many respects the ultimate expression of God's intention for the human race as a whole from the very beginning. This clearly is the thrust of Psalm 8.

This leads to the third major section of the psalm (vv. 6–8) in which God's purpose for humankind's creation is disclosed. This section not only elaborates on what it means for human beings to "be crowned with glory and honor" (v. 5), but it makes the assertion that humankind is of a radically different order from the rest of creation, that difference being, in this psalm at least, primarily a functional one. In language deliberately reminiscent of Genesis 1:26–28, the poet describes humans as being in dominion over all the creatures of earth—land, air, and marine (vv. 7–8). And this is because God created him for this purpose (v. 6). There can be no question in the biblical view as to humankind's nature and function vis-à-vis the rest of creation. He is different from it, stands apart from it, and was created to exercise lordship over it.

Finally, the psalm closes with an enveloping exordium of praise (v. 9), which brings the matter full circle (cf. v. 1). Having celebrated humankind's role as a subregent of almighty God, how can David do other than praise God for his infinite wisdom and grace?

## HUMANKIND IN OLD TESTAMENT CREATION TEXTS

Biblical scholarship correctly identifies Psalm 8 as a commentary on the creation accounts of Genesis, particularly on Genesis 1:26–28. However, whereas the psalm's focus is on the God-ordained mission of humankind, the Genesis record goes beyond that to explore humanity's essential nature. To the "*What* is man?" question must now be added and answered the question, "*Who* is he?" Not surprisingly, the answer appears at the beginning of the sacred record and not just incidentally. A case can be made that the accounts of the creation of the human race in Genesis 1 and 2 constitute one of the most theologically significant themes of the entire Bible.[7]

At the outset, it is important to note that there are not two creation narratives from two originally independent sources as the Documentary Hypothesis would suggest.[8] Rather, there are two ways of looking at creation, specifically the creation of humankind. In the first (Gen. 1:26–28), the human race comes into being as the culmination of six days of creative activity. The narrative is so structured as to point to man's centrality. But it does not stop with a mere statement of his existence. It goes on to delineate the purpose of his creation, the mandate for which he came into being and that he must implement as the vice-regent of God himself.

The narrative of Genesis 2:4–25 gives scant attention to anything but the creation of humanity. In highly anthropomorphic terms, the account speaks of the Lord God busy at work shaping and molding the soil into a human form much like a potter would fashion a vessel of clay. Having brought this form to perfection, God breathed into it his own life, as it were, and the ground plus spirit became a human being. The whole scene speaks of a tender intimacy between the Creator and the creature, a relationship nuanced by the description of the Creator for the first time as YHWH (Gen. 2:4b). As Creator of the whole cosmos in Genesis 1, God is spoken of by the Hebrew epithet Elohim, a term suggesting awesomeness of power and glory but also remote transcendence. It is only when humankind becomes the focus of his interest in chapter 2 that the covenant name YHWH occurs, a name that evokes the idea of participation in human affairs.[9]

### Creation: The Cosmic Account (Gen. 1:26–28)

The second word in the Hebrew Bible is *bārā'*, a verb meaning "create." It is peculiar grammatically in that it never occurs in the Old Testament with a human subject.[10] In other words, only God can create in the *bārā'* sense. Furthermore, it occurs only in Genesis 1:1–2:4 in the creation accounts, that is, in the narrative in which Elohim, the transcendent and cosmic God, is the actor. In the Genesis 2 story, where YHWH is the divine name, other verbs are used. These will be addressed presently. Additionally, *bārā'*, unless qualified grammatically and contextually, connotes *creatio ex nihilo*, the bringing into existence of something out of nothing. This is clearly the intent in Genesis 1:1 ("the heavens and the earth," i.e., everything) and in 2:3 and 2:4, though in the latter two cases the verb is juxtaposed with or is parallel to the verb *'āśāh*, "to make." Here, to make means also to create out of nothing.

The only other uses of *bārā'* in the creation stories are in Genesis 1:21 and 1:27, the creation of the higher life forms of sea, air, land, and humankind, respectively. Besides undercutting any notion of spontaneous generation or macroevolution, the occurrence of *bārā'* in these texts makes a radical disjunction between humankind and all other creatures. Animals are qualitatively different from the rest of creation and humans qualitatively different from and clearly superior to the animals, a point made elsewhere in the passage.

The Genesis 1 account establishes humanity's priority by the pyramidal scheme in which it is shaped (see Figure 1). At the base is the creation of all things, the heavens and the earth (Gen. 1:1–5), what might be called a cosmocentric view. Next (vv. 6–10) is the focus on the earth, a matter of geocentric interest. The next three levels—creation of vegetation (vv. 11–13), of marine and aerial life (vv. 20–23), and of land life (vv. 24–25)—share in common their biocentricity. At the apex of the pyramid is the creation of humans (vv. 26–28), an act to be described as anthropocentric. Again, the ascending order, climaxing with the creation of humankind, establishes humanity's theological and functional supremacy over all else.

**Figure 1: The Creation Pyramid**

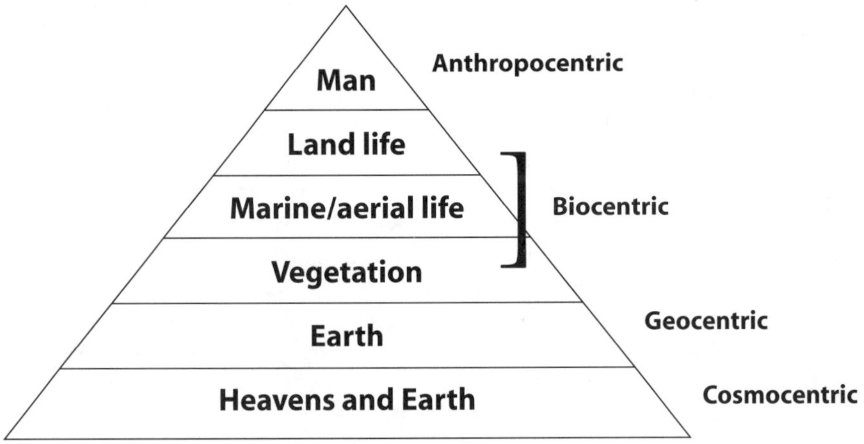

Another clue to the uniqueness of humankind in the created order is the notion of division as seen in the use of the verb meaning "to divide" *(bādal/ hibdîl)* and the noun meaning "kind" *(mîn)*. The verb occurs five times in the Genesis 1 record and each time makes an important theological point.[11] It first speaks of the separation between light and darkness on day one (1:4), then of the division of the celestial from the terrestrial waters on day two (vv. 6–7), and finally between day and night and other time distinctions on day four (vv. 14, 18). The point is that everything has its place and the boundaries established by the Creator have a purpose and must not be violated.

With the creation of living things beginning on day three, the term *mîn* is introduced, occurring a total of ten times in the Genesis 1 record. It bears the meaning "kind, species" and comes as close to the modern biological concept of genetic distinction as ancient Hebrew lexicography could provide.[12] The intent in this creation account is clearly to make the same kind of demarcations as is evident in the use of the verb *bādal* in reference to nonliving materials and objects. The first description of speciation is in the realm of vegetation where *mîn* occurs three times (vv. 11–12) to indicate the several classes of plants and trees. On day five, marine and aerial creatures are created "according to their kinds" (v. 21). And these are not just divisions between these two great life forms but within them. All sea and all air animals were subdivided according to strict biological categories that would certainly not be at odds with modern classifications. Finally, the land animals were created on the sixth day "according to their kinds" (vv. 24–25). All beasts, wild and domesticated, are thus separated from the beginning without the benefit of either aeons of evolution or scientific mutational experimentation.

Striking by the lack of either the verb *bādal* or the noun *mîn* is the description of humankind's creation (vv. 26–28).[13] The reason for the omission is obvious: Humankind is so patently different from all other creatures as not to require further definition or distinction. Furthermore, the formula "and God said," used throughout the narrative to introduce new and different phases of the creation (vv. 3, 6, 9, 11, 14, 20, 24), occurs again in v. 26 to set man's creation off as something of a different category. He is separated and of a different species precisely because he is *sui generis*, the climactic and unique crowning glory of God's creative work.

In light of the intention of the text to draw attention to the uniqueness and significance of humankind, the question, "What is man?" must now be addressed once more. We have seen how David employed the Genesis account in his magnification of the role of humankind in God's redemptive program (Ps. 8). It will now be instructive to look at David's source text on its own terms to see how it sheds light on the subject of biblical anthropology.

The passage (Gen. 1:26–28) lends itself to a straightforward analysis. Verse 26 discloses God's intention, verse 27 the product of that intention, and verse 28 the blessing and reinforcement of the intention. The divine objective is to create a being to represent God as ruler over all his creation. It can be argued that this dominion or kingdom theme dominates the Bible and is a key theological proposition.[14] Humanity's creation appears last in the record because his nature and role culminate and constitute the epitome of God's purpose for the cosmos.

The creation verb employed here in verse 26 ("make"; *'āśāh*) is a synonym of *bārā'*, the verb meaning creation *ex nihilo*, as the fulfillment statement of verse 27 makes clear. The object to be made is humankind ( *'ādām*), that is, the human race, so far without gender distinction. The pattern of creation is for humankind to be "in our image, in our likeness" (v. 26). The terms *image* (*ṣelem*) and *likeness (dᵉmût)* consistently occur in the Old Testament with reference to idols and other representations, usually of pagan deities (cf. 2 Kings 11:18; Isa. 40:18; Ezek. 16:17; 23:14; Amos 5:26). The classical way of understanding the doctrine of the *imago Dei* (humans in the image of God) is that God and humankind share certain common attributes or characteristics such as personality, intellect, emotion, will, and holiness.[15] However, the use of *ṣelem* and *dᵉmût* elsewhere in the Old Testament, as well as the concept of an image representing royal authority in the ancient Near East, points to the meaning here of humankind's standing in God's place in a hierarchy of dominion.[16] The following elaboration of the divine intention supports this understanding.

This intention is that humankind should rule over all the rest of creation. The order of his subjects is quite revealing: marine life, aerial life, and land life, the very sequence of the creation events as listed in verses 20–25. Again, the position of humanity at the apex of the pyramid of creation activity is unmistakable. Humanity is created last, and only humanity exists *as* (not *in*) the image of God, for to us alone is bestowed the privilege and responsibilities of dominion.

The verb that speaks of humanity's exercise of divine authority (*rādāh*) usually occurs in contexts where rule is carried out by force (Lev. 25:43, 46, 53; 1 Kings 4:24; Ps. 72:8; 110:2; Ezek. 34:4).[17] That is not its nuance here, at least on the surface, but it may reflect a somewhat proleptic anticipation of the Fall, an effect of which would be dominion by coercion (see Gen. 9:1–7). The use of this verb in Psalm 110:2 is also interesting inasmuch as David is charged with ruling over YHWH's enemies as YHWH's earthly and human representative. The blessing of God's intention in verse 28 reinforces this possibility of necessary force.

The implementation of the intention in Genesis 1:27 introduces some important advancements in defining the human race and its role under God. The verb *bārā'* appears again, reminding the reader that humankind is not the end product of an evolutionary change but, in fact, is a brand new idea, an entity produced wholesale out of nothing. Also, there is a double reminder that humans are the image of God: "So God created man in his own *image*, in the *image* of God he created him" (emphasis added). Admittedly, this structure is rather typical of ordinary Hebrew poetic form, but the repetition of *image* here also has authorial purpose. One should never forget what humans are, the very representative of the King of Kings on earth!

More significant is the articular form of *man* in verse 27. Verse 26 says, "let us make man," but verse 27 says, "So God created *the* man" (emphasis added). In the former instance, the whole human race is in mind; in the latter, the solitary being—Adam (and Eve as it turns out)—is front and center. The rather amorphous abstraction humankind gives way to the singular, concrete pair, the father and mother of the human race. Identifying the individual in this manner paves the way for the introduction of gender. Humankind is not hermaphroditic sexually but bifurcated into gender, male and female. Nor did the female evolve from or grow out of the male. She as well as he was created, as the last line of verse 27 makes clear. Ruling, then, is a shared responsibility, but gender distinctions exist and must be retained, a truth that admittedly is pernicious to many modern minds.

The transition to individuality and then to plurality (or, better, duality; i.e., male and female) leads to the plural object of God's mandate in verse 28: "God blessed *them* and said to *them*" (emphasis added). The meaning here is not that God blessed the man and woman and then said something. Rather, what God goes on to say is the content or essence of the blessing. One could render the beginning of verse 28, "God blessed them by saying to them," and so on. Verse 26 had stated God's intention for humankind that they rule over all things. That intention is by no means forgotten here, for the latter half of the verse puts into imperatival form (*rᵉdû*) what verse 26 had framed in an optative form (*yirdû*). "Let them rule" has now become "(you) rule." The subjects to be ruled are identical in both places except for the curious omission of the "livestock," or land animals, in verse 28. The LXX adds the missing element but it is also possible to include them in the phrase "every living creature that moves along the ground" (v. 28b).

In any case, the blessing of the divine intention is expanded beyond the initial statement of intention of verse 26 by the addition of four other imperatives in verse 28a.[18] The first of these commands is to "be fruitful" (*pᵉrû*). Though this may convey the idea of prosperity or abundance in some settings, here its juxtaposition to "increase" (*rᵉbû*) suggests that fruitfulness is measured in terms of population growth. As the earth itself became overrun with animal life, humankind must multiply in order to carry out the dominion mandate.

The other two verbs, "fill" (*mil'û*) and "subdue" (*kibšû*), also are mutually informing. As for the latter, its usual sense is that of forcible subjection of one party to another (cf. 2 Sam. 8:11; Zech. 9:15). As with *rādāh*, it may be used here in anticipation of a day when rule by force would be necessary. It is possibly, however, just a standard cliché employed in the semantic field of dominion without either negative or positive overtones. To exercise dominion is to reduce someone or something else to subservience. If so, to fill the earth suggests not only population growth but, in connection with subduing, to take over the earth. Support for this understanding may be found in various texts where the Lord's spirit fills an individual (Deut. 34:9), the Lord himself fills the tabernacle (Exod. 40:34) and temple (1 Kings 8:10), and his glory fills the whole earth (Jer. 23:24; cf. Hab. 2:14).[19] Here, to fill means more than merely to occupy space; it has also the clear connotation of control and dominion.

The four verbs of dominion in rapid sequence are summarized by the fifth, *rādāh*, which, as we have noted, was the only one used in the initial statement of intention in Genesis 1:26. Humankind was created to rule, and now, having been created, he is mandated to do so.

## Creation: The Anthropocentric Account (Gen. 2:4–25)

As already suggested, the narrative of creation in Genesis 2 differs from that in chapter 1 not only in its almost exclusive interest in humans but in its highly anthropomorphic way of describing the Lord God and his creative work. It will be important to bear those twin ideas in mind in this part of the discussion because the focus now is not so much on what humanity does but who humans are. That is, there is a shift from the functional aspect to the ontological, from what humanity does to what humanity is. The implications for modern biological, anthropological, and sociological ways of understanding humanity should be quite apparent.

If Genesis 1 speaks of the dominion of humankind, chapter 2 speaks of our domain, the pristine and original arena of our sovereignty. Our importance, according to this rendition, is immediately apparent in that no plant life had emerged on the earth because there was no one to "work the ground" (Gen. 2:5). This statement of function is matched by that in verse 15 where the same Hebrew verb (*'ābad*) is found, this time with specific reference to the garden as the focal point of worldwide responsibility for care and management. The garden and all the details of its location and contents form the subject matter of verses 8–17. Thus, the key passage for understanding the nature of humankind, verse 7, is sandwiched between two texts describing humans as the ones to "work the ground." Who are these who are to undertake such an awesome task, and what is there about them that qualifies them to do so? We have learned that humankind is the image of God, that is, that we represent God, but so far we are left ignorant as to humanity's physical and spiritual constitution.

So great is the mystery and complexity of God's creation of humans that it has to be related metaphorically. The Lord God, we're told, "formed man from the dust of the ground" (v. 7a), a scene reminiscent of the potter's shop. The raw material is dust (*'āpār*), a rather surprising choice it would seem. Why would not mud or clay or loam be used? The answer perhaps is that dust is light and fine, so fragile and of such loose consistency as to be blown away by the slightest gust of wind. Humankind is mortal, the body subject to rapid disintegration and decay. That clearly is the idea in Genesis 3:19 where YHWH curses the ground (*'ădāmâ*) and then says to Adam "for dust you are and to dust you will return."[20] In such a metaphorical text, one should not look for scientific and technical precision. Of course the first human was not made of literal dust nor are human bodies constituted of soil. To read the Bible in such a way is to misread its poetic as well as theological intention. Neither its friend nor foe can derive much comfort from such a hermeneutic. Yet, it is worth noting that the physical body consists of the very same chemicals, minerals, and other raw materials found in the natural environment of human life.

The verb chosen to speak of human formation *(yāṣar)* is also conducive to ceramics imagery. In fact, the most common term to describe a potter is *yôṣēr,* a participial form of the verb meaning "a former."[21] God, then, took dust and like a potter, formed it into a human shape. Besides its value in helping our limited minds to penetrate the mysteries of creation, this imagery conveys something of the tenderness and intimacy of God's work of bringing the human race into existence. Humankind is not simply a product of blind chance or even of undifferentiated divine fiat. Each individual is important because each, like a clay vessel, is shaped to a specific form and purpose pleasing to the Master Potter (Isa. 29:16; 45:9; Jer. 18:6; Rom. 9:21).

Humankind is more than body, however, despite materialistic claims to the contrary. A consistent nontheistic evolutionary theory would indeed necessitate an exclusively physical definition of humankind because there is no way to account for a spiritual dimension in purely developmental terms. The biblical witness insists on something more, however, and, in fact, denies the possibility of nonspiritual human existence. Thus, our text informs us that once God had formed Adam's body, he undertook the process of animating that body, of taking lifeless dust and making it the vehicle of personhood.

The process by which this was done is, again, couched in graphically anthropomorphic description. There is a divine action that produces a supernatural result. The action is conveyed by the verb "breathe" *(nāpaḥ),* a verb that communicates here a kind of mouth-to-mouth (literally mouth-to-nostrils) resuscitation. The difference is that Adam is not being brought back to life but is becoming a living being for the first time. The verb occurs with God as subject in Ezekiel 37:9 where dead Israel is said to have come alive in the end of the age by virtue of the divine inbreathing.[22]

What is breathed is God's *nᵉšāmâ,* a breath that gives life *(ḥayyîm).* The same idea appears in Job 33:4, Proverbs 20:27, Isaiah 42:5, and Isaiah 57:16. This by no means implies that humankind partakes of divinity, that we are godlike in some way or other. It does suggest, however, that human animation is a result of direct divine impartation of life and is not merely the final stage of a natural developmental process.

The combination of the physical form and the divine inbreathing is what the text calls a *nepeš ḥayyâ,* a "living being." A great deal of confusion results from understanding *nepeš* in the classical sense of "soul" as though Adam, by virtue of God's inbreathing, had received a soul. The passage is clear: Adam *became* a *nepeš.* Since he was obviously more than an invisible entity, *nepeš* means more than soul in this setting. The fact that even the animals are denominated by the term *nepeš ḥayyâ* ("living being," v. 19) indicates that the purpose here is not that of a description of humankind as trichotomous (body, soul, and spirit) but the simple equation of a *nepeš* with a human being.[23] The Old Testament anthropology, then, is quite simple as far as the constitution of a human being is concerned—body plus divine inbreathing equal a person.

Inasmuch as lower forms are also designated *nepeš ḥayyâ,* what makes humankind different? The answer is in the process and its implications. The record is clear that the animals came into existence in the same manner as the material universe as a whole: "God said . . . and it was so" (Gen. 1:24). Only of human beings is it said that God imparted into them something of himself, his $n^e\check{s}\bar{a}m\hat{a}$.[24] But it is that very element that makes humankind unique and of inestimable significance. Only we are the image of God, fit to be such by both the special nature of our creation and the heavenly mandate by which we have been assigned to have dominion over all things.

## CONCLUSION

This attempt to address Old Testament anthropology as a backdrop to current issues springing from genetics research suggests the following major conclusions.

First, the biblical view is that of fiat creation of all things including the human race. If a case can be made at all for naturalistic, materialistic macroevolution, it finds no corroboration in Scripture. To the contrary, the relevant accounts go out of their way to underscore the uniqueness of humankind and to distance us from all other forms of life. Far from developing from them, we stand apart from them in both the process by which we came to be and the relationship we are to sustain with them, that of dominion as the image of God. Genetics research that presupposes a commonality between human beings and all other biological forms can find no aid or comfort in the Old Testament texts. Experimentation in these areas that are ignorant of or insensitive to these biblical distinctions run the risk of violating God-given principles of human dignity and worth.

Second, humankind was created *as* (not *in*) the image of God. This means we enjoy at least derivatively, a divine prestige and authority. We are not a link, even if the last, in a zoological chain connecting all the animal world. Rather, we were made to stand outside that world and to view it as a stewardship, under God, for which we have God-ordained responsibility. For us to be a mere subject of genetic manipulation like any other biological specimen is to rob us of our inherent likeness to God. With all our post-Fall imperfections the human being still retains all that is meant by the *imago Dei*. The perfections of his original creation are there, at least vestigially, and we furthermore embrace the hope of complete renewal and regeneration in the age to come. This is not to be expected as a benefit of continuing biological research but as a divine recreation.

Third, biblical and scientific understandings of humankind need not and should not be antithetical. God is author of both the Bible and the cosmos, and as such fully comprehends each in all his or her complexity. But only he can do so. The human hubris that assumes that enough study and enough experimentation can unlock the secrets of the universe without access to the mind of its Creator is doomed to delusion and ultimate disappointment. It is high time that biblicists, ethicists, and biological scientists begin to look at the human condition through the same sets of lenses, those unclouded by exegetical or naturalistic presuppositions, in order to see the world as God sees it. Then and only then will humankind's nature and function be clearly understood and the boundaries of scientific experimentation properly defined.

## ENDNOTES

1. Walther Eichrodt, *Theology of the Old Testament*, trans. J. A. Baker (Philadelphia: Westminster, 1967), 2:147–50.
2. Thomas A. Shannon and James D. Digiacomo, *An Introduction to Bioethics* (New York: Paulist Press, 1979), 95–103.
3. For concerns in this area, see Bernard D. Davis, ed., *Storm over Biology: Essays on Science, Sentiment, and Public Policy* (Buffalo: Prometheus Books, 1986), 216–36.
4. Matthew 21:16; 1 Corinthians 15:27; Ephesians 1:22; Hebrews 2:6–9.
5. For an excellent analysis of the psalm, see Willem A. VanGemeren, "Psalms," in *The Expositor's Bible Commentary*, ed. Frank E. Gaebelein (Grand Rapids: Zondervan, 1991), 5:109–14.
6. G. H. Ahlstrom, "אַדִּיר *'addîr*," in *Theological Dictionary of the Old Testament*, ed. G. Johannes Botterweck and Helmer Ringgren (Grand Rapids: Eerdmans, 1974), 1:73–74.
7. Eugene H. Merrill, "A Theology of the Pentateuch," in *A Biblical Theology of the Old Testament*, ed. Roy B. Zuck (Chicago: Moody Press, 1991), 13–16.
8. The Documentary Hypothesis suggests that the Torah was written by numerous authors. Therefore, the Torah has been divided into four major sections: J (Jahwistic), E (Elohistic), P (Priestly), and D (Deuteronomistic). The hypothesis suggests that J and P present two views of the creation account. See "Torah" in *The Anchor Bible Dictionary*, vol. 6, ed. David Noel Freedman (New York: Doubleday, 1992), 609–21.
9. Umberto Cassuto, *A Commentary on the Book of Genesis*, trans. Israel Abrahams (Jerusalem: Magnes Press, 1961), 1:84–88.
10. Jan Bergman, Helmer Ringgren, Karl-Heinz Bernhardt, and G. Johannes Botterweck, "בָּרָא, *bārā*," in *Theological Dictionary of the Old Testament*, 1:246–47.
11. Victor P. Hamilton, "The Book of Genesis Chapters 1–17," in *NICOT* (Grand Rapids: Eerdmans, 1990), 119–20.
12. On the other hand, the Bible knows of no speciation that follows all modern taxonomical principles. The term *mîn* speaks of very general categories and yet categories that are clearly defined. Mark D. Futato, "מִין," in *New International Dictionary of Old Testament Theology and Exegesis*, ed. Willem A. VanGemeren (Grand Rapids: Zondervan, 1997), 2:934.
13. Kenneth A. Mathews, "Genesis 1–11:26," in *NAC*, vol. 1A (Nashville: Broadman & Holman, 1996), 153.
14. Eugene H. Merrill, "Covenant and the Kingdom: Genesis 1–3 as Foundation for Biblical Theology," *Criswell Theological Review* 1 (1987): 295–308.
15. So, e.g., Augustus H. Strong, *Systematic Theology* (Philadelphia: Judson, 1907), 515–15.
16. Claus Westermann, *Genesis 1–11: A Commentary*, trans. John J. Scullion (Minneapolis: Augsburg, 1984), 151–54. Westermann himself rejects this interpretation.
17. Philip J. Nel, "רדה," in *New International Dictionary of Old Testament Theology and Exegesis*, 3:1055.
18. These may constitute two pairs of hendiadyses in which the second element in

each explains the first. One could thus translate, "Be fruitful by multiplying and subdue the earth by filling it." For this grammatical form see Bruce K. Waltke and M. O'Connor, *An Introduction to Biblical Hebrew Syntax* (Winona Lake, Ind.: Eisenbrauns, 1990), par. 32.3b.

19. M. V. VanPelt and W. C. Kaiser Jr., "מלא," in *New International Dictionary of Old Testament Theology and Exegesis*, 2:940.

20. Mathews, *Genesis 1–11:26*, 196.

21. A. H. Konkel, "יצר," in *New International Dictionary of Old Testament Theology and Exegesis*, 2:503–6; and Stephen M. Hooks, ibid., 2:429–31.

22. Hans Walter Wolff, *Anthropology of the Old Testament* (Philadelphia: Fortress, 1974), 33.

23. Ibid., 21.

24. Hamilton, *The Book of Genesis Chapters 1–17*, 159.

## An Overview

If genes are responsible for the color of one's eyes and hair and for the diseases that threaten our very lives, might they also be responsible for antisocial and criminal behavior? Is it possible that genes (mutated or otherwise) *cause* certain individuals to live lifestyles that society terms deviant and, if so, does a genetically determined behavior relinquish these individuals from moral accountability? In a social climate that longs to place personal responsibility for one's behavior on anything other than self, J. Daryl Charles discusses the iconization of the gene as the successor of social constructionism for the determination of an individual's traits and behavior. The many potential dangers that are likely to surface if humanity's "complex biopsychosocial system" is reduced to its genes are outlined in detail. In the face of growing crime and violence, will America become a therapeutically based tolerant people who have succumbed to determinism at the expense of free will?

# Chapter Sixteen

# BLAME IT ON THE BETA-BOOSTERS

*Genetics, Self-Determination,
and Moral Accountability*

## J. Daryl Charles

MODELS OF CRIMINAL LAW IN OUR TRADITION . . . based on the concept of rehabilitation or that of retribution . . . have failed to achieve their stated objective. Neuroscientific research . . . suggests the propriety of turning to a medical approach to crime. . . . What we call "free will" is the activities of the brain in controlling the somatic nervous system. . . . Since behavior is dependent on the serotonin levels of the brain, whether or not one is rational depends on the serotonin levels of the brain. . . . My moral self is thus defined by my serotonin level.

—C. Ray Jeffery
*The Neurotransmitter Revolution*

We are now on the verge of a revolution in genetic medicine. . . . The future will be to understand the genetics of aggressive disorders and to identify those who have greater tendencies to become violent. . . . You could ask parents whether they consider their infant high-strung or hyperactive. Then screen more closely by challenging the infants with provocative situations. . . . [Y]ou could do careful neurologic testing and train the family how not to goad and fight them. . . . And when these things don't work, consider medical interventions, such as beta blockers, anticonvulsants or lithium.

—Stuart Yudofsky
*Scientific American*

To gain a hearing in our culture, theology has often assumed a voice not its own and found itself merely repeating the bromides of secular intellectuals in transparently figurative speech. . . . Meanwhile, secular intellectuals have largely stopped paying attention. . . . The explanation for the eclipse of religious ethics in recent secular moral philosophy may therefore be . . . that academic theologians have increasingly given the impression of saying nothing atheists don't already know.

—Jeffrey Stout
*Ethics After Babel*

## INTRODUCTION

In the ongoing debate over nature versus nurture, nature currently has the upper hand. Biology is destiny, at least, the scientific pendulum is swinging in that direction.[1] Given recent advances in genetic research—e.g., mapping the human genome, DNA identification of criminals, and gene splicing[2]—the gene is becoming, if it has not already become, a cultural icon.[3]

This development can be measured not only by the gene's iconic status in scientific and medical journals but also in popular culture and political discourse. In outlining the contours of this cultural phenomenon, one writer observes that

> the whole culture is metaphorically awash in genes, which are depicted as pervasive and powerful agents central to understanding both everyday behavior and the secret of life. Foraging through countless specialty periodicals and mass-culture sources, [one uncovers] references to selfish genes, pleasure-seeking genes, violence genes, gay genes, couch-potato genes, celebrity genes, depression genes. Everything but the kitchen-sink gene.[4]

Increasingly, diverse social critics maintain that we stand on the threshold of the "biological century." While physics has dominated the present century, advances in other laboratories suggest a noteworthy shift. Writes Gregory Benford, a professor of physics at the University of California, Irvine:

> Just as the 1890s hummed with physical gadgetry, our decade bristles with striking biological inventions. Conceptual shifts will surely follow. Beyond 2000, the principal social, moral, and economic issues will probably spring from biology's metaphors and approach, and from its cornucopia of technology. Bio-thinking will inform our world and shape our vision of ourselves.[5]

But what shall we make of the vaunted biogenetic advances at the threshold of the twenty-first century? What place shall they be accorded? And what do they portend?

Volumes such as *The DNA Mystique: The Gene as a Cultural Icon*[6] and *Refiguring Life: Metaphors of Twentieth Century Biology*[7] represent attempts to assess the exalted status of molecular and medical genetics. Ongoing progress in the biomedical field confronts contemporary society with inherent and perplexing ethical dilemmas—dilemmas that will need to be addressed against the backdrop of scientific materialism and moral skepticism. In the view of the authors of *The DNA Mystique*, the gene has become an explanation for human behavior that is too readily appropriated, too seldom criticized, and too frequently misused in the service of socially destructive ends. In the end, the gene is not *merely* a cultural metaphor; it holds sway over scientific assumptions and theory, both of which trickle down to drive common culture.[8]

The relationship between biology and free will, fully apart from recent advances in science, has long occupied scientists and philosophers. Are human beings capable of moral reason and free choice and thus responsible for their actions? Is there a dimension of human existence that transcends the gene and biology, thereby allowing humans to define themselves morally and spiritually? Is human behavior determined by one's genetic makeup?

In light of the more recent progress in medical genetics (notably the mapping of the human genome), the stakes are raised significantly with regard to human beings' giving account of their behavior. Identifying the genetic basis for an ever-growing number of diseases has been a particular focus of medical genetic research. Of equal interest among many scientists has been the attempt to explain the interplay between genes and behavior. Are human beings truly capable of self-determination whatever their gene-based physiological and psychological predispositions? Or are humans mere robots programmed by their genes and thus not to be held morally accountable for their actions? Writing in *Ethics and Medics*, Renee Mirkes summarizes the critical issues that stand before us with the new genetic twist to the question of human behavior and moral self-responsibility:

> According to chemical reductionism central to biological determinism, the causal laws of the tightly structured nexus of human biology—a nexus that is becoming ever more refined through the advances of human genetics—dictate human behavior. It is illogical within this view of human behavior to require personal responsibility for the moral quality of one's actions; moral accountability makes sense only if actions [proceed] from a free agent.[9]

The biological metaphor, then, which is no mere metaphor, would appear to have the potential of allowing us to re-conceive the entire realm of human behavior. What indeed does biology tell us regarding human activity? And, perhaps more importantly, what does it *not* tell us?

## ASSUMPTIONS OF MOLECULAR GENETICS

For much of this century, human behavior has been explained by its relationship to social environment, that is, in accordance with its "social construction." Thus, it is understood that the relative absence of Black, Hispanic, and Asian females in the hard sciences or among construction workers is not a question of inherited predisposition; rather, dominant culture has created "stereotypes" that preclude and exclude these members of society from such vocational opportunities. Social scientists today, as Francis Fukuyama notes, are still in thrall to the notion that one's identity and behavior are socially constructed.[10] By way of example, what passes as contemporary "multiculturalism" is largely premised on modern anthropology's fascination with and celebration of non-Western cultural practice and "diversity."[11]

Curiously parallel to the entrenchment of the "social construction" model has been the accumulation of biogenetic evidence suggesting that human identity and behavior are less socially constructed or manipulated than social theorists have led us to believe. Molecular biologists, through their mapping, classification, and analysis of the human genome, posit an entirely different model for understanding human behavior.[12]

Like medical research in general, medical genetics operates on the principles employed in the natural sciences. Modern science will seek to objectify reality, quantify what is observed, establish causal relationships among those things observed, and formulate corresponding models.[13] This methodology—the methodology of abstraction—can be observed to undergird scientific investigation of the organization and structure of human hereditary information. Given the fact, not always expressly or tacitly conceded, that science and technology issue out of a particular paradigm (i.e., a certain way of viewing life and the universe), crucial questions are raised. On a presuppositional level, what is the implicit, and possibly hidden, philosophical nature of these new developments?[14] What worldview is being presupposed? Correlatively, what are the implications of these assumptions for ethics? What significant ethical dilemmas are thereby posed?

According to the central dogma of molecular genetics, hereditary information is stored in DNA, transcribed into RNA, and then translated into specific proteins that specify human traits and characteristics.[15] The flow of genetic information is understood to occur in one direction—from DNA via RNA and proteins to individual traits. *The gene is thus defined as the unit of heredity*. This governing model for genetic research suggests, at the very least, a deterministic view of human identity and human behavior.[16] One scientist expresses what for many behavioral theorists is axiomatic, namely that "the assumption that most human behavior is adaptive in neo-Darwinian terms of inclusive fitness . . . has yet to be falsified."[17] Critics of an evolutionary explanation for human behavior point out two problems in the new biology: the shaky philosophical ground on which some science is proceeding and a public eager for simple explanations that absolve people of responsibility for their actions.

The reductionistic and deterministic character of presuppositions that undergird genetic research invites scrutiny. Very much needed is a critique that is applied, on a broader level, to the scientific model of abstraction governing molecular investigation and, on a narrower level, to the central dogma of molecular genetics itself, by which particular traits are understood to be a fixed identity.[18] Both the general methodology and the genetic formula impersonalize, indeed, depersonalize an individual creature for the purposes of investigation. The consequence is that only what can be observed sensorily is taken into consideration.

It is disturbing to consider the implications of potential biogenetic "discoveries." If the discovery of genes or gene groups correlates not merely with acknowledged disease conditions but also with normal personality traits such as shyness, impulsiveness,[19] or aggressiveness, it is not difficult to extrapolate how overzealous or impatient behavioral theorists and criminologists might utilize these findings.[20] Erik Parens cautions against the mistaken theoretical moves common both to genetic researchers and those who interpret such research:

> When speaking about the contribution that genetics can make toward understanding . . . complex behaviors, it is enormously important to remember that genes are but one component of fabulously complex biological, and ultimately biopsychosocial, systems. Even if there are strong correlations between single-gene defects and certain dispositions to some complex behaviors, such correlations will never provide anything approximating a full account of those behaviors. . . . And as genetics always will be only one important part of biology, biology always will be only one important part of any richer human behavior.[21]

The fundamental tendency to conceptualize human existence in terms of a division between body and soul (or mind) can be traced both to Cartesian and Kantian assumptions. For Kant, the realm of the natural or phenomenal (the physical) was to be understood as distinct from the noumenal (the soul). This basic dichotomy is implicit in most discussions of genetics and human behavior.

Inasmuch as the starting point of modern science tends toward reductionism and determinism, late twentieth-century approaches to genetic-scientific research are utilitarian and instrumental in nature. Questions such as the origin and meaning of life, which are eminently philosophical and theological issues, are transmuted into questions of functionality and material cause and, tragically, economics.

A further danger lies in the potential wedding of biomedical technology to political power. In an important book recently translated into English, French political and moral philosopher Michele Schooyans warns against the markedly undemocratic character of the considerable achievements in the fields of reproductive technology and biomedical science. In *Maitrise de la vie—domination des hommes*,[22] Schooyans cautions that the ambiguous relationship existing between science and political power—what he calls "biopolitics"—does not bode well for Western democracy. Our present recourse to scientific and biomedical techniques, undergirded by our corresponding recourse to political power in ethical matters, has the effect of nurturing a de facto control over both the quality and the existence of human life.

On a biotechnical level, this recourse both to politics and ethics-by-committee in the end prevents the application of universally binding moral principles. Laws that define the parameters within which acceptable biotechnological and genetic research are to proceed reflect the goals and preferences of particular social as well as economic interest groups. Propelling any discussion of ethical matters that may surface is, at best, a firmly ensconced relativism. When moral governance proceeds by ethical committees, as is generally the case in scientific research, all that is needed is a consensus. Who and what shapes this consensus is of critical importance. The twentieth century alone suggests that consensus is frequently molded by strictly utilitarian interests—interests that are wedded to the exigencies of the political moment.

In a society governed by consensus, everything becomes negotiable—from abortion and fetal-tissue research to mechanical procreation and eugenics to euthanasia. All forms of bioethical discrimination and manipulation can be justified, not merely *for the sake* of quality of life but *against* life itself.

The reticence among scientists, academicians, and politicians to identify transcendent and definitive moral markers in biogenetic research parallels another social phenomenon pandemic to Western democracy (i.e., a breakdown in social morality reflected in the ascendency of deviant behavior and criminal violence). Increasingly, behavioral scientists have a stake in both biogenetics and criminal justice. Both spheres are characterized by calls for biology to supply "solutions" to social need. While the relationship between biology and free will in the laboratory may seem relatively innocuous (or even nonexistent), in the streets and neighborhoods and in the prisons of our land the interpretation of this relationship is far from academic.

## GENES, BIOGENETICS, AND CRIMINAL JUSTICE

With a growing number of pundits and politicians citing crime as the political issue of the 1990s, it is guaranteed a preeminent place in our national discourse as we move toward the third millennium. Thoughtful social commentators such as James Q. Wilson,[23] John J. DiIulio Jr.,[24] and D. D. Polsby[25] join other cultural critics in warning that American society, within the next fifteen years, is headed for a deluge of violent crime perpetrated by young predatory males, the likes of which this culture has not known.[26] The prognosis of DiIulio is rather bleak: "[W]hat is really frightening everyone from D.A.s to demographers, old cops to old convicts, is not what's happening now but what's just around the corner—namely, a sharp increase in the number of super-prone young males."[27]

As American society becomes increasingly violent and loses its patience with the criminal justice system in its present form, behavioral scientists are coming to a consensus that deviant behavior has a biological explanation. We are currently witnessing what historian Christopher Dawson with prophetic insight observed thirty-five years ago. In a small but important volume titled, *Progress and Religion,* Dawson wrote tellingly about the contradiction of the secular mind-set. Dawson noted that the most enthusiastic supporters of the doctrine of human progress in Western culture have been the very people who are most impatient with the purported injustices of existing social institutions.[28]

At the end of the twentieth century, this insight is finding validation in unsettling ways. Charting trends in behavioral science, Wayt Gibbs reports in the March 1995 issue of *Scientific American* on the optimism among a growing number of social theorists that science will identify markers of maleficence which, in ten years, could revolutionize our criminal justice system. One of those interviewed, psychologist and author Adriane Raine, believes that after seventeen years of biological research on crime that the following scenario could be with us in the near future. Given the breadth and accuracy of available statistical measurements, we will be able to predict with 80 percent certainty that someone's son will become seriously violent within twenty years. Therefore, as a society, we are under obligation to offer a series of biological, social, and cognitive intervention programs on his behalf.[29]

Does Raine represent an isolated minority in holding this view? Stuart Yodofsky, chairman of the psychiatry department at Baylor College of Medicine, is one of those who welcomes this development: "[W]e're going to be able to diagnose many people who are biologically brain-prone to violence."[30] Yodofsky worries less about the dangers intrinsic to prediction models than he is encouraged by the opportunities for prevention.

While a growing chorus of behavioral scientists contends that American society should trade its traditional system of criminal justice based on guilt and punishment for a "medical model" based on prevention, diagnosis, and treatment, there are some who have grave reservations. Ronald Akers, director of the Center for Studies in Criminology and Law at the University of Florida, points out the danger in this approach to social pathologies. Out of desperation, Akers warns that we can readily succumb to the temptation of premature or inappropriate use of knowledge. Such a precedent is found in the eugenics movement of the 1930s, when criminality and mental illness were considered to be inherited. By 1931, Akers points out, twenty-seven states had passed laws allowing compulsory sterilization of the feebleminded and the habitually criminal (see Edward J. Larson's chapter in this volume).[31]

In his 1993 book, *The Psychopathology of Crime*, Raines states that "a future generation *will* reconceptualize nontrivial recidivistic [repeated] crime as a 'disorder.'"[32] A frightening eventuality presents itself: When the "disease" reaches a socially intolerable level, will "treatment" become compulsory even for those who are innocent? Florida State University's Ray Jeffery, one of several criminologists interviewed by *Scientific American*, is indicative of many who are looking to psychiatrists, neurologists, and geneticists to provide answers to nagging questions, ready or not: "Science must tell us what individuals will or will not become criminals . . . and what law enforcement strategies will or will not work."[33]

Untangling the mystery of the genetic code creates for many scientists a "moral imperative" to use that knowledge; to ignore it would be indefensible. Yet to replace the justice in criminal justice with forced biomedical therapy based on the evaluations of scientific experts surely is to invite greater, indeed, catastrophic injustices. If science is being pressed to provide sociological and biological answers to pathological behavior, whence will come the necessary moral constraints that hold bad science in check? And if a consensus regarding crime in the public mind is not molded by a view that sees human beings personally responsible for their actions, what prevents the reign of social anarchy?

Given the sobering demographic realities of the present and future crime problem, it is not premature to be thinking about responses to the tide of violence that lies directly ahead. On a theoretical level, are we indeed willing to accept the conclusion that science "must tell us what individuals will or will not become criminals . . . and what law enforcement strategies will or will not work"? Is biology in fact destiny? Are individuals genetically predisposed to crime and deviant behavior?[34]

## FREE WILL IN THE HISTORIC CHRISTIAN TRADITION

When Richard Berendzen, former president of American University, resigned his post in 1991 in an uproar after having admitted to making obscene phone calls from his presidential office, a physician by the name of Kenneth M. Grundfast argued subsequently in the *Washington Post* that Berendzen deserved public sympathy. The reason, according to Grundfast? Berendzen was the victim of "an obsessive-compulsive disorder," which was frequently "caused more by abnormal DNA sequences within an individual's chromosomes than by the moral lapses commonly described as wickedness, hostility or turpitude."[35] In breathtaking fashion, Grundfast shifted the locus of scrutiny with these words: "I feel that the tragedy does not lie in what the man did or is accused of doing. Rather the tragedy is ours more than his. We may be the weak and misguided, not Berendzen."[36]

Following his death sentence by a Georgia jury in connection with the murder of a Domino's Pizza store manager, Stephen Mobley had tattooed on his back the word *Domino* and hung a pizza box on the wall of his prison cell. At the same time that Mobley was celebrating in prison, his lawyers set in motion an appeal of his case to the state supreme court, submitting a controversial defense that argued that Mobley's genes may have predisposed him to commit crimes.[37]

Roughly concurrent with the Mobley case, a team of five scientists at Harvard Medical School, led by neuroscientist Xandra Breakefield, released a study that purported to have identified a genetic mutation in a middle-class family prone to violence. According to Breakefield, a female member of the family had approached one of the researchers out of concern about incidents of aggression, arson, attempted rape, and exhibitionism occurring among her male relatives.[38]

Are cases such as the aforementioned an aberration? What do they suggest, both in legal culture and in civil society? And what might they portend, both in legal culture and in civil society? What concerns not a few social critics is that advances in genetic research, coupled with the disturbing trend of therapeutic society to deny moral agency, will have the effect of creating a social environment that denies that people act of their own volition. When behavioral deviancy has reached pandemic proportions, will our society respond therapeutically by defining away the moral disease, on the one hand,[39] and biologically by negating free will, on the other?

The Judeo-Christian tradition, by means of natural law in accordance with reason and revealed truth in concert with informed faith, historically has affirmed what pre-Christian philosophers in the main had concluded, i.e., human moral freedom and the capacity to manifest virtue or vice.[40] Socratic as well as Christian moral philosophers since have stressed the freedom to choose and to be held accountable for the moral consequences of one's action. *Only late in the twentieth century has the notion entered civilization that people are not responsible for their own behavior.*[41]

Both pre-Christian and Christian philosophical traditions hold the relationship of natural law to freedom, reason, and conscience to be one of harmony. In accordance with biblical revelation, writings of the church fathers attest to the human capacity for free choice. Irenaeus is representative of patristic thought:

> God made man free from the beginning, so that he possessed his own power just as his own soul . . . to follow God's will freely, not being compelled by God. For with God, there is no coercion, but a good will is present with him always. He, therefore, gives good counsel to all. In man as well as in angels—for angels are rational—he has placed a power of choice, so that those who obeyed might justly possess the good things which, indeed, God gives but which they themselves must preserve.[42]

Thomas Aquinas further expounds the essence and implications of natural law and moral freedom. In Thomistic thought, natural law, like every law, is ordered by reason, yet it is a law interior to humans. As a law, it refracts into five natural inclinations: a desire for the good, the instinct of preservation, procreation and the rearing of children, seeking the truth, and cultivation of the social life.[43] As a shadow of divine law, natural law serves as a foundation for civil law.[44] Thomas defines justice in eminently moral terms: It is the virtue that is a constant and firm resolve to render what is due to all humans.[45]

In the important encyclical of John Paul II, *Veritatis Splendor,* released in 1994, the essential link between freedom and truth is confirmed and accented. This link, elucidated by reason, allows human beings to discern between good and evil both for ourselves and for others.[46] In confirming the classical Christian tradition expressed by Thomist exegesis, *Vertatis Splendor* locates the natural human inclinations in the realm of the spiritual and not the biological order, yet at the same time insists, in full accord with the classical Christian philosophical tradition, on the profound unity of body and soul—of the material and immaterial—in a "unified totality" of the human person. It is not permissible to "dissociate the moral act from the bodily dimensions of its exercise;"[47] biological and moral planes are indivisible.

Thus understood through the lens of the Christian moral-philosophical tradition, natural law is an emanation of the eternal divine law, taking on a special mode in human beings via reason, which renders the human capable of self-direction and free action. Accomplishing what is good and virtuous is *the product of discernment through reason and conscience*, thereby qualifying humans as moral agents. The flip side of the capacity for free choice, as Renee Mirkes has pointed out, is personal responsibility for the moral character of what one freely chooses. Historically, the Christian church has taught that when an action is *freely undertaken*, i.e., when it is performed with no coercion from within or without as well as with *sufficient* knowledge (which is to say, the person has reflected on and understands the moral quality of what he or she is choosing), the agent is accountable for the good or evil that is generated as a result of the act.[48]

To view human behavior in accordance with our inherited moral-philosophical tradition—tradition extending over two millennia—is to reject a view of human nature as purely biological raw material subject to the procedures of science and technology, by which the body is understood as a mechanism divorced from reason and freedom. Judeo-Christian anthropology acknowledges the primacy of the person as a moral subject, created in the image of God and ordered by God. This understanding reestablishes the preeminence of ethics over technology.[49]

## CONCLUDING REFLECTIONS ON BEING MORAL CREATURES

While a biophysical and biochemical relationship can be said to exist between particular sequences of DNA and the structure of particular proteins, the precise relationship between specific proteins, the expression of particular traits of an organism, and an explanation of *how* this occurs remain a mystery. Genetic information can be described as an essential *precondition* for biological life. This information, however, neither describes nor determines the life of the organism as a whole.[50] Whereas biophysics and biochemistry constitute the level of molecular interaction, they do not explain the identity of a moral subject on the level of consciousness, which is dependent, for example, on the presence and activity of the central nervous system. Nor do they account for the mental, social, and spiritual development of human beings that are foundational to human identity.[51] Questions that belong to the domain of science must be distinguished from those that do not or cannot. In this regard, whether applied to social-scientific or biomedical disciplines, the authority of science must be constantly scrutinized; scientific imperialism has gone largely unquestioned.[52]

The relationship between biology and free will, particularly in the last century, has been an ongoing focus of study by behavioral scientists, philosophers, and ethicists. With the breakdown of civil norms in common culture, the question of this relationship takes on new urgency. Given society's relative helplessness in dealing with deviant and violent behavior through the criminal justice system in its present form, requests for biological solutions will be taken much more seriously as we head toward the twenty-first century. As a result, genetic research will be endowed with new authority to assist us in dealing with our social pathologies and in responding to our social need of public safety.

From the point at which society denies the role of free will and moral agency, there is only one path, and that is a descent into cultural barbarity.[53] That descent, however, is not inevitable. The cultivation (or absence) of a moral consensus in society fundamentally depends on two criteria: (1) the correspondence of moral theory and practice to reality, and (2) the integrity and resilience of those advocating such moral theory.

Presupposed in all moral theory and ethical practice is a particular view of human nature. Nowhere are the implications of one's anthropology more critical than in the realm of bioethics, for anthropological assumptions will inform ethical responses to the questions of the origin of life, the unity and totality of human existence, human suffering, and death. It is here that a biblically informed anthropology—one that posits human creation in the *imago Dei*, a divinely ordered structure in this creation, and a moral universe in which humans function in community—must be brought to bear.[54]

It is useful to compare the time-tested assumptions of our inherited moral-philosophical tradition with the sort of moral reasoning—or, shall we say, moral madness—exhibited by Mr. Grundfast as well as American University itself. In the aftermath of his resignation, Richard Berendzen was to receive a $1 million settlement from the school, authorized by the board of trustees, for giving up his tenure as a professor (his salary, which reflected both administrative and teaching duties, had been $140,000). Following an uproar among both faculty and students, however, the settlement was rescinded by the board.[55] Subsequent to his resignation, it should be noted, Berendzen continued to draw his $140,000 salary. In December of 1991, not quite two years after the episode, Berendzen was in a reflective mood: "1990 was for me just hell. But 1991 has been very restorative, healing—quite an exceptional year."[56] (Adding to this sordid state of moral affairs, Berendzen was invited to appear on ABC's *Nightline*, where before a nationwide audience he recounted the abuse of his childhood, opting for the "social construction" alibi rather than genetic predisposition.[57] According to his testimony, the abuse, inflicted by "a woman very close to me," started when he was eight.[58] Asked by Ted Koppel why, during the two years of obscene phone calls, he never reached out for help, Berendzen replied that a Ph.D. who was a university president should not have needed help.)

But let us consider the advice of Kenneth Grundfast, the key player in the American University fiasco. Assessing the role of biology in the initiation of obscene phone calls, the good doctor writes: "Stress plays a role in causing individuals with a genetic predisposition to actually behave abnormally. When a certain stress level is reached, then some biological and molecular systems that control behavior break down, and people can be forced to do things that they ordinarily would not want to do."[59] Note the backbone of the doctor's argument: Genetic predisposition not only causes us to act, it does so *against our wills*. On this level, Grundfast wishes to instruct us.[60]

But this is not all. Grundfast intends to exonerate the university president—and in this exoneration *we all* are exonerated from the consequences of the evil that we perpetrate. Consider his twisted line of thinking.

I feel that the tragedy does not lie in what the man did or is accused of doing. Rather the tragedy is ours more than his. We may be the weak and misguided, not Berendzen. . . . Whatever phone calls he might have made and whatever he might have said over the phone appear to be actions motivated from a compulsion. Recent research on obsessive-compulsive disorders is revealing that genetic factors and biochemical imbalances can predispose certain individuals to behave in abnormal ways.[61]

Chances are quite high that the reader of the above citation who is allergic to biomedical nonsense might be experiencing a violent reaction to Grundfast's explanation. And rightly so.

Columnist Charles Krauthammer, trained as a psychiatrist, poignantly summarizes how this genetic exculpation, rooted in moral promiscuity, works.

Not very long ago, when someone did something awful, a loud liberal chorus would explain that because of childhood deprivation, poverty or racism, the criminal was not truly responsible for his actions. Society—a sick society— made him do it. This environmental exculpation, popular in the guilt-ridden '60s and '70s, is now in decline. We have now a new model of exoneration, shiny, scientific and designed for the guilt-free '80s and '90s: Nature made me do it. The beauty of this excuse is that it is adaptable to middle-class malefactors whose white-collar crimes cannot be blamed on a wretched environment. They are blamed instead on disease. . . . By this logic, when a pedophile rapes a child, it is the disease raping. The rapist, like the child, is a victim. It takes little effort to relate almost any punishable misbehavior to some . . . syndrome.[62]

Because there exist genetic tendencies toward aggressive responses, we do not, at least yet, let a serial killer off the hook on the grounds that he was dealt a bad hand genetically or that he had an unfortunate childhood. The day, however, when murderers and pedophiles are exonerated may not be that far removed, given their excellent chances (presently) of a reduced sentence, parole, and return to society. The opposition between determinism and responsibility raises the issue of justice, and justice in its essence requires that people be held responsible for their behavior—responsible, that is, if human behavior is at all predictable. If it is unpredictable and unaffected by what behavioral theorists call "reinforcement contingencies," there is no point to punishment or *any other form of behavioral control*, since it would have no predictable effect.[63]

In the end, the unwillingness to hold ourselves morally accountable for our actions can take on countless forms. That unwillingness may express itself through social construction, which has been extraordinarily effective in the hands of social scientists, and it may express itself through an opposite extreme that contends that biology is destiny. Either way, the chief motivation is to obfuscate, becloud, and deny any sort of moral intuition with which humans are born; such can be achieved by ideological, political, or economic means.

Today I can claim, with the backing of science, that "society made me do it." Tomorrow a new vista offering new potentialities spreads itself before me, anointing the claim that "my genes made me do it" and bolstering my case with stubborn biological evidence. Who will prevent me from relinquishing my moral autonomy?

## ENDNOTES

1. The received wisdom of the behavioral sciences concerning the importance of nature (genetics) and nurture (environment) in explaining human behavior has changed dramatically in the last two decades. In 1992, for example, the American Psychological Association identified genetics as one of several themes best representing the present and future of psychology. See R. Plomin et al., eds., *Nature, Nurture, and Psychology* (Washington, D.C.: American Psychological Association, 1993).
2. Only several years ago, scientists would spend weeks searching the library for gene sequence and protein information. Thanks to the Internet, however, scientists presently can access innumerable databases of technical information on the structure, sequence, and function of genes and proteins. See, e.g., M. Hendricks, "Presto! Genetic Sequencing Information at Your Fingertips," *Johns Hopkins Magazine* (September 1994): 33; and I. Peterson, "NSF Funds New Computing Partnerships," *Science News* 151 (April 1997): 204. On new quantitative and molecular genetic techniques as they contribute to behavior correlation, see R. Plomin et al., "The Genetic Basis of Complex Human Behaviors," *Science* 264 (June 1994): 1733–39.
3. Thus, for example, D. Nelkin and M. S. Lindee, *The DNA Mystique: The Gene as a Cultural Icon* (New York: W. H. Freeman and Co., 1995); and J. Reid, "The DNA-ing of America," *Utne Reader* (September–October 1995): 26–28.
4. Reid, "DNA-ing," 26.
5. Gregory Benford, "Biology 2001: Understanding Culture, Technology, and Politics in 'The Biological Century,'" *Reason* (November 1995): 23.
6. See n. 3.
7. E. F. Keller, *Refiguring Life: Metaphors of Twentieth Century Biology* (New York: Columbia University Press, 1995).
8. This is forcefully argued by Keller, *Refiguring Life* (see n. 7).
9. Renee Mirkes, "Programmed by Our Genes?" *Ethics and Medics* 16, no. 6 (1991): 1.
10. See the critique of twentieth-century social-scientific and biological-scientific assumptions contained in Francis Fukuyama, "Is It All in the Genes?" *Commentary* (September 1997): 30–35 (esp. 30–32).
11. This premise is conveniently applied to issues of gender and sexuality, to which proponents of "multiculturalism" inevitably graduate.
12. Roger Masters, director of an annual seminar at Dartmouth College on biological perspectives in the social sciences, notes that most university departments of social science have few members who are aware of research in the life sciences. In 1993, that gap prompted the Gruter Institute for Law and Behavioral Research in Portola Valley, California, and Dartmouth's Nelson Rockefeller Center for the Social Sciences to begin cosponsoring annual seminars to bring together the two disciplines. On the emerging conversations between social scientists and evolutionary biologists, see K. A. McDonald,

"Biology and Behavior," *Chronicle of Higher Education* (September 1994): A19–21.

13. U. Eibach, *Gentechnick—Der Griff nach dem Leben* (Wuppertal: Brockhaus Verlag, 1986), 54; and H. Jochemsen, "Medical Genetics: Its Presuppositions, Possibilities and Problems," *Ethics and Medics* 8, no. 2 (1992): 18.

14. For a frank discussion of the role of philosophical assumptions in the biotechnological field, see H. Jochemsen, "Medical Genetics," 18–31. A similar critique has been applied to broader scientific (and academic) culture by P. E. Johnson, *Reason in the Balance: The Case Against Naturalism in Science, Law, and Education* (Downers Grove: InterVarsity, 1995), but not without considerable backlash.

15. See V. A. McKusick, "Mapping and Sequencing the Human Genome," *New England Journal of Medicine* 320 (1989): 910–15; also, D. Suzuki and P. Knudtson, "Maps and Dreams: Deciphering the Human Genome," in *Genethics: The Clash Between the New Genetics and Human Values* (Cambridge: Harvard University Press, 1989), 316–40.

16. Such is implicit in the statement of G. J. V. Nossal in the introduction to the volume *Human Genetic Information: Science, Law, and Ethics* (Ciba Foundation Symposium; Chichester: Wiley, 1990), 2: "DNA is iconic for the new biology, a biology that seeks to explain phenomena not . . . at the level of the whole organism . . . but at the level of the cell, of the individual protein molecule with its near-magical powers as molecular machine. . . ."

17. M. Dickeman, "Human Sociobiology: The First Decade," *New Scientist* 1477 (1985): 42.

18. Worthy of note is the assessment offered by L. Foss, "The Challenge to Biomedicine: A Foundation Perspective," *Journal of Medicine and Philosophy* 14 (1989): 165–91; and H. Jochemsen, "Medical Genetics," 18–31. Jochemsen is director of the G. A. Lindeboom Instituut, a center for the study of medical ethics in the Netherlands.

19. Consider the effects on parenting and governing society of a discovery that would identify genetic roots of an inability to defer gratification.

20. For examples of exploration into this sort of correlation, see R. D. Masters and M. T. McGuire, eds., *The Neurotransmitter Revolution: Serotonin, Social Behavior, and the Law* (Carbondale/Edwardsville: Southern Illinois University Press, 1994); and Plomin et al., "The Genetic Basis," 1733–39.

21. E. Parens, "Taking Behavioral Genetics Seriously," *Hastings Center Report* (July–August 1996): 13.

22. Michele Schooyans, *Maitrise de la vie—domination des hommes*, trans. J. H. Miller (St. Louis: Catholic Central Verein of America, 1996).

23. James Wilson is James Collins Professor of Management and Public Policy at UCLA. His books include *Thinking About Crime*, rev. ed. (New York: Vintage Books, 1985); with R. J. Herrnstein, *Crime and Human Nature* (New York: Simon & Schuster, 1985); *On Character* (Washington, D.C.: American Enterprise Institute Press, 1991); and *The Moral Sense* (New York/Toronto: Free Press/Maxwell Macmillan, 1993).

24. John DiIulio is professor of politics and public affairs at Princeton University, director of the Brookings Institution Center for Public Management, an adjunct fellow at the Manhattan Institute, and codirector of issues research for the Foundation for the American Family. His books include *No Escape: The Future of American Corrections* (New York: Basic Books, 1991); *Rethinking the Criminal*

*Justice System: Toward a New Paradigm* (Washington, D.C.: U.S. Department of Justice/Bureau of Justice Statistics, 1992); *Performance Measures for the Criminal Justice System* (Washington, D.C.: U.S. Department of Justice/Bureau of Justice Statistics, 1993); and *Deregulating the Public Service: Can Government Be Improved?* (Washington, D.C.: Brookings Institution, 1994).

25. D. Polsby is the Kirkland and Ellis Professor of Law at Northwestern University and an affiliated scholar at the Heartland Institute, a nonprofit public-policy institute in Chicago.

26. See, e.g., J. J. DiIulio Jr., "The Coming of the Super-Predators," *The Weekly Standard* (27 November 1995): 23–28. This forecast transcends political labels of "liberal" and "conservative." At the opposite end of the spectrum from Wilson and DiIulio, politically and ideologically speaking, is James Alan Fox, dean of the College of Criminal Justice at Northwestern University. Fox's studies of homicide lead him to conclude that the United States is headed for a crime wave: "Hidden beneath the overall drop in crime is this tremendous surge in youth crime." The surge predicted by Fox can be seen in the murder rate among fourteen to seventeen year olds. Between 1985 and 1994, the rate escalated from 7 to 19.1 per 100,000. Presently, ca. 40 million people of the baby-boom generation are under the age of ten. In the next decade this "baby boomerang," as Fox calls it, will enter the most crime-prone years. Barring any sort of miraculous interference, the next crime wave, in Fox's opinion, "will get so bad that it will make 1995 look like the good old days." See P. Yam, "Catching a Coming Crime Wave," *Scientific American* (June 1996): 40–44.

27. DiIulio, "Super-Predators," 24. To the degree that DiIulio's prediction is grim, his understanding of the root cause is clear and supported both by the best social science and common sense. DiIulio cites "abject moral poverty" as the prime contributing factor (pp. 25–26).

28. James Q. Wilson's *The Moral Sense* set off a veritable firestorm of reaction among criminologists, social scientists, and behavioral theorists following its publication in 1993, though not because of a failure to interact with interpretative paradigms in philosophy, biology, and social science—indeed the book is an ambitious synthesis of philosophical, biological, and social-scientific insight. Rather, its assumptions about moral philosophy appear to have been the cause of most controversy. Wilson takes the position that moral judgments begin with intuitions about what one ought to do (hence "*the* moral sense," as the title has it). This implies what for most philosophers and scientists amounts to a scandal, i.e., that it is possible to arrive at a valid moral judgment about any given act.

   Social-scientific reaction to Wilson's book is exemplified by the summer/ fall issue of the journal *Criminal Justice Ethics*, which is devoted to a very spirited symposium on *The Moral Sense*. Invited to respond were three philosophers, three anthropologists, two political scientists, a psychologist, and a criminologist. The tone of the responses is indicative of how various social- and behavioral-scientific disciplines tend to react to the notion of a posited normative standard of morality. Ironically, it is the criminologist who dissents most strongly from Wilson's thesis of a "moral intuition." Sensing in Wilson a sympathetic note toward religious commitments in undergirding moral intuition, the criminologist trots out past missionary atrocities on indigenous peoples—the "hammer" in any skeptical anthropologist's toolbox. And waxing critical of Wilson's unsympathetic critique of ritual cannibalism in some cultures, he observes that the consumption of human flesh also can be "a physical channel for communicating social value," since it "ties together one generation to the other by virtue of sharing certain substances." In the end, he laments, "Christianity spoils our feasts." Indeed, the criminologist's entire critique of Wilson is drenched in a biting sarcasm reminiscent of the comedian Don Rickles.

29. W. W. Gibbs, "Seeking the Criminal Element," *Scientific American* (March 1995): 101.
30. Ibid.
31. Ibid.
32. A. Raines, *The Pyschopathology of Crime: Criminal Behavior as a Clinical Disorder* (San Diego: Academic Press, 1993), 319. Chapter 12 of this volume poses the central question in its title: "Is Crime a Disorder?" to which an affirmative answer is given, based on sociobiological and psychosocial factors (see the author's conclusions as stated on pp. 318–19).
33. Gibbs, "Criminal Element," 104. Impatience with the criminal justice system leads criminologist Jeffery to call for the integration of law and biology in the future. In his contribution to the volume *The Neurotransmitter Revolution* (see n. 20), Jeffery writes: "We must shift the emphasis from punishment to treatment and prevention. Crime prevention must replace the police-courts-prison system" (p. 174).
34. In mid-1993, researchers in the Netherlands reported discovering what they believed to be a gene for aggression. Similarly, in their book *Altered Fates: Gene Therapy and the Retooling of Human Life* (New York: W. W. Norton, 1995), researchers Jeff Lyon and Peter Gorner seek to establish genetic patterns in the occurrence of alcoholism, divorce, and other social ills in their study of twins.
35. K. M. Grundfast, "Bring Back Berendzen," *Washington Post* (4 May 1990), A27. Berendzen is one of countless examples in a hit parade of extraordinary "victims" critiqued in an essay by John Taylor that is at once supremely entertaining and sobering. See J. Taylor, "Don't Blame Me! The New Culture of Victimhood," *New York* (3 June 1991), 27–34.
36. Grundfast, "Bring Back," A27. Consider Grundfast's choice of words in his Berendzen *apologia*—"the president of the university *allegedly* has made obscene phone calls" (emphasis mine). This sort of duplicity is advanced in spite of the fact that Berendzen pleaded guilty to charges and offered "anguished" accounts of how he felt after having made pornographic phone calls to a Fairfax County (Virginia) woman who ran a day-care service. (Police had traced the calls to the university president's office. Berendzen entered the sexual disorders clinic at Johns Hopkins University in Baltimore and later pleaded guilty to two misdemeanor counts. He received two thirty-day prison sentences, which were suspended on the condition that he remain in outpatient psychological treatment.) At the time of his op-ed piece in the *Post*, Grundfast was chairman of the Department of Otolaryngology at Children's Hospital and studying molecular biology at the National Institutes of Health.
37. E. Felsenthal, "Man's Genes Made Him Kill, His Lawyers Claim," *Wall Street Journal* (15 November 1994), B1.
38. Reported in Ibid., B1.
39. This sort of moral leveling has been variously described by Daniel P. Moynihan, in his much-acclaimed essay, "Defining Deviancy Down," *The American Scholar* (winter 1993), 17–30, who writes: "I proffer the thesis that, over the past generation, . . . the amount of deviant behavior in American society has increased beyond the levels the community can 'afford to recognize' and that, accordingly,

we have been re-defining deviancy so as to exempt much conduct previously stigmatized, and also quietly raising the 'normal' level in categories where behavior is now abnormal by any earlier standard" (p. 19). Columnist Charles Krauthammer, in "Defining Deviancy Up," *The New Republic* (22 November 1993), 20–25, affirms Moynihan's thesis but contends that this is only half the story: "There is a complementary social phenomenon that goes with defining deviancy down. As part of the vast social project of moral leveling, it is not enough for the deviant to be normalized. The normal must be found to be deviant. . . . Large areas of ordinary behavior hitherto considered benign have had their threshold radically redefined up, so that once innocent behavior now stands exposed as the true home of violence and abuse and a whole catalog of aberrant acting and thinking" (p. 20). Date rape, politically incorrect speech, and "thought crimes" are but several examples cited by Krauthammer as part of this upward movement.

40. For helpful reflections on the nature of justice in Christian and pre-Christian philosophical concepts, see T. Rebard, "Justice: Moral Virtue in Society," *Ethics and Medics* (December 1994), 1.

41. Even in ancient cultures where astral configurations were studied for the purposes of guidance and deterministic fate governed people's lives, crimes against humanity were punished, reflecting at minimum a tacit acknowledgment that humans were responsible for their actions in the context of community.

42. *Adv. Her.*, 2.4.4.

43. *Summa Theologica*, 1–2, Q. 90, Art. 108.

44. Ibid.

45. *Summa Theologica*, 2–2, Q. 58, Art. 1.

46. *Veritatis Splendor*, no. 43. For the English text of the encyclical, see *"Veritatis Splendor,"* *Origins* 23, no. 18 (1993): 297–336.

47. Ibid., nos. 48–50.

48. Mirkes, "Programmed," 2.

49. Thus S. Pinckaers, *"Veritatis Splendor:* Human Freedom and the Natural Law," *Ethics and Medics* (February 1995), 3–4.

50. For an informed critique of biomedical assumptions that guide medical genetics, see Jochemsen, "Medical Genetics," 22–24.

51. Moreover, research amply confirms that variances in personality and one's emotional state contribute to the onset of—and healing from—certain diseases.

52. In a thoughtful essay appearing in *The Atlantic Monthly*, John Staddon has pressed this argument as it relates to the study of human behavior and criminal justice. See J. Staddon, "On Responsibility and Punishment," *The Atlantic Monthly* (February 1995), 88–94.

53. Members of the Christian community normally tend to respond to "negative" cultural critique in one of two ways. On the one hand there are those whose prophetic timetables dictate that the church, literally, is shortly to be removed from its earthly venue, and thus, should withdraw from cultural participation. This noninvolvement is often implicit, the fruit of faulty theological assumptions, and not expressly propagated. These individuals generally fail to inculcate among their own the necessity of formulating—and transmitting—a robust, philosophically sound, and biblically faithful worldview. On the other hand, there are also those who, due to a sense of inferiority and the deep-rooted need to be taken seriously by secular culture, uncritically adopt secular assumptions into their view of life and the universe—this frequently with a view

of becoming more "socially relevant." Both of these responses, it should be emphasized, fall short of what the church has historically understood to be its cultural mandate; both require a measure of repentance and turning.

54. On the broader application of biblical anthropology to bioethical matters, see D. A. du Toit, "Anthropology and Bioethics," *Ethics and Medicine* 10, no. 2 (1994): 35–41.

55. Berendzen, in being restored to the faculty two years later, was assigned to teach two sections of Astronomy 220, an elective course for freshmen and sophomores, and Physics 370, an introduction to quantum mechanics required of physics majors.

56. Cited in A. Goldstein, "Berendzen Set to Teach at AU," *The Washington Post* (9 December 1991), C3.

57. May 23, 1990.

58. D. L. Brown, "'I Thought I Had It Under Control,'" *The Washington Post* (24 May 1990), A40.

59. Grundfast, "Bring Back," A27.

60. News accounts of the AU episode were prone to describe Berendzen's problem in terms of an "addiction," as science has been perfectly willing to do. The medicalization of vice, for example, is on display in A. I. Leshner, "Addiction Is a Brain Disease, and It Matters," *Science* 278 (October 1997): 45–47. Leshner, who works with the National Institutes of Health, is upset because "many, perhaps most, people see drug abuse and addiction as social problems" rather than as "brain problems." He concludes: "Understanding addiction as a brain disease explains in part why historic policy strategies focusing solely on the social or criminal justice aspects of drug abuse or addiction have been unsuccessful. . . . If the brain is the core of the problem, attending to the brain needs to be a core part of the solution" (p. 47).

61. Grundfast, "Bring Back," A27.

62. C. Krauthammer, "Illness Made Me Do It? The Excuse Is Criminal," *St. Louis Post-Dispatch* (15 May 1990), 3B.

63. The objective case for personal responsibility, as J. Staddon ("On Responsibility," 93) observes, rests on the beneficial *collective* or *communal* effects of just punishment, which minimize the sum total of human suffering.

*An Overview*

Doug Kenny (Michael Keeton) found himself overworked and tired and in need of rest. He came across a geneticist who offered him a "simple" solution. "Multiply yourself through the cloning process." In the movie, *Multiplicity*, Doug reduplicated his "adult" self three times and the comedy of look-a-likes, each with separate personalities, lived happily ever after. *Jurassic Park* was created to show the horrible consequences of science when its development of technologies goes unchecked. Raymond G. Bohlin separates fact from fiction in this historical and scientific evaluation of where cloning has been and where it is likely to go. The difference between artificial twinning (Stillman and Hall) and cloning is delineated, and the usefulness and "successes" of animal and human cloning are described in the context of their practical and ethical considerations. It is interesting to note that the same ethical argumentation that surrounds the abortion issue also surrounds embryonic cloning: When does human life begin?

Chapter Seventeen

# THE POSSIBILITIES AND ETHICS OF HUMAN CLONING

Raymond G. Bohlin

### A BRIEF HISTORY

To clone a human involves the production of an exact copy of a previously existing individual. This is different from producing identical twins. Identical twins begin as the same fertilized egg. When the cell divides for the first time, instead of the two cells remaining in one embryo, the two cells split apart and begin developing independently. Therefore, since both individuals arose from the same fertilized egg, they share all the same genetic material. This, of course accounts for their sameness in appearance and even in a few behaviors.

But cloning is different. If I were to hire someone to clone me, I would first of all, supply some of my cells (probably white blood cells or skin cells). These cells would probably be grown in culture apart from my body for a while and then several would be selected and the nucleus removed. The nucleus contains all my chromosomes and therefore nearly all of the genes that make me who I am. The nucleus from one of these cells would then be placed in an enucleated egg cell (egg cell with its nucleus removed). Depending on the procedure being used, the egg cell would be treated to cause it to begin dividing as an embryo normally would. If successful, the new embryo would be implanted into a woman so it could develop normally. If successful at this stage, my identical twin would be born around nine months later. This identical twin would have been formed by an entirely different process than normal and would have been born with the same adorable face as me but forty-four years later! While this is not yet feasible, I'm afraid it is not too far away. Recent advances in sheep and cattle cloning make the application to human beings easier than ever.

Cloning from adult cells was long thought to be extremely unlikely if not impossible. The more we learned about cell nuclei, chromosomes, and DNA the less likely cloning appeared to be. The fully differentiated cells of adults perform very limited functions. Outside of some basic functions all cells need to perform, liver cells only produce proteins from DNA to perform liver functions, skin cells for skin functions, bone cells for bone functions, and so forth. Though the cells of adult organisms contain all the DNA necessary to construct a complete organism, *most of this DNA is inactive*. Activating this DNA was the big mystery. Scientists could only guess whether it was even possible.

The first crude attempt to clone animals came in 1952. Researchers Robert Briggs and Thomas King cloned frogs, starting with nuclei from the cells of early blastula embryos.[1] Frogs were used because the large size of their eggs made manipulation easier and because amphibians possess the mysterious ability to regenerate limbs. Researchers reasoned that if amphibians can regenerate entire limbs from just a few cells, perhaps they could be enticed to regenerate a complete organism from just one cell. Ten years later, J. B. Gurdon produced adult frogs from the intestinal cells of tadpoles.[2] Later, in 1975, Gurdon reported only partial success starting with the cells of adult frogs. None of the embryos developed to the tadpole stage, but nuclei from cells of these embryos could be used to produce clones of swimming and advanced tadpoles. No adults could be coaxed from embryos starting with adult cell nuclei. Gurdon, however, did speculate that the inactivation of DNA in adult specialized cells was not irreversible.[3]

About this time, cloning of a different variety was in the news—the cloning of pieces of DNA. Molecular biologists discovered they could create numerous copies of a segment of DNA by manipulating the DNA at the molecular level in bacteria. *Molecular cloning*, though initially halted by a self-imposed voluntary moratorium,[4] has since become a nearly ubiquitous technique in biology labs around the world.

The ability to manipulate and clone DNA, the hereditary material, at the molecular level, together with the somewhat successful attempts to clone frogs, announced the possibility of cloning mammals and eventually humans. Indeed, before much progress had been made in the laboratory toward the first human clone, a work of literary fiction masquerading as historical fact burst on the scene in 1978. David Rorvik's, *In His Image: The Cloning of a Man*,[5] purported to tell the story of the first successful cloning of a human being. In the book, a wealthy industrialist arranged and financed to have himself secretly cloned. Though Rorvik assured his publisher that the story "is true"[6] and claimed that "complete documentation of this accomplishment will be forthcoming,"[7] documentation never came, and his account was not only blasted as a hoax by scientists in the press but also eventually labeled a work of fiction by a United States district judge.[8]

This same year marked the release of the film, *The Boys from Brazil*, based on the best-selling book by Ira Levin.[9] This fictional tale relates how the famous Nazi, Dr. Josef Mengele, attempts to clone Adolf Hitler. Mengele succeeds in cloning ninety-four Adolf Hitlers and attempts to have them all raised in family situations resembling Hitler's to recreate Hitler as accurately as possible. The film contains an excellent scene detailing how human cloning was thought to be achievable at that time. Needless to say, the public's curiosity was peaked. Many truly believed that human cloning was just around the corner.

However, as the years went by, cloning was pushed aside by the advances of in vitro fertilization.[10] Human cloning slipped from the public's consciousness until 1993.

## THE CLONING TECHNOLOGY OF *JURASSIC PARK*

The movie, *Jurassic Park*, released in the summer of 1993, brought cloning technology, once again, to the forefront of public attention. Based on the riveting novel by Michael Crichton, the film left many dazzled by the dinosaurs. Others, however, were left with questions and new views of science and nature.

*Jurassic Park* was intended to warn the general public concerning the inherent dangers of biotechnology, first of all, and also of science in general. Listen to this comment from the author, Michael Crichton: "Biotechnology and genetic engineering are very powerful. The film suggests that [science's] control of nature is elusive. And just as war is too important to leave to the generals, science is too important to leave to scientists. Everyone needs to be attentive."[11] Overall, I would agree with Crichton. All too often, some *scientists purposefully refrain from asking ethical questions concerning their work* in the interest of the pursuit of science.

But now listen to director Steven Spielberg from the pages of the *Wall Street Journal*, "There's a big moral question in this story. DNA cloning may be viable, but is it acceptable?"[12] And again in the *New York Times*, Spielberg said, "Science is intrusive. I wouldn't ban molecular biology altogether, because it's useful in finding cures for AIDS, cancer and other diseases. But it's also dangerous and that's the theme of *Jurassic Park*."[13] So, Spielberg openly states that the real theme of *Jurassic Park* is that science is intrusive.

While I agreed with much of the movie's concern over biotechnology, the movie *Jurassic Park* directly attacked the scientific establishment. Throughout the movie, Ian Malcolm voiced concerns about the direction and nature of science. In one scene, Malcolm says, "Genetic power is the most awesome force the planet's ever seen, but, you wield it like a kid that's found his dad's gun."[14] Genetic engineering rises above nuclear and chemical or computer technology because of its ability to restructure the very molecular heart of living creatures, even to create new organisms. Use of such power requires wisdom and patience. Malcolm punctuated his criticism in the same scene when he said, "Your scientists were so preoccupied with whether or not they could, they didn't stop to think if they should."[15]

These lines should hit a raw nerve in the scientific community. As Christians, we ask similar questions and raise similar concerns when scientists want to harvest fetal tissue for research purposes or experiment with human embryos. *It is the worldview of the culture that determines how computers, biotechnology, or any other technology is to be used.* The problem in *Jurassic Park* was the arrogance of human will and the lack of humility before God, not technology.

## THEY CLONE DINOSAURS, DON'T THEY?

Prior to the release of *Jurassic Park*, magazines and newspapers were filled with speculations concerning the real possibility of cloning dinosaurs. The specter of cloning dinosaurs was left too much in the realm of the eminently possible.

Scientists are very reluctant to use the word *never*. But this issue is as safe as they come. Dinosaurs will never be cloned. The positive votes come mainly from Crichton, Spielberg, and the public. Reflecting back on his early research for the book, Michael Crichton said, "I began to think it really could happen."[16] The official *Jurassic Park* souvenir magazine fueled the speculation when it said, "The story of *Jurassic Park* is not far-fetched. It is based on actual, ongoing genetic and paleontologic research. In the words of Steven Spielberg: 'This is not science fiction; it's science eventuality.'"[17] No doubt spurred on by such grandiose statements, 58 percent of 1,000 people polled for *USA Today* said they believe that scientists will be able to recreate animals through genetic engineering.[18]

Now contrast this optimism with more sobering statements from scientists. The *Dallas Morning News* said, "You're not likely to see *Tyrannosaurus rex* in the Dallas Zoo anytime soon. Scientists say that reconstituting any creature from its DNA simply won't work."[19] And *Newsweek* summarized the huge obstacles when it said:

> Researchers have not found an amber-trapped insect containing dinosaur blood. They have no guarantee that the cells in the blood, and the DNA in the cells, will be preserved intact. They don't know how to splice the DNA into a meaningful blueprint, or fill the gaps with DNA from living creatures. And they don't have an embryo cell to use as a vehicle for cloning.[20]

These are major obstacles. Let's look at them one at a time.

First, *insects in amber*. DNA has been extracted from insects encased in amber from deposits as old as 120 million years.[21] Amber does preserve biological tissues very well. But only very small fragments (~200 base pairs) of a single gene were obtained. The cloning of gene fragments is a far cry from cloning an entire genome (all 100,000 genes nested within $3 \times 10^9$ base pairs). Without the entire intact genome, organized into the proper sequence and divided into chromosomes, it is virtually impossible to reconstruct an organism from gene fragments.

Second, *filling in the gaps*. The genetic engineers of *Jurassic Park* used frog DNA to shore up the missing stretches of the cloned dinosaur DNA. But this is primarily a plot device to allow for the possibility of amphibian environmentally induced sex change. It is also very far-fetched to suppose that an integrated set of genes to perform gender switching, which does occur in some amphibians, could actually be inserted accidentally and be functional.

Third, *a viable dinosaur egg*. The idea of placing the dinosaur genetic material into crocodile or ostrich eggs is preposterous. You would need a real dinosaur egg of the same species as the DNA. Unfortunately, there are no such eggs left, and we can't recreate one without a model to copy. So don't get your hopes up. There will never be a real Jurassic Park!

While the technology involved in the cloning of extinct organisms is significantly different than that of cloning living creatures, people were primed for what came next.

## THE FIRST HUMAN CLONES?

Right on the heels of the release of *Jurassic Park* came reports of human cloning in early October 1993, by researchers Robert Stillman and Jerry Hall from George Washington University. The media reaction was swift and the controversy heated. If nothing else, this announcement raised serious questions about the ethical legitimacy and potential abuses that could result from the cloning of human beings.

In one respect, I sympathize with the scientists involved who naïvely felt their work was nothing unusual but who suddenly found themselves the subjects of *New York Times* and *Time Magazine* cover stories as well as live appearances on *Good Morning America, Nightline,* and *Larry King Live.* The spotlight did not suit them very well. Some aspects of the media hoopla were drastically overplayed, but other concerns are very real.

Stillman and Hall, rather than cloning humans, actually just performed the *first artificial twinning* using human embryos. A similar procedure had been performed in mice successfully for twenty years and in cattle for ten years. Identical twins are produced when a fertilized egg divides for the first time and, instead of remaining as one organism, actually splits into two independent cells. Stillman and Hall were able to achieve this same effect by removing the protective layer around the developing embryo (zona pellucida), splitting the cells apart, and replacing the outer coating with an artificial shell. Where there was once one embryo, there was now two identical one-celled embryos.

It is possible to create as many as eight identical embryos from one single embryo if you simply wait until the embryo reaches the eight-cell stage before teasing the cells apart. The procedure was pursued to assist couples who still had trouble conceiving by in vitro fertilization. Many women are unable to produce multiple eggs. This becomes very expensive when each in vitro attempt can cost from $5,000 to $8,000, or more. Once fertilized, the resulting embryos only implant 10 to 20 percent of the time. If you have two to eight identical embryos, all formed from one original embryo, you can implant one and freeze the rest. If the first implant is unsuccessful, you can thaw one of the frozen twins and try again.

To call this cloning, as the media had done, is a bit misleading. The more usual meaning of cloning an individual, as explained earlier, would be to take a cell from an adult individual, remove the nucleus, and implant it in a fertilized egg that has had its nucleus removed. Strictly speaking, this was not possible with human beings at this time.

## THE ETHICAL DILEMMAS OF ARTIFICIAL TWINNING

Many within the field had recognized, for quite some time, that artificial twinning would be possible with human embryos. But they knew that such experiments would raise a host of ethical concerns that they were unwilling to face. It is unfortunate that Stillman and Hall were so unprepared for the controversy because it reinforces in some people's minds that all scientists are blind to the ethical ramifications of their work. It is clear from interviews that Stillman and Hall care deeply but just didn't think ahead.

Jerry Hall was asked if he feared that his work would create a public backlash toward this kind of research. He said: "I respect people's concerns and feelings. But we have not created human life or destroyed human life in this experiment."[22] What this statement implies is that Hall and Stillman do not consider the embryos they were working with as human life. The embryos used in this research project were doomed from the start because they were fertilized with more than one sperm. The extra genetic material precludes the possibility of normal embryonic development. But does this mean that these embryos are not human?

Many individuals carry a death sentence because of congenital conditions or genetic disease, but they are certainly human. We will all die eventually. The timetable is not important. I believe that these embryos were human beings and further experimentation was performed on them that added an additional risk to their already imperiled condition. Human experimentation was performed without informed consent.

Stillman and Hall defended their work by saying they consider it only a logical extension of in vitro fertilization. These efforts were driven by a desire to relieve human suffering—in this case the suffering of infertile couples. I know of many couples who have battled infertility, and I know that their pain is real and deeply rooted. But I also believe that this is a case where our desire to live in a painless world is clouding our ability to make moral decisions. One woman who had undergone eight unsuccessful in vitro attempts was asked if she would be willing to try artificial twinning. She said: "It's pretty scary, but I would probably consider it as a desperate last attempt."[23] She is clearly frightened by the moral and ethical implications, yet if nothing else worked, she'd do it! Unfortunately, *our decisions are often based more on the tug of our hearts and pocketbooks than on sound ethical principles.*

## WHAT ARE THE POTENTIAL
## ABUSES OF ARTIFICIAL TWINNING?

There are several scenarios that should receive attention. One concerns couples who are known to be at risk for a hereditary disease such as cystic fibrosis. If from a single fertilized egg, two to four identical embryos could be created by the artificial twinning process, then one could be tested for the genetic marker, and the others held in frozen storage. The genetic testing may require the destruction of the initial embryo. If the test is negative, then one of the reserve embryos could be thawed, implanted, and brought to term. If the test confirms the presence of the genetic disease, all embryos could be destroyed. This process is hardly respectful of human life.

Another suggestion is that the artificial twins could be kept frozen as an insurance policy even after the original child is born. If the original child dies at an early age, a frozen twin could be thawed, and you could have the identical child to raise again. Another suggestion has been to keep the frozen twins available in case the original twin needs a bone-marrow transplant or some other organ. The tissues would match perfectly. In 1991, a couple in California has already set a precedent by electing to have another child to provide bone marrow for their older daughter who had contracted leukemia. Fortunately for them, the tissues matched and both children are doing fine.[24] (See Scott Rae's chapter in this book for further detail into this case.)

A final scenario suggests that frozen twins can be kept in reserve as the salable stock for children catalogs. A catalog could be set up offering pictures and descriptions of the original twin and offering prospective parents the opportunity to have the very same child. This may sound foolish to you, but there are many in our society who would be willing to pay for just such a service. If you truly respect human life, then none of these possibilities should make sense.

## WHAT CAN CONSTRAIN SCIENTIFIC RESEARCH?

I have to admit that as a scientist myself, I am wary of giving the public a free voice to approve or disapprove what kinds of research are pursued by qualified scientists. Scientists themselves are usually the best judges of whether a particular project is worth doing on its scientific merits. Only other scientists can judge the worthiness of a research proposal based solely on its ability to contribute significantly to our body of scientific knowledge. In a society deeply rooted in the Judeo-Christian heritage, scientists could be trusted to make the correct moral decisions about their research as well. But this is not the case in our society today. We are a culture that is without a moral compass. One of the consequences of this lack of direction is that many scientists and ethicists believe that scientists should be free to pursue their research goals regardless of what some in society believe the long-term consequences might be.

John Robertson is a professor of law at the University of Texas. In a recent editorial, he said:

> As long as the research is for a valid scientific purpose, embryos that would otherwise be discarded can, with the informed consent of the couple whose eggs and sperm produced the embryos, be ethically used in research. Neither the lack of guidelines, the moral objections of some people to any embryo research, nor the fears about where cloning research might lead justify denying researchers the ability to take the next step.[25]

Essentially professor Robertson has insulated himself from any criticism from outside the scientific community. As long as informed consent can be obtained from the parents, the sole criteria is a valid scientific purpose. Questions concerning the sanctity of human life are not allowed. Questions concerning the potential abuses are not allowed. In other words, scientists exist in some kind of a moral vacuum.

## THE LITTLE LAMB THAT MADE A MONKEY OUT OF US ALL

In 1993, I wrote, "There are so many roadblocks to the successful cloning of an adult human that I don't expect it any time soon. However, I am afraid our current culture will pursue it as long as there is potential profit and a perceived scientific benefit."[26] Like so many others, I was caught totally flat-footed and astonished by the announcement of the successful cloning of an adult sheep, Dolly.

Cloning was thought to be so difficult because as stated earlier, while the genetic material is the same in all cells of an organism (except the reproductive cells, sperm and egg, which have only half the full complement of chromosomes), differentiated cells (liver cells, stomach cells, muscle cells, and so forth) are biochemically programmed in their DNA to perform limited functions, and most of the DNA is turned off. Most scientists felt that the reprogramming was next to impossible based on cloning attempts in frogs and mice.

So what did the scientists in Scotland do that was successful? Well, they took normal mammary cells from an adult ewe and starved them of critical growth nutrients to allow the cells to reach a dormant stage. This process of bringing the cells into dormancy apparently allows the cell's DNA to be deprogrammed. Apparently most, if not all, of the programming for specific functions of the mammary cells were turned off and the DNA made available for reprogramming. The starved mammary cells were then fused with an egg cell that had its nucleus removed and was stimulated to begin cell division by an electric pulse. Proteins already in the egg cell somehow altered the DNA from the mammary cell to be renewed for cell division and embryological functions.[27]

As might be expected, the process was inefficient. Out of 277 cell fusions, twenty-nine began growing as embryos in vitro or in the petri dish. All twenty-nine were implanted into thirteen receptive ewes, only one became pregnant and one lamb was born as a result; a success rate of only 3.4 percent (see Table 13–1). The success rate is even less, .36 percent when you calculate from the 277 initial cell fusions attempted. In nature, somewhere between 33 and 50 percent of all fertilized eggs develop fully into newborns.

**Table 13–1: Dolly**

| PROCEDURE | NUMBER |
|---|---|
| Cell Fusions | 277 |
| Growing Embryos | 29 |
| Ewes Implanted | 13 |
| Pregnancies | 1 |
| Live Births | 1 |

Altogether the procedure was rather nontechnical, and no one is really sure why it worked. The experiments still need to be repeated. Previously, all attempts to clone mice from adult cells have failed.[28] But clearly, an astounding breakthrough has been made. You can be sure that numerous labs around the world will be attempting to repeat these experiments and trying the technique on other mammalian species.

As the weeks and months passed following Dolly's announcement, skepticism began to publicly appear. In January 1998, Vittorio Sgaramella of Italy and Norton D. Zinder published a letter in *Nature*[29] questioning Dolly's authenticity. They believed that the genetic tests performed were not sufficient to establish, beyond doubt, that Dolly was identical to the ewe that donated the mammary gland cells for nuclear transfer. More significantly, they suggested that Dolly may actually have been cloned from a fetal cell. The six-year-old ewe, from which Dolly was allegedly cloned, was pregnant at the time the cells were harvested. Fetal cells are known to circulate in their mother's blood stream which would make it possible for Dolly actually to have been cloned from one of these cells rather than from an adult cell. What looked even more suspicious to Sgaramella and Zinder was the fact that no one had as yet succeeded in cloning another sheep, or anything else for that matter, using the same procedure, although various labs had been successful in cloning sheep and cattle from fetal cells. While Ian Wilmut acknowledged the remote possibility that Sgaramella and Zinder were right,[30] the group from PPL Therapeutics affirmed confidence in the original claim or findings.[31] However, all doubts concerning Dolly's authenticity should be laid to rest by two articles published in the July 23, 1998, issue of *Nature*.[32] Two different genetic analyses were performed (DNA microsatellite analysis and DNA fingerprinting) comparing Dolly, her donor's cells, and other sheep from the same flock. In both tests, Dolly's DNA was significantly different from the other sheep, but identical to her donor's cells. This confirms that Dolly was cloned from an adult somatic cell rather than from a fetal cell as Sgaramella and Zinder have suggested.

## WHY CLONE ANYTHING?

The purpose of these experiments was to find a more effective way to reproduce already genetically engineered sheep for production of pharmaceuticals. Sheep can be genetically engineered to produce a certain human protein or hormone in its milk. The human protein can then be harvested from the milk and sold on the market. This is accomplished by taking the human gene for production of this protein or hormone and inserting it into a sheep embryo. Hopefully the embryo will grow into a sheep that will produce the protein. This is not a certainty, and while the process may improve, it will never be perfect. Mating the engineered sheep is also not foolproof because even mating with another genetically engineered sheep may result in lambs that have lost the inserted human gene and cannot produce the desired protein. Therefore, instead of trusting the somewhat unpredictable and time consuming methods of normal animal husbandry to reproduce this genetic hybrid, cloning more directly assures that the engineered gene product will not be lost. Indeed, on July 24, 1997, the Roslin Institute and PPL Therapeutics, the two institutions that cloned Dolly, announced the birth of five more lambs cloned from fetal cells. These animals, however, actually carry extra genes, some of them human genes, that the researchers introduced into the cells before they were cloned.[33]

There may be other benefits to cloning technology. If further research is able to uncover the biochemical mechanisms of the genetic reprogramming, this could be put to very practical medical use. Reprogramming the nucleus of other cells, such as nerve cells, could lead to procedures to stimulate degenerating nerve cells to be replaced by newly growing nerve cells. Nerve cells in adults do not ordinarily regenerate or reproduce. This could have important implications for those suffering from Parkinson's and Alzheimer's.

If the process can actually be perfected to the extent that production costs are reduced and the quality of the eventual product is improved, then this would be a legitimate research goal. The simplicity of the technique, though still inefficient, makes this possible. But there are still questions that need to be answered.

One critical question is the life span of Dolly. All cells have a built-in senescence, or death, after so many cell divisions. Dolly began with a cell from a ewe that was already six years old. A normal life span for a ewe is eleven years. Will Dolly not live to see her sixth birthday?[34] Actually, most cell divisions are used up during embryological development. Dolly's cells may peter out even earlier. This is critical because a ten-year-old sheep is considered elderly and lambing and wool production decline in sheep after their seventh year.[35] My guess, though, is that since Dolly's genes were reprogrammed from mammary cell functions to embryological functions that the senescence clock was also reset back to the beginning. I expect Dolly to live a normal life span.

It is also uncertain as to whether Dolly will be reproductively fertile.[36] Frogs cloned from tadpole cells are frequently sterile. It is possible that while Dolly is normal anatomically, the cloning process somehow interferes with the proper development of the reproductive cells. If this is the case, there may be other problems not immediately detectable. These problems may arise from the fact that Dolly's genes are from a differentiated cell that may have been perfectly normal for its mammary-cell functions, but may have hidden mutations in genes not expressed in mammary cells.[37] Mutations occur naturally in all cells but will be silent in genes that are not being used. A mutation in a gene for a skin-cell protein in a mammary cell cannot be detected. But when this gene is needed in a developing embryo, survivability may be comprised. This may be part of the reason why there was only one lamb born from 277 cell fusions. Some may have died from lethal mutations in silent genes in the mammary cells.

While animal cloning indeed appears doable and potentially useful and profitable, there may be an additional drawback. Livestock that have been cloned from early embryonic cells have been larger than normal and somewhat delicate, requiring extra care to ensure survival.[38] In addition, the leader of the Scottish research team that produced Dolly has reported that many animals pregnant with clones are miscarrying, and some of the surviving fetuses show evidence of subtle genetic abnormalities.[39]

## CAN WE CLONE HUMANS?

While animal cloning may be permissible and even scientifically useful, what about cloning humans? First of all, is it feasible? Second, just because we can do it, should we? Should we even try?

At this point, it is reasonable to assume that because the procedure works with sheep and possibly with cattle (it has since been announced that, Gene, a Holstein calf, was produced by two rounds of fusion with an enucleated egg from cells grown in culture after removal from a thirty-day-old embryo by a firm in Wisconsin[40]), it should be perfectible with humans. This does not mean, however, that there may not be unique barriers to cloning humans as opposed to cloning sheep.

Some suggest that using the particular procedure used by the researchers in Scotland, mice and humans may not be clonable. The reason is that sheep embryos do not employ the genes located on the chromosomes in the nucleus until after three to four cell divisions. This may give the egg cell sufficient time to reprogram the DNA from mammary-cell functions to egg-cell functions.[41] (It is significant to note that this is just an educated guess. The researchers in Scotland don't really know why their experiment worked!) Human and mouse cells employ the nuclear DNA after only the first cell division. Therefore, the molecular environment of the egg cell has significantly less time to reprogram the genes for development. This may be why similar experiments have not worked in mice. Therefore, human and mouse cells may not be capable of being cloned.

A research team from the University of Hawaii apparently circumvented these potential barriers when they published the successful cloning of mice by nuclear fusion.[42] Not only were more than fifty clones produced, but several generations were created. In other words, the "granddaughters" were identical twins themselves as well as of their "grandmother." Wakayama and colleagues transferred the nuclei of cumulus cells (cells which surround an egg cell in the ovary, meaning only females were cloned) into enucleated egg cells and allowed them to sit for one to six hours before activating the egg cells. Some suspect that this waiting period may have allowed time for the cumulus DNA to be reprogrammed to embryonic functions by the egg cell cytoplasm. Once again, there is uncertainty as to why this technique worked when so many others failed. Since other cell types failed to successfully produce cloned mice, it may just be that cumulus cells are, for some as yet unknown reason, better suited for cloning than other tissue types. With a success ratio of only 2–3 percent, this technique would be wildly wasteful of human life if applied to human cells. But, as many have suggested, this technique may be more applicable to humans than the procedure that produced Dolly.[43]

If a barrier does indeed exist, it is not necessarily insurmountable. The news of a cloned sheep was surprising enough—no one, including myself, is now going to step out on the same sawed-off limb and predict that it *can't* eventually work with humans. This procedure is so startlingly nontechnical that there are numerous laboratories around the world that could immediately begin their own cloning research program with a minimum of investment and expertise. While I fully expect that many labs will begin studies on cloning other mammalian species besides sheep, I'm not so sure about humans.

Many countries have already either completely banned experimentation in human cloning, or at least imposed a temporary moratorium so that the ethical questions can be properly investigated before stepping ahead. Even the researchers in Scotland responsible for Dolly *have plainly stated that they see no reason to pursue human cloning and are personally repulsed by the idea.*

There are some in the scientific community who feel that the ability to do something is reason enough to do it. But in this case, I believe that this is the minority. Molecular biologists imposed a moratorium of their own in the 1970s when genetic technology was first being developed until critical questions could be answered. Also, while nuclear weapons have been produced for over fifty years, only two have been used and that was over fifty years ago. Many are now being dismantled.

So while it is reasonable to believe that humans can be cloned and somewhere, someone may try, the overall climate is so against it, I don't think we will see it announced anytime soon.

## WHY CLONE HUMANS?

Overall, the public reaction to human cloning has been negative, and this is rather curious. In an admittedly post-Christian culture, it is interesting that while few have expressed concerns over sheep cloning, many still want to draw a distinction between animals and humans by forbidding human cloning. Shortly after the announcement of the cloning of Dolly, I was in the newly independent country of Slovenia of the former Yugoslavia. After a public lecture on the possibilities and ethics of human cloning, a college student frankly stated that while she disagreed with me that God exists, she did agree that we should not clone humans. I pressed her a little by asking: If she did not believe in God, then are we just another animal species? If so, then why is it all right to clone sheep but not humans? Her response pointed to our track record with technology that is not very good. There is too high a probability that we will trample over people with this new technology. Clearly she had no moral reason, just fear. If her fears could be relieved, would she change her mind? I believe that she would eventually agree that changing her mind would make sense, but she would not. The reason is, I believe, that most men and women still want to act as if there are real differences between humans and the rest of the animal world.

As Christians, we assert that humans are made in the image of God and therefore, there is a clear demarcation between animals and humans. But in an evolutionary view, humans are nothing special—just another animal species. The expected reaction to Dolly was offered in an editorial in the *Dallas Morning News* by Tom Siegfried,[44] which he titled "It's Hard to See a Reason Why a Human Dolly Is Evil." He summarized his perspective when he said: "The ability to clone is part of gaining deeper knowledge of life itself. So Dolly should not be seen as scary, but as a signal that life still conceals many miracles for humans to discover." To the naturalist, any knowledge is valuable and the means to obtain it is justified essentially by its benefit to society.

Shortly after the announcement of the cloning of Dolly in February 1997, people from inside and outside the scientific community railed both for and against human cloning. An editorial in *Nature*[45] spoke for the majority of the scientific community by arguing that any attempt to block scientific progress is misguided and futile. *Nature* proclaimed that legislators needed to balance the maintenance of the maximum scientific freedom with society's perceived dignity of human life. This sounds rational and reasonable until they pontificated that human cloning does not inevitably compromise human dignity. If that is the case, then the only concern is maintaining maximum scientific freedom with few if any constraints. This self-serving, pragmatic approach was echoed by Harold Varmus, the director of the National Institutes of Health (NIH) when he warned a congressional subcommittee against legislating "precipitously" on cloning techniques that may result in the impediment of new avenues of research.[46] *Some clearly lose sight of the fact that research is not an inalienable right.* Some things are right and some are wrong. If there are sound moral principles that would prohibit human cloning, then we should refrain from cloning research that has as its goal the asexual reproduction of human beings. President Clinton's adoption of the National Bioethics Advisory Commission's recommendation that all human cloning be banned, needs to be watched carefully. First, the bill introduced to Congress only bans research that leads specifically to the development of embryos that will be implanted to produce a baby. It says nothing about producing cloned embryos that will be used for research apart from the intent to produce a child.[47] Second, the commission recommends that the decision be reviewed in three to five years. This allows the possibility for safety concerns to be addressed and, therefore, the primary reason for the ban may be removed. The ban was motivated, not by any steadfast moral principle, but by temporary safety concerns.

Nathan Myhrvold, chief technology officer at *Microsoft*, proclaimed: "A person's basic humanity is not governed by how he or she came into this world, or whether somebody else happens to have the same DNA."[48] He goes on to deride people's attempts to turn back research because of their ignorant fears. What Myhrvold misses is that *a clone doesn't just happen to have the same DNA* as someone else, as in an identical twin, but was planned that way. This means that while they will indeed be a unique individual from the original, they will always know that they technically do not have a father and mother as everyone else does and that they were made with a particular purpose in mind—not just from the desire by two people to have a child. Alex Kahn, the director of the INSERM Laboratory of Research on Genetics and Molecular Pathology, rightly states:

One blessing of the relationship between parents and children is their inevitable difference, which results in parents loving their children for what they are, rather than trying to make them what they want. Allowing cloning to circumvent sterility would lead to it being tolerated in cases where it was imposed, for example, by authorities. What would the world be like if we accepted that human "creators" could assume the right to generate creatures in their own likeness, beings whose very biological characteristics would be subjugated to an outside will![49]

## FREQUENTLY ASKED QUESTIONS

Before drawing a conclusion to this discussion, I would like to answer some frequent questions and explore some prominent scenarios that this new technology presents if applied to humans.

*Will humans be cloned for spare parts?* While this is certainly possible, I consider it very unlikely that this would be sanctioned by any government. If we are just talking about tissue for a bone-marrow transplant or a skin graft or even a kidney, there might not be much controversy. But if one needs a heart or lung, this flies in the face of most peoples' sense of human dignity and worth. That doesn't mean however, that someone won't try.

*Will humans be cloned to replace a dying infant or child?* This is certainly a possibility, but we need to ask if this is an appropriate way to deal with loss. Might unrealistic expectations be placed on a clone that would not be placed on a normally produced child that was unique? A variation on this theme was recently offered in *Scientific American.*[50] Suppose both parents have a genetic disease, such as sickle-cell anemia, which guarantees that all their children will be affected. Cloning technology could allow cells from an early embryo (fertilized in vitro by sperm from the father and an egg from the mother) to be cultured and the normal hemoglobin gene introduced into the cells. A genetically corrected cell from the culture could then be used for nuclear transfer into an enucleated egg cell from the mother to create a genetically healthy child. What isn't expressly spelled out in this article is that the original unhealthy baby is destroyed so a genetically healthy twin can be created.

*Will humans be cloned to provide children for otherwise childless couples?* This is the most often given reason for human cloning. This argument is unpersuasive in the face of so many children who need to be adopted. Also, this further devalues children to the level of a commodity. If in vitro fertilization is expensive, cloning will be more so.

*Will human clones have a soul?* This frequently asked question has a rather simple answer. In my mind, they will be no different than an identical twin or a baby that results from in vitro fertilization. In the case of identical twins, how a single fertilized egg splits in two to become two individuals with distinct identities and destinies is a similar mystery, but we all accept twins as individuals.

*Does cloning threaten genetic diversity?* Excessive cloning may indeed deplete the genetic diversity of an animal population, leaving the population susceptible to disease and other disasters. But most biologists are keenly aware of these problems, and I would not expect this to be a major concern unless cloning was the only means available to continue a species.

*If the technique is perfected in animals first, will this save the tragic loss of fetal life that resulted from the early human experimentation with in vitro fertilization?* In vitro fertilization was perfected in humans before it was known how effective a procedure it would be. This resulted in many wasted human beings in the embryonic stages. The success rate is still only 10 to 20 percent. Still less than the success rate of normal fertilization and implantation (33 to 50 percent). While animal models will help, there will be unique aspects to human development that can only be known and overcome by direct human experimentation that disrespects the sanctity of human life.

*Will human cloning technology provide a means for lesbians to have a child?* Yes, one partner supplies the nucleus and the other provides the egg. The egg does contain some unique genetic material in the mitochondria that are not contributed by sperm or nucleus. Therefore, each partner makes both a genetic and biologic contribution to the child. But the technological hoops that must be jumped through for any gay couple to have children should be a clear warning that something is wrong with the whole arrangement.

*Will human clones be unique individuals?* Even identical twins manage to forge their own identities. The same would be true of clones. In fact, this may argue strongly against the usefulness of cloning since you can never reproduce all the life experiences that have molded a particular personality. The genes will be the same but the environment and the spirit will not.

## CONCLUSION

All together, I find the prospect of animal cloning potentially useful. But I wonder if the procedure is as perfectible as some hope. It may end up being an inefficient process to achieve the desired result. John Kilner, the director of the Center for Bioethics and Human Dignity, offers three reasons to stop the cloning of humans: (1) The research necessary to develop human cloning will cause the death of human beings. Even if the 1 in 277 odds for the successful cloning of a sheep comes down to 1 in 10 for humans, that still means that human embryos will be sacrificed on the altar of scientific progress. (2) Since cloning usually involves genetic copying for the sake of preserving some desirable trait, such utilitarian approaches may be fine for cows and corn, but human beings, made in the image of God, have a God-given dignity that prevents us from regarding other people merely as means to fulfill our desires. (3) Though technology is neither good or evil, only the human hands that employ the technology can fulfill that dichotomy. Nevertheless as C. S. Lewis argued, "technology never merely represents human mastery over nature; it also involves the power of some people over other people. . . . When human cloning becomes technically possible, who will control who clones whom and for what ends?"[51] Human cloning is fraught with too many possible difficulties, from the waste of human fetal life during research and development to the commercializing of human babies with far too little potential advantage to individuals and society. What there is to learn about embryonic development through cloning experiments can be learned through animal experimentation. The cloning of adult human beings is an unnecessary and unethical practice that should be strongly discouraged if not banned altogether.

## ENDNOTES

1. Robert Briggs and Thomas King, "Transplantation of Living Nuclei from Blastula Cells into Enucleated Frog Eggs," *Proceedings of the National Academy of Sciences* 38 (1952): 455–63.
2. J. B. Gurdon, "Adult Frogs Derived from Nuclei of Single Somatic Cells," *Developmental Biology* 4 (1962): 256–70.
3. J. B. Gurdon, R. A. Laskey, and O. R. Reeves, "The Developmental Capacity of Nuclei Transplanted from Keratinized Skin Cells of Adult Frogs," *Journal of Embryological and Experimental Morphology* 34 (1975): 93–102.
4. Paul Berg et al., *Nature* 250 (1974): 175; *Science* 185: 303.
5. David, M. Rorvik, *In His Image: The Cloning of a Man* (New York: J. B. Lippincott, 1978).
6. Ibid., v.
7. Ibid., 176.
8. Kerby J. Anderson, *Genetic Engineering* (Grand Rapids: Zondervan, 1982), 101–2.
9. *The Boys from Brazil*, Martin Richards and Stanley O'Toole, producers (ITC Entertainment, Ltd., 1978).
10. The first test-tube baby, Louise Brown, was born in England in 1978 under the direction of Drs. R. G. Edwards and Patrick Steptoe.
11. Sharon Begley, "Here Come the DNAsaurs," *Newsweek* (14 June 1993), 61.
12. Patrick Cox, *Jurassic Park*, a Luddite Monster, *The Wall Street Journal* (9 July 1993).
13. Steven Spielberg, quoted by Patrick Cox, *Wall Street Journal* (9 July 1993).
14. *Jurassic Park*, Kathleen Kennedy and Gerald R. Molen, producers (Universal City Studios, Inc. and Amblin Entertainment, 1993).
15. Ibid.
16. Michael Crichton, "Crichton's Creation," in *The Jurassic Park Official Souvenir Magazine* (Brooklyn: The Topps Company, Inc., 1993), 4.
17. "Welcome to Jurassic Park," *The Jurassic Park Official Souvenir Magazine*, 2.
18. American Opinion Research poll of 1,000 adults from May 7–24, 1993, cited in *USA Today* (11 June 1993), 2A.
19. Graphic inset, "How Real Is Jurassic Park?" *The Dallas Morning News* (14 June 1993), 10D.
20. Begley, "Here Come the DNAsaurs," 60–61.
21. Raul J. Cano et al., "Amplification and Sequencing of DNA from a 120–135-Million-Year-Old Weevil," *Nature* 363 (1993): 536–38.
22. Elmer-Dewitt, "Cloning: Where Do We Draw the Line?" *Time* (8 November 1993), 67.
23. Ibid., 67.
24. Andrew Kimbrell, *The Human Body Shop: The Engineering and Marketing of Life* (New York: HarperCollins, 1993), 50.
25. John Robertson, "Editorial," *Chronicle of Higher Education* (24 November 1993), A40.
26. Raymond G. Bohlin, "Human Cloning: Have Human Beings Been Cloned?" *Probe Radio Perspective* (Richardson, Tex.: Probe Ministries, 1993), 5–6.

27. I. Wilmut et al., "Viable Offspring Derived from Fetal and Adult Mammalian Cells," *Nature* 385 (1997): 810–13.
28. Colin Stewart, "An Udder Way of Making Lambs," *Nature* 385 (1997): 769–70.
29. Vottorio Sgaramella and Norton D. Zinder, "Letters," *Nature* 279 (1998): 635–37.
30. Keith H. S. Campbell, Alan Colman and Ian Wilmut, "Letters," *Nature* 279 (1998): 637–38.
31. J. Madeleine Nash, "Was Dolly a Mistake?" *Time* (2 March 1998), 65.
32. David Ashworth, M. Bishop, K. Campbell, A. Colman, A. Kind, A. Schnieke, S. Blott, H. Griffin, C. Haley, J. McWhir, and Ian Wilmut, "DNA Microsatellite Analysis of Dolly," *Nature* 394 (23 July 1998): 329; and S. N. Signer, Y. E. Dubrova, A. J. Jeffreys, C. Wilde, L. M. B. Finch, M. Wells, and M. Peaker, "DNA Fingerprinting Dolly," *Nature* 394 (23 July 1998): 329–30.
33. Elizabeth Pennisi, "Transgenic Lambs from Cloning Lab," *Science* 277 (1997): 631.
34. J. Travis, "Ewe Again? Cloning from Adult DNA," *Science News* 151 (March 1997): 132.
35. Sue Goetnick, "Biological Mysteries Still Surround Cloning," *Dallas Morning News* (3 March 1997), 8–9D.
36. Karen Hopkin, "Cloned Sheep: Where's the Beef? Dolly raises—and answers—some scientific questions," *The Journal of NIH Research* 9 (April 1997): 25–7; and Delcan Butler and Meredith Wedman, "Calls for Cloning Ban Sell Science Short," *Nature* 386 (6 March 1997): 8–9.
37. Sharon Begley, "Little Lamb, Who Made Thee?" *Newsweek* (10 March 1997), 59.
38. Elizabeth Pennisi and Nigel Williams, "Will Dolly Send in the Clones?" *Science* 275 (1997): 1415–16.
39. Meredith Wadman, "Cloning for Research 'Should be Allowed,'" *Nature* 388 (1997): 6.
40. Constance Holden, "Calf Cloned from Bovine Cell Line," *Science* 277 (August 1997): 903.
41. Pennisi and Williams, "Will Dolly Send in the Clones?" 1416.
42. T. A. Wakayama, C. F. Perry, M. Zucotti, K. R. Johnson, and R. Yanagimachi, "Full Term Development of Mice from Enucleated Oocytes Injected with Cumulus Cell Nuclei," *Nature* 394 (23 July 1998): 369–74.
43. Adam Rogers, "The Mice That Roar," *Newsweek* (3 August 1998), 54–55.
44. Tom Siegfried, "It's Hard to See a Reason Why a Human Dolly Is Evil?" *Dallas Morning News* (3 March 1997), 9D.
45. Editorial, "Human Cloning Requires a Moratorium, Not a Ban," *Nature* 386 (6 March 1997): 1.
46. Wadman, "Cloning for Research," 6.
47. Eliot Marshall, "Clinton Urges Outlawing Human Cloning," *Science* 276 ( June 1997): 1640.
48. Nathan Myhrvold, "In Vitro Veritas," *Wired* ( June 1997), 109–10.
49. Alex Kahn, "Clone Mammals . . . Clone Man?" *Nature* 386 (March 1997): 119.
50. Steve Mirsky and John Rennie, "What Cloning Means for Gene Therapy," *Scientific American* ( June 1997), 122–3.
51. John F. Kilner, "Stop Cloning Around: In the Flurry of Scientific Boundary Breaking, Let's Remember That Humans Are Not Sheep," *Christianity Today* (28 April 1997), 10–11.

*An Overview*

The ethical issues connected with the cloning of human embryos are many and varied and demand serious reflection to ensure that this science benefits humanity. Scott B. Rae carefully details the potential benefits that human embryonic cloning provides for couples who are struggling with infertility and the moral problems that must not be ignored—problems involved with handling leftover embryos, informed consent, genetic screening and research, and the unconscionable temptation of commercial marketing. An informed understanding regarding the application of human embryonic cloning delineates its values and threats and diminishes fears related to ignorance.

Chapter Eighteen

# ETHICAL ISSUES AND CONCERNS ABOUT HUMAN CLONING

## Scott B. Rae

### A CLARIFICATION OF CLONING TERMINOLOGY

On October 13, 1993, at the annual meetings of the American Fertility Society, held in Montreal, George Washington University infertility researchers Dr. Jerry Hall and Dr. Robert Stillman announced that they had successfully cloned a human embryo for the first time. The scientific community was electric with excitement at what they had accomplished, and Hall and Stillman were thrilled with the prospects that their achievement held out for infertile couples. Although presented in a very low-key fashion at the meeting, news of their discovery spread quickly around the world, bringing the strongest reaction and most intense debate on any issue in medical ethics since in vitro fertilization in the late 1970s.

Shortly after the release of their research, Hall and Stillman were invited to be guests on *Nightline, Good Morning America*, and *Larry King Live*. Particularly on *Larry King Live*, as the calls poured in, they were caught off guard, astonished at the amount of criticism they received for their work. Interestingly, the disapproval they encountered came from both religious and nonreligious people. Many people who called in that evening had an intuitive reaction to their work that it was not right but were unable to pinpoint reasons why. Others had strong reactions based on religious beliefs that cloning was "playing God" with life in the lab—something that was inherently objectionable. Still others were supportive of the progress of science that their work represented and were critical of those who sought to place moral and religious restrictions on scientific research that was clearly well intentioned. Polls taken around this time showed that roughly three out of four Americans disapproved of the idea of embryo cloning.[1]

The November 8, 1993, issue of *Time* captured the visceral reaction of many people when they heard of this research. It was the cover story that week, and the cover of the magazine was a modified reproduction of Michelangelo's painting of the creation, in which the finger of God touches Adam's finger and through that touch God extends the breath of life into him and he becomes alive. *Time* artists altered the painting and instead of

God's touching one person, he is touching five identical clones of Adam at the same time. The point clearly was that there was "something wrong with this picture," implying that there is similarly something wrong with human beings' taking the liberty of copying in the lab what God had already created in the body. It also called into question a fundamental Judeo-Christian assumption about human beings being unique creations of God, since that presumably unique genetic design was now capable of being copied outside of the body.

Concerns about cloning in general arose again in 1997 with the publication of research in which scientists from Scotland successfully cloned an adult sheep, not just an embryo, by copying a strand of its DNA and placing it in an egg in which the nucleus had been removed. A surrogate sheep mother carried the cloned sheep to birth successfully. At the time the research was published, the cloned sheep was roughly nine months old.[2] This set off rounds of media and academic debate that culminated in a presidential commission report in June 1997, that set parameters and encouraged further discussion of cloning.[3] The commission recommended that human cloning, in which the process is allowed to produce a fully grown cloned human being, should be a criminal offense, with the ban to be reevaluated in three to five years. *But more difficult questions remain on the use of cloned embryos in embryo research.* Although the specter of human cloning has captured the imagination of the public, it is embryo cloning for use in research that is the real controversial issue and is the focus of this chapter.

For many people, human cloning is the stuff of which science fiction is made. From its beginning in Aldous Huxley's *Brave New World* to the midseventies novel by Ira Levin and later a movie, *The Boys from Brazil*, in which a group of neo-Nazis attempt to clone a whole host of Hitlers, to the most recent example in the blockbuster movie, *Jurassic Park*, cloning has never been viewed as something that society would actually have to face. It has always been something that is, at best, a distant remote possibility. In fact, the speculation that has accompanied cloning has been widespread enough to warrant an extended entry on the subject in *The Encyclopedia of Science Fiction*. It is no longer accurate to put it in the realm of science fiction.

In light of all the science fiction and the way people's imaginations tend to get carried away when discussing cloning, it is important to recognize exactly what Hall and Stillman accomplished. Perhaps more significantly, it is key to realize what they did not accomplish. To be precise, they cloned a human embryo, that is, they made an exact genetic duplicate of an embryo that had been previously fertilized in vitro in the lab. They essentially reproduced in the lab the same process that occurs in the body when identical twins (or triplets in some cases) are produced. Most of the embryos were cloned once. In some cases, they made two duplicates of the same embryo. Two copies of the same embryo appears to be the limit of what their process can accomplish. They began the experiment with seventeen different embryos, and produced a total of forty-eight in all.

However, *they did not clone a person.* They only copied the genetic material of a human embryo. Cloning a person involves much more than simply copying his or her genes. It also involves duplicating the developmental environment and experiences that inevitably shape the personality of the person. That is what the neo-Nazis were trying to do in *The Boys from Brazil.* Cloning a person is very different, and truly belongs in the realm of science fiction. But more importantly, they did not clone adult cells, also the raw material of science fiction. They did not take tissue from a mature adult and copy the DNA code. This is what the Scottish researchers who produced the cloned sheep Dolly accomplished. Hall and Stillman cloned human embryos, not adult cells. Researchers can do either of these processes today.

Lest you think that these cloned embryos had started the process of becoming a baby that could grow if implanted in a woman's uterus, that was not quite the case. Because the original embryos were defective, they were incapable of developing for more than a few days. Hall and Stillman were not trying to produce cloned embryos that could be implanted and develop to a full-term pregnancy (still two to three years away, they estimate). They only wanted to see if the cloning process could be done. They were not attempting to set up embryo production lines or create any of the more outlandish scenarios that critics of their work fear.

Actually, embryo cloning is neither new nor particularly difficult, though cloning of human embryos does contain some complicated aspects. Researchers have been cloning certain types of animal embryos since the late 1970s. For example, sheep embryos were successfully cloned to produce adult sheep in 1979, and the same result was produced with cattle in 1980. In addition, certain types of food plants such as corn are capable of being copied. Animal cloning has not become a widespread commercial practice simply because it is too expensive. In fact, the firm that developed and patented the cattle-cloning process is now out of business.[4]

The technical process of cloning embryos does not appear to be that complicated, though it does contain a complex procedure. Scientists who work with animal embryos suggest that there is no reason why human embryos could not be cloned in the same way it is done with animals. Dr. Arthur Caplan, director of the Center for Bioethics at the University of Pennsylvania, commented that "it doesn't take a Nobel Prize team with a million dollar lab [to accomplish human embryo cloning]. It's fairly simple."[5] There are many other scientists who were capable of accomplishing Hall and Stillman's feat, but chose not to do so for fear of the criticism they would receive and the ethical Pandora's box that they would open. Dr. Leeanda Wilton, director of the world renown Monash In Vitro Fertilization Center in Australia, where much of the pioneering work in IVF was done, suggested that *the reason why many qualified researchers have not pursued embryo cloning is that they fear opening up ethical issues that society is not equipped to resolve.* She stated: "They haven't done so [cloned embryos] because it opens up a can of worms."[6]

Cloning of human embryos as well as adult human beings does indeed open up a world of complicated ethical questions. Some countries around the world have elected not to allow human cloning in any form. For example, what Hall and Stillman did would be a federal crime in the countries of Germany, Great Britain, and Japan. Germany has strict regulations on cloning and other reproductive technologies, for understandable reasons, given their recent experience with the Nazi eugenics program. In Britain, researchers who want to attempt cloning must obtain a government license to do so, and to date, the government refuses to issue them. Most European countries have passed laws making cloning of human beings from adult cells a crime. The real ethical issues revolve around the use of cloned human embryos for research.

The ethical dilemmas in cloning human embryos revolve around two areas. The first concerns the question of whether embryo cloning per se is morally allowed. That is, can scientists ethically clone embryos of human beings, irrespective of the uses envisioned for the clones. Is it something that is inherently morally objectionable? There are questions about scientists' playing God with the basic substance of life in its beginnings. Additionally, there are questions about the unique personal identity of each individual person. Does the prospect of cloning, even at the embryonic stage, compromise the right that each individual has to his or her own unique individual identity?

The second set of ethical dilemmas concerns the potential uses of cloned embryos. Whether or not cloning is morally allowed depends on how the cloned embryos will be used. In other words, why would someone want to clone human embryos in the first place? Are there legitimate reasons for cloning embryos that do not include some of the more extreme scenarios that critics of cloning fear? It may be that some uses of cloned embryos would be ethically acceptable and others would not. That is, cloning of human embryos would not be objectionable per se, and the morality of cloning would be determined by the uses to which the cloned embryos would be put. These same questions can be put to someone who is considering cloning human beings from adult cells instead of embryos. The process is different, but the moral issues are very similar.

## EMBRYO CLONING PER SE

First, is cloning of human embryos inherently an ethical problem? Is it an example of scientists' playing God in the laboratory, taking creative prerogatives that belong only to God? Many people who are uncomfortable with the whole notion of embryo cloning use the idea of playing God as the overarching criticism of the process. But is it a valid charge? Objectors to embryo cloning might argue that cloning would be similar to fertilization outside the womb in in vitro fertilization (IVF), an unjustified manipulation in a divinely ordained process. However, it would not be consistent to accept IVF and reject cloning per se because they are two aspects of the same process. There is little difference between creating embryos in the lab and copying those creations. Both are unnatural in that they do not occur naturally within the body. Both are reproductive interventions that create life. Both processes reproduce in the lab that which the body does naturally. Of course, one can reject IVF and cloning and be consistent. But is that necessary from the perspective of Christian ethics?[7]

Science and technologies that generally improve the lot of humankind and specifically help alleviate the effects of the Fall (of which infertility is one) are part of God's revelation to the human race unveiled outside of Scripture.[8] Of course, most technologies can be put to immoral uses, the result of sinful human beings implementing them. But technology that improves the state of affairs in creation can be seen as a part of the mandate that God originally gave man at creation—to have dominion over the earth. Certainly this task was made more difficult by the entrance of sin into the world, but sin did not and does not today disqualify humanity from continuing to exercise dominion over creation. A significant part of that dominion is the human race's gaining an increasing degree of control over itself, namely over the body. The advances of medicine over the centuries are examples of humanity's increasing dominion over the pinnacle of creation—man and woman themselves. The ability of human beings to discover, synthesize, and apply new information that results in advances in the sciences and technology comes from God's common grace, or is made known by his general revelation. Human beings are continuing to fulfill the creation mandate of Genesis 1–2 by searching out and applying those things that God has revealed in the creation. God's general revelation is not limited to those who know God; it is available generally, to everyone who applies himself or herself. To be sure, not everything that science or technology discovers is an example of general revelation. If such discoveries are proven false later or contradict Scripture, then Scripture is the final umpire to resolve the dilemma. If Scripture and general revelation conflict, it may be because our biblical interpretation is incorrect. Or, it may be that we must reject what is coming from outside Scripture and conclude that because it contradicts Scripture it cannot be a legitimate form of general revelation.

Advances in medical technology that alleviate disease, a result of the Fall, can surely be seen as a part of God's general revelation. Humanity's increasing mastery over the human body has increased our life span, decreased infant mortality, and generally improved the quality of life for most patients. Certainly in some cases, the availability of life-sustaining medical technology has resulted in people's living with a very low quality of life, but in medicine in general, those are the exceptions and not the rule. Medicine has rarely been viewed as playing God with the human body. Since infertility is a result of the Fall, similar to disease, *reproductive medicine in general is to infertility what medicine is to disease, a part of God's general revelation and common grace* that can be used within limits set by Scripture. If reproductive medicine in general is not playing God with life in the lab, then it would seem to follow that cloning human embryos per se is not playing God with life in the lab either.

## THE QUESTION OF IDENTITY

A second objection to cloning per se is that it violates the idea of a person's individual identity. Since cloning produces exact genetic duplicates, that practice calls into question the unique genetic identity that individuals have, and to which, some suggest, they have a right. Daniel Callahan of the Hastings Center, the preeminent bioethics think tank in the United States, questioned the advisability of cloning this way: "I think we have a right to our own individual genetic identity. I think this [cloning of embryos] could well violate this right."[9] Imagine that a couple underwent IVF, had embryos cloned, implanted some, and kept some in storage for later, anticipating a second child. But they implanted one of the cloned embryos five years later, so that they had an identical twin born five years after the sibling was born. The older child now has a sibling that is an exact genetic duplicate of him or her. This scenario causes some moral discomfort for many people as they wonder about the effect on the older child of seeing a genetic duplicate for a little brother or sister. When asked if they would have liked being a clone, 86 percent of people surveyed responded negatively, and only 6 percent indicated that they would be comfortable with that.[10] The objection goes deeper when harm beyond the cloned person is considered. It may be that we harm ourselves as well. Theologian and ethicist Richard McCormick put it this way:

> It is increasingly easy to shatter our wonder at human diversity and individuality, especially in the era of the Human Genome Project, when we are tempted to collapse the human person into genetic data. It would be ironical were this to happen in an era that prides itself on [the] treasuring of uniqueness and diversity of all kinds.[11]

It may be that cloning will cause us to lose our sense of appreciation for the wonder of God's creation and the uniqueness of each individual human being. As McCormick rightly points out, it would be ironic if that happened at the same time that society is emphasizing multiculturalism.

However, there is much more to one's unique personal identity than simply genetics. A person is born with his or her genetic identity, but *the identity of the person develops over time.* The personality is formed, dispositions are developed, and the experiences and the environment shape the whole person throughout life. In fact, the dominant aspects of one's personal identity are the personality and character traits that are learned and developed over time. We should be very careful about reducing a person's uniqueness to his or her genetic makeup alone, especially in view of the Christian doctrine of the soul. What makes individuals unique from a Christian perspective is ultimately the soul. However one views the transmission of the soul, whether it is directly created by God with each new conception or mediated through the parents, it does not appear that the soul presents a problem with embryo cloning. The reason for this is that, again, cloning in the lab duplicates a natural bodily process that occurs when identical twins or triplets are produced. However one would resolve the problem of the soul if those natural cases would be the same in dealing with cloned embryos.[12] In addition, even if a person had a right to a unique genetic identity, particularly if that is seen as the gift of God, then identical twins or triplets, when produced naturally in the body, would violate that right. But that is logically problematic, and calls into question the assumption that people have the right to a unique genetic identity when God himself may violate that right from time to time when identical twins are produced. From a biblical perspective, our genetic identity is entirely the gift of God and not something to which we have a unique right. God affirms that we do not have this right each time identical twins or triplets are born. The fact that most people do have a unique genetic identity does not mandate that it is our right. Thus, embryo cloning does not appear to be playing God in the lab nor does it violate our notion of individual personal identity. However, we may run the risk in the long run of losing the proper valuation of human diversity and individuality. That concern is worth taking seriously, but by itself is not sufficient to warrant prohibiting embryo cloning per se.

Embryo cloning was developed by infertility specialists to help couples increase their chances of having a baby. The most commonly mentioned and least controversial uses for cloned embryos are for enhancing IVF and keeping the costs down. Imagine that you and your spouse are patients in the infertility clinic. To your disappointment, after an entire cycle of expensive hormone treatments, only four eggs can be retrieved—far fewer than normal. When it comes time to have embryos implanted, you are told that only two of the eggs have been fertilized. You know that the best chances for achieving one pregnancy come from having four embryos implanted. So, instead of risking the entire expensive procedure with only two embryos, the clinic offers to clone two more, giving you statistically the best odds at becoming pregnant.

A second scenario is perhaps more likely to occur. Since couples routinely fail to achieve pregnancy in any given round of IVF, frequently they face the decision whether or not to try again. This means another cycle of hormone treatments, egg retrieval, laboratory fertilization, and implantation, all involving considerable expense that must be borne again. It is not uncommon for some couples to go through the cycle repeatedly, spending tens of thousands of dollars. Couples who wish to avoid the expense and physical demands on the woman that superovulation involves could have one cycle that produces a number of embryos, some of which are implanted with clones made of one of the rest to be kept in storage. Should the treatment fail to produce a pregnancy after all the noncloned embryos were implanted, the cloned embryos would still be available for implantation. This would enable the couple to attempt implantation again without egg retrieval. A variant of this scenario is that the couple may decide to try for another child at a later date. If there are no noncloned embryos left after the cycle that achieves the first pregnancy, there would be cloned embryos available for subsequent children. Thus, cloned embryos could be used to help infertile couples avoid a second egg retrieval procedure should the first implants fail or should they want another child in the future.

For example, suppose that during the initial cycle of egg retrieval, the couple produced five embryos suitable for implantation. Four are implanted and the one that is left is cloned to produce three more embryos. Should the original implants fail to produce a pregnancy, three more embryos are waiting in storage to be used when the couple wants to try again. If they become pregnant during the first implants and want another child three years later, then embryos are waiting to be implanted at that time.

The problem with these scenarios is no different than with IVF in general. With both of these procedures, as many eggs as possible are harvested and fertilized to keep in storage in order to keep the costs down. Should the couple become pregnant, the excess embryos are routinely discarded, or, in some cases, they are donated. The same would be true of cloned embryos used for infertility enhancement. Any clones that are not needed would be discarded. That raises the same problems that IVF raised. Intentionally ending the lives of embryonic persons is the moral equivalent of abortion. The proper way to use cloned embryos is the same way that embryos are used in IVF. A couple should only authorize the number of embryos cloned (instead of created with IVF) that they intend to implant and are prepared to raise. A couple should not put themselves in the position of having leftover embryos in storage, whether cloned or produced by IVF. In addition, *a couple should avoid the prospect of selective termination should more embryos, cloned or not, be implanted than they are prepared to carry or raise.* In other words, use of cloned embryos for infertility enhancement should be subject to the same guidelines as IVF.

One objection to using cloned embryos for infertility does not apply to IVF. Should a couple use them and more than one pregnancy occurs, they have deliberately created identical twins. In this case, there does not seem to be any significant moral difference between that and what takes place naturally when identical twins are conceived. It would not seem to be any different than a scenario in which twins or triplets are conceived by IVF. When more than one pregnancy develops, technology has duplicated what takes place in the body naturally. The only difference is that the twins created through natural means are identical, not fraternal as are created by IVF.

There is a bit more discomfort when the twin is born later, the result of a second round of implants. But there is a problem only if one reduces personal identity to genetics. The second child's personality, character, environment, and experiences will be different from his earlier-born twin. Since the process of development is the dominant part of one's identity as a whole person, it is difficult to see how having a genetic duplicate can be problematic, since the younger twin will become a much different person, though sharing some of the same physical traits and predispositions.

## BENEFITS AND RISKS: ETHICAL CONSIDERATIONS

In 1990, the Ayala family of Orange County, California, made the national headlines when their teenage daughter contracted leukemia and needed a bone-marrow transplant.[13] A donor whose bone marrow was compatible with hers could not be found, so the family decided to conceive a child in the hope that he or she would be a match and could contribute the bone marrow necessary to save their daughter's life. They were able to discover in utero whether or not the baby was a match for the daughter. The family maintained that they would not abort the pregnancy should the unborn child not be a tissue match, and they would love the child and welcome it into their family. This story had a happy ending since the child turned out to be a match and in 1993 donated the bone marrow that enabled her sister to make great progress in her fight against leukemia.

Had the Ayala's had a clone of their older daughter's embryo in storage, they would have been assured of a tissue match. They would have thawed the embryo and implanted it and waited for the child to reach the age at which she could be a bone-marrow donor. Or to take it a step further, if their older daughter had died of leukemia, her cloned embryo could be implanted and actually "replace" her. That is, in the first case, the embryo provided health insurance for the family, and in the second, it provided life insurance.

Imagine the pressures that the Ayala's little daughter would have faced to donate her bone marrow. You have been conceived primarily to be a bone-marrow donor, though your parents valued you and welcomed you into the family. They made it very clear that had you not been a tissue match for your older sister, your parents would not have aborted you. However, it would have been very difficult for you to say no to your older sister's request for tissue. Donating bone marrow can be a painful experience, one that most people would not undergo for a stranger. But family relationships often create pressures to do things that people ordinarily would not do. Situations like these raise the question of informed consent. That is, all medical treatment, particularly organ and tissue donation, must proceed with the consent of the patient or donor. It must be informed consent, consent that is based on adequate information. In other words, the donor must know exactly what he or she is getting into and cannot be in any way coerced or manipulated into granting consent. Most minors are presumed incapable of giving consent because of their age, and the bone-marrow donor in the Ayala case would surely be asked to donate while still a child, likely at an age where he or she is incapable of understanding all that is necessary to give informed consent. Parents are usually authorized to give consent for treatment for their children, but parents' authorizing organ and tissue donations on behalf of their children is something quite different. Normally, society does not ask children to be organ or tissue donors, unless they have died tragically. Then parents as next of kin can authorize organ donation. But informed consent is such an important value in medicine that society has been very hesitant to ask children to donate, even for family members. To clone and save embryos for the purpose of tissue compatibility, or health insurance, raises serious questions regarding the consent of the donor. This issue is more questionable when the donor has been implanted, borne, and raised for the primary purpose of donating tissue.

A second problem with this kind of health insurance involves the way society would view this person. It is axiomatic among civilized people that human beings are not to be treated as means to accomplishing other ends but as ends in themselves. They are valued because as persons, they are inherently valuable, irrespective of what they accomplish. With a scenario such as the above bone-marrow donation, it is hard to escape the conclusion that *these donors have instrumental as opposed to inherent value.* That is, they are valued primarily for their tissue compatibility. Whether or not these two problems, informed consent and viewing the person as a means to an end, are enough to outweigh the obligations to do good and prevent harm when it is in one's power to do so is a difficult question. One way to view it is to weigh the potential benefits to the recipient with the risks to the donor. The greater the risk to the donor and the less the potential benefit to the recipient, the less the obligation to provide the donation. The problem with this kind of weighting is that it assumes that the person making the decision about donation can objectively stand back and make a rational decision. But when you are that person, and you know that you were cloned and implanted for the primary purpose of making this donation, being able to make an objective decision in the midst of family pressures seems unrealistic.

A second, and perhaps unlikely scenario is that couples would use cloned embryos as a form of life insurance; that is, to replace a child who has died a tragic and premature death. Although the thought of replacing children with genetic twins is an interesting thought, especially for couples grieving the loss of a child, this use of cloned embryos is improbable. The only way this could be done is by the couple's setting aside some embryos in in vitro fertilization for cloning and storage. Though it is possible that couples could undergo IVF in order to provide such a backup, that would be rare because of the cost involved. However, it may be that the couples already undergoing IVF would welcome the chance to store cloned embryos just in case the unthinkable happens. In addition, couples using IVF usually want to maximize the number of embryos available for implantation, and it is again possible, though unlikely, that they would set some aside for such life insurance. Furthermore, it is hard to imagine couples' planning in advance to replace a child who might, by some chance, die tragically. In fact, having a genetic twin as a replacement for a deceased child would probably increase the sadness and sense of loss for the child who had died. Every day of that twin's life would be a reminder to the parents that another child who looked like him or her had died in his or her youth. It would surely make it more difficult for the parents and other siblings to appropriately grieve their loss and get on with their lives.

## CLONING IN GENETIC SCREENING
## AND EMBRYONIC RESEARCH

Embryo cloning could also enhance the efficiency of both genetic screening and embryonic research. Imagine a couple with a family history of genetic disease, say Down's syndrome for example. Instead of trying to conceive naturally and rolling the "genetic dice" so to speak when it comes to their children, they may decide to conceive in the lab through IVF and have the embryos screened for the gene for Down's syndrome. Those embryos found with the gene for the disease would be discarded and only those that did not receive it would be considered for implantation. On the one hand, this looks like a great benefit to the couple who genuinely wants a healthy child and desires to avoid the prospect of giving birth to a handicapped baby. On the other hand, this type of screening could also be used for sex and trait selection. Only embryos with the desired gender or traits would be candidates for implantation.

Some clinics can already do this type of genetic screening of embryos with IVF. But in some cases, embryos are damaged or even destroyed by the screening process. Cloning helps increase the chances that a couple will have embryos without the genetic disease they fear because it is not a significant setback if some embryos are damaged in the process when exact cloned duplicates are available.

As significant a benefit as this use of cloned embryos appears, there are problems involved. First, if one takes the position that personhood begins at conception, then any process that damages, destroys, or results in embryos being discarded is problematic. This happens both in the process of screening and as a result of information gained from the screening. In the latter case, there does not seem to be any morally significant difference between discarding the defecting embryos and aborting a defective fetus when the defect is discovered during pregnancy. Second, most acknowledge that any kind of sex selection is morally troubling because of the gender bias toward boys and against girls. For example, in China, which has had restrictive population control policies, it is common for families to abort female fetuses and keep male ones. In addition, trait selection is viewed as playing God and moving society down the road toward *eugenics*, the term used to describe the use of technology to produce a specific type of human beings—also called *preferential breeding*. This is often considered a flight into science fiction, but there are already sperm banks of Nobel Prize winners and other similarly gifted people from which couples can select a sperm donor for their child.[14]

Using cloned embryos for research and experimentation has the potential for producing great scientific advances in our knowledge of embryonic life. But such research usually damages or destroys the embryos involved and as such, is problematic for the person who holds that personhood begins at conception. In research of this sort, wholesale discarding of embryos damaged in the experiments is highly likely, and this presents a moral problem. Embryo research is moving ahead at full speed with the endorsement of the current administration. Even if one does not hold that personhood begins at conception, at the least, one must acknowledge that the embryo should be given high value because of their potential to become fully functioning human beings. In the right setting in the womb, embryos become babies, and given their potential to do so, they are entitled to respect beyond their use as morally neutral objects for research and experimentation.

Finally, imagine the possibilities if there were a market for embryos. People could shop around for the right combination of genetic traits to produce a "designer child." Embryo banks would spring up where prospective parents could select a child with all their desired traits. Bioethicist and law professor George Annas remarked in the aftermath of Hall and Stillman's announcement that "without regulation, it will only be a matter of time before some entrepreneur tries to market embryos derived from Michael Jordan or Cindy Crawford."[15] The appeal of embryos with the genetic material of superstar athletes or supermodels is not hard to imagine, nor is the potential for profit in such a market. A commercial market in human embryos is the nightmare that most experts in this field fear.

However, upon further thought, it may be less likely to develop than people fear, for several reasons. First, it is highly probable that any governing body that oversees embryo research will prohibit the purchase and sale of human embryos. Right now such a body does not exist, but with embryo research scheduled to move forward, it will not likely move forward without a board of scientists and ethicists to set guidelines for the research. All indications from the debate at the National Institutes of Health in Washington, D.C., point to the government's prohibiting a commercial market in embryos from developing. Of course, the degree to which that can be enforced is another question. For example, most state law makes purchasing a child in adoption illegal, that is, prospective adoptive parents cannot pay a birth mother a fee beyond reasonable expenses for her child. But there is a thriving black market for adoptable children in which children are undoubtedly bought and sold. It is clearly difficult to enforce adoption laws that prohibit such a market. It may be that enforcing a prohibition against the sale of embryos will be similarly difficult. However, the presence of black-market adoptions does not justify shutting down all adoptions because of the good produced. But the potential in embryo research is clearly not yet proportional to that in adoption, and some argue that it is not overkill to prohibit cloning entirely because of the prospect of a commercial market in human embryos.

A second reason that fears of a commercial market may be overstated is that the demand for cloned embryos may not be as great as people suspect. Granted, it may appeal to some to have a child with the genetic endowment of a superstar athlete or model, but most prospective parents desire a child with their genetic material, not someone else's, irrespective of who it is. Most couples who could afford to purchase cloned embryos and who could have their own children would probably choose to have a child of their own, that is, with their genetic materials. It is true that they may want to have some control over the process through genetic screening or even through embryo screening if necessary. Although there may be many potential sellers of embryos in the market, it is debatable how many potential buyers there would be. Surely couples or single people, particularly single parents, who are in poverty might view a child from a cloned embryo of a gifted athlete or model as their ticket out of poverty. But with the technology needed to clone embryos being so costly, it would probably put the price of these cloned embryos out of their reach.

Society should avoid a market for embryos for the same reason it should avoid a market for human beings and for body parts.[16] Persons are not inherently objects of barter. They are not commodities to be bought and sold on the open market. The inherent dignity of the individual person made in God's image should prevent people from being viewed as market commodities.

## CONCLUSION

Cloning of human embryos is a cutting-edge technology with promise to help infertile couples undergoing IVF. Since the process essentially duplicates in the lab what the body does naturally when it produces identical twins, as a technology per se it poses no problems. The moral problems come when the clones are used in certain ways. There are the same issues related to the disposition of leftover embryos as in IVF. There are problems of informed consent when clones are contemplated for health insurance, and it is unlikely that they would be used for life insurance. There are problems with using the clones for genetic screening and research since they are often damaged or destroyed in the process. And there are serious problems with a commercial market for cloned embryos, for the same reason that there are problems with the sale of babies and body parts. As long as there are no embryos left over to be thrown away and none destroyed in the process, there is no reason why cloned embryos cannot be used to enhance infertility treatments.

## ENDNOTES

1. See for example the *Time/CNN* poll in Philip Elmer-Dewitt, "Cloning: Where Do We Draw the Line?" *Time* (8 November 1993), 65–70.
2. See the cover stories in *Time* (10 March 1997), and *Newsweek* (10 March 1997), for further information on human adult cloning.
3. Christine Gorman, "To Ban or Not to Ban?" *Time* (16 June 1997), 66.
4. That company is Granada Biosciences, who sold the rights to the technology that enables cattle embryos to be cloned and went out of business in 1992.
5. Quoted in Gina Kolata, "Doctor Clones Human Embryos, Creates Twins," *New York Times* (24 October 1993), 1.
6. Elmer-Dewitt, "Cloning," 70.
7. I have argued that in vitro fertilization is not inherently objectionable. There are limits that a couple should place on its use, such as insuring that there are no leftover embryos that are discarded after the process is finished. See Scott B. Rae, *Brave New Families: Biblical Ethics and Reproductive Technologies* (Grand Rapids: Baker, 1996), 123–46.
8. Not everyone views technology as being so positive. From a more secular perspective see Neil Postman, *Technopoly* (New York: Vintage, 1992).
9. Cited in Elmer-Dewitt, "Cloning," 68.
10. Ibid., 65.
11. Richard A. McCormick, "Blastomere Separation: Some Concerns," *Hastings Center Report* 24 (March–April 1994): 14–16.
12. The technical terms for the ways in which people view the transmission of the soul are "traduceanism," whose advocates hold that the soul is mediated through the parents, and "creationism," whose advocates hold that each soul is directly created by God. For more on the doctrine of the soul, see J. P. Moreland, "A Defense of a Substance Dualist View of the Soul," in *Christian Perspectives on Being Human: An Interdisciplinary Approach*, ed. J. P. Moreland and David M. Ciocchi (Grand Rapids: Baker, 1993): 55–79.
13. For more on this story, see the *Orange County Register* (31 August 1990), B1.

14. The most notable one of these is Robert Graham's clinic called the Repository for Germinal Choice in Escondido, California.
15. Cited in Elmer-Dewitt, "Cloning," 69.
16. There is some debate, however, on both a market for babies in adoption and a market for body parts. For the merits of an open adoption market see Elisabeth M. Landes and Richard A. Posner, "The Economics of the Baby Shortage," *Journal of Legal Studies* 7 (1978): 323–48. For the discussion of a market for body parts, a California Court of Appeals (upheld by the state supreme court) ruled that human beings have a property interest in their own body parts. The court did not rule on the right to financial compensation however. See *Moore v. Regents of the University of California*, 249 Cal Rptr. 494 (1988).

*An Overview*

Too often throughout history, Christians have hastily resisted technologies created to provide health and healing to humanity for fear that its acceptance would be an affront to genuine faith in God. Dennis Hollinger differentiates between illegitimate and legitimate intentions for the use of genetic engineering in order to determine which uses are inappropriate from a Christian perspective and which are appropriate. Genetic engineering *can be* a divine instrument in the battle for life in a world tormented by the intrusion of death.

Chapter Nineteen

# A THEOLOGY OF HEALING AND GENETIC ENGINEERING

## Dennis P. Hollinger

OUR INTENTIONS MAKE A DIFFERENCE in ethics. Right and wrong are not determined only by particular actions or by a given set of principles and virtues utilized in determining a course of action. Ethical judgments also include the intentions of our actions. Two people may follow the same moral rules and perform the same human behavior, but the moral judgments on their conduct may be vastly different due to what they intended.

Intentionality in ethics is not a mere weighing of the results or consequences of our actions, as in utilitarian ethics. In fact, the intentional dimension can be applicable to principle- and rule-based ethics, consequentialist ethics, or character ethics. Intentionality focuses on the purposes for using certain means and actions at our disposal, and the particular intentions we have in mind as moral actors may well determine whether our endeavors are morally praiseworthy or morally culpable.

When it comes to genetic engineering, intentionality is crucial. While several different scientists may be performing exactly the same genetic procedure, what they are intending to do in that procedure makes all the difference in the world. As we know from the popular and scholarly literature, the possibility of genetic manipulation raises the potential of great misuse. But the enterprise also carries with it potential for much good. The moral judgment depends largely on the objectives in mind.

In genetic engineering there is one intention that must be the focus and primary motivation of the entire enterprise—the healing of human disease and sickness. Most other aims of this sophisticated technology should be called into question, not because the procedures themselves are unethical, but because *the intentions* are ethically suspect. The morally suspect intentions are not themselves universally wrong but are questionable with regard to the enterprise at hand.

This chapter will first examine some of the suspect intentions that have been or might be espoused in genetic engineering. Second, it will examine the one intention that is legitimate healing by attempting to show that genetic engineering can fit within a theology of healing.

## MORALLY SUSPECT INTENTIONS IN GENETIC ENGINEERING

Though the scientific procedures of genetic engineering might be identical from one scientist to another, the intentions can differ significantly. As the new technologies have dawned, it is evident that they are being used for many different reasons, some of which are morally suspect, especially when taken alone.

### Monetary Gain

There is potential for big money in genetic engineering, just as there is in many applications of scientific knowledge. The understandings of science are quickly adapted to technological procedures that then become commercialized and consumed by the society at large.[1] This became particularly evident in the 1970s with the first form of genetic manipulation—recombinant DNA. Very quickly these "new forms of life" were patented and became part of a commercial enterprise. In and of itself this was of course not a problem, but the potential for misuse of new forms fueled by economic interest was of great concern. This was especially true in light of concern over possible bacteria that might escape the laboratory and cause serious damage to humans or the ecosystem. Many felt that the economic factors were overriding these safety issues. Similarly, with the development of somatic gene therapy and germ line therapy, there is intense commercial interest.

Making money through genetic engineering is not in itself ethically wrong, since payment for services rendered is a good and natural part of life. We could hardly expect that genetic services would be any different from other medical services provided for the consumer. From a Christian standpoint, money and economic exchange is a good gift from God. It is not money that is the root of all evil, but as 1 Timothy 6:10 says, "the love of money is a root of all kinds of evil. Some people, eager for money, have wandered from the faith and pierced themselves with many griefs." The costs for genetic research and, subsequently, for genetic engineering are very high, and we can only expect that services will be very expensive. Payment for those services in line with supply and demand, the expertise of the provider, and the vast overhead expenses is a moral responsibility.

The problem comes, however, when moneymaking becomes the driving force of genetic engineering and is isolated from the primary intent—the restoration of health. In one sense, this is no different than other medical services or any human endeavor for that matter. But because genetic engineering has the potential to drastically reshape the human person and human race, our moral antennas must be fully extended to keep track of related commercial implications and leanings.

### Eugenics

Another potential intention of genetic engineering is eugenics, the development of so-called good genetic types. There are essentially two forms of eugenics, positive and negative. Positive eugenics is the breeding in of good genes through some sort of selective breeding, such as artificial insemination with a highly desirable sperm donor. Negative eugenics is the breeding out of bad genes, which could be accomplished by the sterilization of certain individuals or by genetic engineering that would remove a defective gene that could be passed on to offspring.

At the heart of eugenics is the desire to build so-called superior types of people and limit the offspring of so-called inferior types. While the very notion of eugenics sparks images of a brave new world that emanates from scientific sophistication, the idea is very old. Plato in his *Republic* said, "If we want to prevent the human race from degenerating, we shall take care to encourage union between the better specimens of both sexes and to limit the worse."[2] In the nineteenth century, Sir Francis Galton, a cousin of Darwin, became known as the father of modern-day eugenics with his assertions about "superior European stock" and his call for careful mate selection. In the twentieth century, it was not only Nazism that pushed a eugenics agenda, there was also a widespread interest in the topic throughout Europe and the United States.

Genetic engineering could be utilized in a eugenics program as an attempt to breed out undesired genes with the ultimate hope of developing a superior stock of people and limiting the reproduction of inferior genetic types. Eugenics is at its heart a form of human degradation and discrimination, even though contemporary forms of eugenics proclaim a desire to improve the genetic constitution of the human race, not enhance one race or class over another, as in earlier forms. But at its core, eugenics is an affront to the Christian understanding that all human beings are created in God's image and thus have value, worth, and dignity regardless of genetic or external characteristics. Attempting to limit or enhance the reproduction of individuals or groups because of their genetic constitution contradicts that dignity.

The line between the healing of genetic diseases and a eugenics agenda is not visible at first glance. For this reason, motives and intentions must be sorted out during the decision-making process. If anyone suggests that eugenics be a primary consideration or an intentional aspect of genetic engineering, we must say no. Eugenics can never be an acceptable motive in genetic engineering because it is the attempt to direct human history as if we were God, but *without God's wisdom, justice, and nondiscriminating love*. The eugenics intention undermines God's love for us as the basis for our value as human beings. As Arthur Dyck put it, "Being loved by God is . . . our only realistic hope that our lives will be regarded as lives, worthy of life, and all of us equally worthy of life."[3]

## Scientific Knowledge

The genetics revolution has generated huge amounts of new understanding about human life, heredity, and genetic diseases. Such knowledge is indispensable in our attempts to deal with genetic diseases and bring healing. It is possible, however, to isolate such knowledge from its noble uses and to make scientific knowledge a questionable end in itself. While knowledge per se is not morally suspect, the pursuit of knowledge for its own merit can raise serious ethical questions.

For starters, we do well to recall that at the heart of the human fall into sin was a desire to know beyond the limits of human finitude in order to be like God. In the garden, the Tempter told Adam and Eve to disregard the divine orders that prohibited their eating from the tree of the knowledge of good and evil. "You will not surely die. . . . For God knows that when you eat of it your eyes will be opened, and you will be like God, knowing good and evil" (Gen. 3:4–5). Believing that by the tree's fruit they would gain wisdom beyond their natural limitations, Adam and Eve ate, and their moral innocence turned to moral evil. The problem of course is not that certain kinds of knowledge are wrong. The wrongness is the *hubris* in using that knowledge to play God and rule the world.

Though the scientific enterprise and the fruits of its labors are good gifts from God, they, like all human endeavors, bear the marks of the Fall. As such, it is very possible to use scientific knowledge as a means of human pride and power in which we transcend the limits of our own moral capabilities and sensitivities. When knowledge becomes an end in itself, it is very difficult to place moral limits on its usage. The limits of knowledge can only emerge when we recognize a higher purpose for that knowledge and when we operate out of a transcendent frame of reference that places a check on our scientific pursuits. Science is knowledge, and it is quite tempting to use that knowledge to argue that we have a moral right to do what is scientifically possible. But such a perspective will allow for no moral limits on the scientific agenda.

Genetic engineering can procure significant amounts of insight about human life that until recent years was unfathomable. The temptation is to play God, believing that our eyes will be opened and that scientific knowledge will embody its own moral limitations; thus "knowing good and evil." Human history should teach us what Scripture so clearly teaches; that *even our noblest endeavors are fraught with self-centeredness and the potential for grave abuse.* Therefore, knowledge alone can never be the primary intention of genetic engineering. Knowledge, humbly accepted from the hand of our Maker, is a gift to be used for a specific and honorable end.

## Enhancement

One way that genetic engineering could potentially be used is personal enhancement of one's physiological or even emotional state. There is no one gene that determines things such as physical appearance, height, weight, or strength, but there is the potential of discovering a cluster of genes that provide a proclivity in a particular direction on these matters. Hence, there is the possibility that genetic engineering could intend to provide personal enhancement that would make one a better athlete, a more beautiful person, or even a more appealing personality.

The realities of genetic enhancement were brought home with clear force to Scott McIvor, who oversees the gene-therapy program at the University of Minnesota. He is working on injecting healthy new genes into patients with genetic diseases but recently received an inquiry to genetically change a person's skin color. Similarly, Christopher Evans of the University of

Pittsburgh, who is working on therapy for muscle diseases such as muscular dystrophy, received an inquiry from a sports doctor regarding genetic treatment to help athletes grow bigger muscles. McIvor never even responded to the skin change request, and Evans said no to genetically growing muscular athletes.[4] But these requests indicate that there is already a growing interest in using genetic engineering for personal enhancement.

The line between enhancement and therapy is of course not always easy to draw. For example, would the reduction of weight through genetic engineering be therapy or enhancement? It could be either, depending on motivation and particular circumstances. And as one writer put it, "Disease is a spectrum, spanning from what we all clearly believe to be disease . . . to someone like me who would clearly benefit from a hair transplant."[5] We already use medicine for cosmetic purposes that clearly have no healing value.

Though the line between genetic enhancement and genetic therapy is not always clear, we need to always be cautious regarding genetic enhancement and, in some cases, render a clear moral objection. Cosmetic enhancement through gene therapy is perhaps a frivolous use of the technology but would not carry the same ethical concerns as muscle enhancement for athletes. The latter is a clear violation of the very nature of sports with its built-in ethic of fair competition. The same would hold for a cosmetic enhancement that might engender unfair competition in a beauty contest. Using the technology to enhance racial characteristics would also need to be judged morally culpable because such use would seem to always embody some form of racism and ethnocentrism. Some types of genetic enhancement then are morally unpraiseworthy, but are not so serious in nature that they would warrant a clear policy prohibiting them. Other forms of enhancement are of such a nature that the medical and scientific communities should agree to self-policing measures or even larger public policy measures to preclude their use.

## HEALING: THE MORALLY GOOD INTENTION OF GENETIC ENGINEERING

Though there are potential misuses in genetic engineering and though some intentions are ethically suspect, there is an intention that deserves our moral praise. It is this intention that can not only be accepted but be encouraged because of the significant good that it would embody and bring to humanity. This is the intention of genetic healing. Because some diseases (such as Cystic Fibrosis and Huntington's disease) are caused by deleterious genes, gene therapy is the only way of bringing healing to these conditions. Moreover, Francis S. Collins, director of the Human Genome Project, notes that "for many common diseases that afflict us, including heart disease, hypertension, breast cancer, prostate cancer, and schizophrenia, a genetic contribution is evident since these diseases tend to run in families."[6]

But is such healing compatible with a Christian understanding? Can we make a case for genetic therapy with this specific intention on biblical and theological grounds? We know of course that "Jesus went through all the towns and villages, teaching in their synagogues, preaching the good news of the kingdom and healing every disease and sickness" (Matt. 9:35). But can this serve as a basis for genetic healing? I believe that it can if we rightly understand the nature of healing.

From a biblical and theological standpoint, all healing is divine healing.[7] But divine healing doesn't always come in the same form. There are at least four ways in which God brings healing, and genetic engineering can be included in one of these ways.

## The Natural Process

One of the means through which God heals is through the natural processes of our bodies and minds. God has created us in such a way that there are built-in mechanisms to bring health and healing. This natural process of healing is not happenstance, nor the fortunate flukes of nature, nor the lucky bounces of the evolutionary ball. Rather, it comes from our Creator and thus constitutes a form of divine healing.

For example, when we have a wound or cut, the blood normally clots or coagulates to stop the bleeding. It is a built-in mechanism of the body. When an infection invades a body, a built-in combatant in the form of white blood cells goes into action. Paul Brand and Philip Yancey describe it this way:

> Watching the white cells, one can't help thinking them sluggish and ineffective at patrolling territory, much less repelling an attack. Until the attack occurs, that is. . . . an alarm seems to sound. Muscle cells contract around the damaged capillary wall, damming up the loss of precious bloods. Clotting agents halt the flow at the skin's surface. Before long, scavenger cells appear to clean up debris, and fibroblasts, the body's reweaving cells, gather around the injury site. But the most dramatic change involves the listless white cells. As if they have a sense of smell . . . nearby white cells abruptly halt their aimless wandering. Like beagles on the scent of a rabbit, they home in from all directions to the point of attack. Using their unique shape-changing qualities, they ooze between overlapping cells of capillary walls and hurry through tissue via the most direct route. When they arrive, the battle begins.[8]

Our body cells are continually in the process of keeping us healthy. Every minute, three billion cells in our bodies die, and in the same minute, three billion new ones are born to replace them. The entire process is a natural one to keep us healthy, but because it is a part of God's design of creation, it is a form of divine healing.

Of course we recognize that our bodies are also fallen and limited. In this world, disease and ultimately death still hold sway, though they are not the final word. The built-in mechanisms don't heal all ailments and some are never healed in this earthly life. But it is one of the ways God heals and continually reminds us that we are indeed fearfully and wonderfully made.

## Spiritual Resources

Because we are whole beings whose physical, mental, emotional, and spiritual dimensions are deeply intertwined, there is healing that comes from spiritual resources. There are times when the body and emotions experience health and restoration through a spirituality that transcends the physiological and emotional components of the self.

Numerous studies in recent years have demonstrated a significant correlation between spiritual activities, such as prayer, church attendance, and religious ceremonies, with health and rapid healing. David Larson in the *American Journal of Psychiatry* documented numerous studies that, contrary to traditional prejudices in the scientific community, demonstrated a clear association between religious commitments and both physical and mental health.[9] A number of studies recently have found clear correlations between prayer and healing. In one study of 393 patients in a San Francisco critical care unit (CCU), almost half were randomly given intercessory prayer by a prayer group in the hospital. The patients receiving the prayer support interestingly had less congestive heart failure, pneumonia, antibiotics, intubation, and cardiac arrest.[10]

All of this is a form of divine healing. God has created us as spiritual beings who cannot live by bread alone. What happens in prayer, worship, Bible study, Christian fellowship, and divine forgiveness has a profound impact on the human body and the mind. It is one of the ways God brings healing to humanity.

## Direct Intervention

This is the type of healing that is usually designated as divine. Here God directly intervenes into the ailment and brings restoration in a miraculous way. God may still use the natural processes in some way or bypass them, but the intervention comes in a way that is beyond the normal means of healing. This is the type of healing that Jesus performed when he healed the lepers, the blind, the crippled, and the woman with the blood problem. Some, of course, have tried to explain away Jesus' healings, accounting for them on purely natural grounds. But the real issue here is whether we have a supernatural worldview or a naturalistic one. The essential matter is whether we believe that the power of God is greater than the natural patterns that exist within the world, which of course ultimately come from his hand.

C. S. Lewis put it this way, "Unless there exists, in addition to Nature, something else which we may call the supernatural, there can be no miracles. Some people believe that nothing exists except Nature; I call these people naturalists. Others think, that, besides Nature, there exists something else: I call them Supernaturalists."[11] That is the fundamental issue in this form of healing.

Unfortunately, there are some Christians who see this as the only form of true healing. They assert that if we don't experience this form of healing, we are without faith. Such perspectives cannot be sustained biblically and are bankrupt theologically. They fail to embody a theology of creation that allows divine healing to come in various forms, including the built-in natural process as well as the next form of healing, the healing arts.

## The Healing Arts

Throughout history people have discovered insights and realities about the body, the mind, nutrition, and medicine to develop the healing professions. We often fail to recognize that this, too, is a form of divine healing. Traditionally, healing and religion were intimately tied together, not only in Christianity but in various traditions. With the secularization of medicine, health and healing have been divorced from faith and a theistic framework.

From a Christian worldview, all truth is God's truth. The world cannot be divided up into divine truth and secular truth because wherever truth about the world, humans, life, and history are discovered, that truth is ultimately from God. Thus, when physicians, psychologists, and researchers discover new realities about the body, mind, drugs, and genetic patterns they are discovering God's truth. Of course our perceptions of these things are finite and sometimes even distorted. Though science aims to discover indisputable facts about the world, we also understand that our apprehension of those facts hinge on paradigms and historical frameworks. They are never complete, infallible, and without human limitations. Only God can transcend those constraints. But insofar as science and medicine make discoveries that can be used to bring healing to human beings, their breakthroughs are ultimately from God. In this framework, the truth is not dependent on the faith stance of the doctor or researcher. Even an atheist might discover God's truth, for the truth about the world inheres within God's creation. We can discover some of that world because we are created in God's image, and when we do so, we are uncovering a little more of the unfathomable essence of our infinite God. Thus, healing from the medical arts is a form of divine healing, whether or not it is recognized by the participants in the healing process.

It is within this framework that we can understand genetic engineering, rightly used, as a healing that comes ultimately from God. However, there can be misuses in its procedure and unethical intentions in its practice. But this is true of many forms of medicine. New breakthroughs in science and medicine were often at first resisted by Christians for fear that they would undermine some dimension of human nature or Christian faith. Some believers initially even rejected penicillin on the grounds that it was incompatible with the nature of true faith and God's providence. The answer to potential misuses is not to automatically reject a drug or medical technology, but to *harness its good and limit its evil*. This does not imply a blindness to the many dangers that face us in the use of modern technologies, especially ones that have the power to alter human life and even history. But as caretakers of God's garden, we are called to cultivate the good and restrain the ignoble.

If genetic therapy can be a form of healing and a procedure that does not cave in to base intentions or unethical procedures, then we should accept it as a good gift from God. It can then be a form of divine healing, which is a participation in God's actions in history to overturn the effects of the Fall and a sign of the ultimate redemption that will occur one day when "the creation itself will be liberated from its bondage to decay and brought into the glorious freedom of the children of God" (Rom. 8:21). Rightly understood and practiced, genetic engineering can be a sign of that glorious freedom— the ultimate healing of God.

## ENDNOTES

1. See, e.g., Richard Bube, "Crises of Conscience for Christians in Science," *Perspectives on Science and Christian Faith* (March 1989), 11–19. He writes, "Much of scientific research today is motivated by one of two simple questions: (1) does the research promise financial profit in the near future, . . . or (2) does it promise contributions to the military program?" (p. 14).
2. Quoted in John F. Dedek, *Human Life: Some Moral Issues* (New York: Sheed and Ward, 1972), 98. Cf. Plato, *The Republic of Plato* (New York: Oxford University Press, 1966), 158–65.
3. Arthur J. Dyck, "Eugenics in Historical and Ethical Perspective," in *Genetic Ethics: Do the Ends Justify the Genes?*, ed. John Kilner, Rebecca Pentz, and Frank Young (Grand Rapids: Eerdmans, 1997), 37.
4. See Rick Weiss, "Gene Enhancements' Thorny Ethical Traits," *Washington Post* (12 October 1997), A1.
5. Ibid.
6. Francis S. Collins, "The Human Genome Project," in *Genetic Ethics*, 95.
7. While I assert that all healing is divine healing, I recognize that there is the possibility of healing coming from evil sources. The Scripture is clear that Satan has power within the world (though it is not infinite) to bring about things that immediately appear to be good, though their intent is to deceive and mislead. Some healing could fall into such a category.
8. Paul Brand and Philip Yancey, *Fearfully and Wonderfully Made* (Grand Rapids: Zondervan, 1987), 17.
9. David B. Larson et al., "Associations Between Dimensions of Religious Commitment and Mental Health Reported in the *American Journal of Psychiatry* and *Archives of General Psychiatry* 1978–1989," *American Journal of Psychiatry* 149, no. 4 (April 1992): 557–59.
10. R. B. Byrd, "Positive Therapeutic Effects of Intercessory Prayer in a Coronary Care Unit Population," *Southern Medical Journal* 81 (1988): 826–29.
11. C. S. Lewis, *Miracles: A Preliminary Study* (New York: Macmillan, 1947), 10.

*An Overview*

Whenever a new technology becomes available, it is incumbent upon those who hope to use it to pause and evaluate their motives and goals. There are many questions to be answered: Whose struggles are we hoping to remedy? If we identify a genetic mutation or disorder early enough, will we always be able to correct the problem? Can we live with what we discover? Genetic screening has much to offer society, but, like any technology, it can be deployed unethically, selfishly, and often with grandiose claims that border on the miraculous. Sonya Merrill takes an objective look at genetic screening and the suffering it can and cannot, or maybe should not, ameliorate. She challenges each of us to approach genetic technology reasonably and with motives that, at their core, promote the glory of God. No decision should be made that does not take into account the will of a sovereign and compassionate Creator from whom all things have their origin.

Chapter Twenty

# GENETIC SCREENING
## *Suffering and Sovereignty*

Sonya Merrill

AS RECENTLY AS THE EARLY PART OF this century, patients who suffered from severe ailments such as cystic fibrosis or heart disease were unable to have their conditions diagnosed in time to make any difference to the progression of their diseases. With the coming of modern medicine in the mid-1900s, with its armamentarium of antibiotics, batteries of diagnostic X-rays and cultures, and cumulative wisdom drawn from epidemiological and clinical research, patients who displayed the early warning signs of disease were able to be identified and treated with gradually improving degrees of success. For example, persons born with cystic fibrosis are now living productive lives well into their thirties, whereas one generation ago, most died in their teens or early twenties. Successes with heart disease are even more impressive; patients with a constellation of indicators such as high blood pressure, irregular heart beats or murmurs, elevated cholesterol levels, and family history of heart disease are being identified and treated in time to prevent or minimize the occurrence of severe, debilitating disease.

And now the labors of the lab bench promise to usher in a new era, one where past advances in clinical medicine will be informed and supplemented by premonitory knowledge of the sort that will enable patients' conditions to be identified years before symptoms are manifested and perhaps before they are even born. With the discovery of DNA by Watson and Crick, scientists were empowered to understand for the first time the chemical basis of heredity—the inward spiral of deoxyribonucleic acid, its sequence of bases arranged in the distinctive double-helical motif, was determined to encode the structure of proteins, which are present in every cell of the body. This sequence was subsequently discovered to be transmitted from parents to their offspring in the form of genes. These genes undergo seemingly random changes, or mutations, which are then passed on to subsequent generations. The information found in genes is manifested in physical traits, or phenotypes, including the particulars of a person's appearance as well as her or his predisposition to certain conditions such as cystic fibrosis and heart disease.

Not only are scientists learning more about the principles of genetic inheritance, but concomitantly they have been developing diagnostic techniques to identify the genetic structure of individuals. At the center of this effort is the Human Genome Project, an international endeavor to map the entire human genome, or collection of genes, and identify which genes are correlated with which phenotypes. Already, scientists and clinicians collaborate to determine whether a patient is carrying the gene correlated with cystic fibrosis, and when the Human Genome Project is completed, which may occur soon after the turn of the century, they will be able to identify not only genes for serious medical problems such as heart disease *but also* genes associated with more trivial phenotypes such as eye and hair color.

Already, many people are asking questions about how this knowledge can be utilized. Physicians and scientists are excited about the possibilities for identifying genetic predisposition to health-impairing conditions and beginning treatment before the damaging phenotype is manifested. Treatment, they believe, will also be improved as the chemical basis of disease is understood more precisely and drugs are designed that are able to target directly the cellular mechanisms responsible for physiological damage. Gene therapy, the replacement of "defective," mutant genes with normal, "wild-type" genes is touted as the treatment of the future. Persons born with genetic mutations, which would otherwise inevitably produce disease, will thus be able to have its onset arrested or postponed or its severity reduced. Because many diseases, including cystic fibrosis, are manifested at birth or shortly thereafter, *early identification of the corresponding genes is mandatory* in order for therapeutic benefit to be maximized; the earlier a harmful mutation can be detected, the better the outcome for the patient. Therefore, screening a fetus for such genetic "danger areas" would seem to be the ideal way to prevent the development and progression of disease.

But underlying and, therefore, to some extent obscured by the questions about *how* this technology can be utilized is another more fundamental concern. *Why* should genetic screening be developed and implemented in the first place? Should its development be guided by a desire to prevent and ameliorate human suffering? Should genetic screening be part of a wider agenda, the framing of a new society free from disease and deformity? Or is this merely another instance of science's and technology's pushing the limits of the heretofore "natural" world? Understanding our motivation for employing screening techniques is a matter of great importance, particularly for the Christian who seeks to measure all human motives by the standard of God's truth and to place all human efforts within the context of his sovereignty.

## FACTS AND VALUE: SOME PRELIMINARIES

One line of reasoning goes like this: If we have the ability to do something, it is morally permissible to do it. Therefore, since we have the ability to screen people for many genetically determined diseases, it is morally permissible for us to do so. This is admittedly a crude argument and one unlikely to be adopted by very many people when given more than cursory thought. Accepting its validity would commit us to agreeing that the Holocaust, nuclear warfare, and slavery are morally acceptable because these situations are within our ability to create or maintain. Such conclusions are quite simply repugnant and counterintuitive and, therefore, we may suspect that the argument that produced them is dubious. Furthermore, philosophers speak of a distinction between is and ought, between fact and value, such that the descriptive and the normative aspects of a situation cannot be conflated nor can moral conclusions be derived from solely descriptive, or factual, premises. Another moral premise must be invoked in order to arrive at a morally significant conclusion.

Thus, we might refine our original argument as follows: If we have the ability to do something that is *morally good*, or at least morally neutral, then we are morally permitted to do it. If we have the ability to genetically screen people and that technology is either *good or without moral value*, then it is right for us to use it. On its own, this argument appears unproblematic—it eliminates the sort of unpleasant conclusions that our first line of reasoning generated, and it does not commit the philosophers' cardinal sin of deriving values from facts. However, we are now faced with another set of questions: Is genetic screening morally good or at least morally neutral? If it is claimed to be good because it alleviates human suffering, then we must ask whether this is itself the right sort of aim to have. And if it is thought to be morally neutral, we may then ask whether there is any reason to pursue screening technology for its own sake.

## SUFFERING AND SOVEREIGNTY

In many parts of the developed world, screening for certain medical conditions is already mandatory. For example, in some American states newborns must be tested for *metabolic disorders*, those pertaining to the body's biochemical reactions, including phenylketonuria, homocystinuria, sickle-cell disease, and congenital adrenal hyperplasia. The rationale for this mandatory screening is that these conditions do irreversible damage early in life and may be prevented or ameliorated by early detection and treatment. Here the aim, apparently, is to benefit the person who has one of these diseases by diminishing her or his suffering.

For a related reason, namely, the protection of other parties, some states have laws requiring couples to be screened for syphilis before a marriage license may be issued. Many countries require that immigrants be tested for communicable diseases before entry permits are granted. Some people have suggested that the entire population of the United States be tested for HIV. In all of these cases, it may be argued that there is a public interest in preventing the suffering of the state's citizens that is sufficiently important to justify mandatory screening measures.

Parallel arguments may be made in defense of genetic screening. We may reason that an individual—whether preborn, newborn, or fully grown—must be tested so that she or he will not suffer from the effects of a preventable or treatable disease. Or we might argue that a society's interest in eradicating human suffering is sufficiently compelling to require its citizens to undergo genetic screening. But whether attempts are made to justify such screening on the grounds that it will reduce the suffering of the particular individual or of society as a whole, it is important to consider whether this goal of eliminating suffering is one that is congruent with the Christian understanding of suffering and sovereignty.

At first it may appear that this is an unnecessary, if not, a deliberately provocative question. Of course, it is wrong to stand by and watch someone suffer when it is within one's power to render assistance that would reduce or even put an end to her or his agony. Surely it would be inhumane to allow suffering to continue when we can do something about it. If we can screen a fetus for cystic fibrosis or a child for hereditary vascular disease, genetically linked disorders that cause much suffering, *surely we are morally obliged to utilize this technology*. This, perhaps, was the motivation behind Simon Peter's instinctive defense of his friend, Jesus Christ, that night on the Mount of Olives: How can I stand by and watch him suffer and not do something to prevent it? And yet Jesus gently remonstrated with Peter, "shall I not drink the cup the Father has given me" (John 18:11)? Again, after his resurrection, Christ appeared to his disciples and placed his suffering in the wider context of God's destiny: "This is what is written: The Christ will suffer and rise from the dead on the third day" (Luke 24:46). While I hesitate to draw perfect parallels with this most exceptional man in this most unusual of circumstances, namely, the eternal redemptive plan of God carried out through his only Son, Jesus' response to Peter's desire to prevent his suffering is instructive.

There appear to be some occasions in which the prevention of suffering is not the right course of action; in this case, Jesus' suffering was necessary for God's salvific purposes to be fulfilled. While this is obviously a unique sort of situation in the respect that Christ's passion and death occurred only once and its import is far more significant than that of any other person's suffering, *I do not believe it is unreasonable to suggest that God's purposes might include human suffering*. If this is correct, then suffering is not without purpose; it is not a meaningless experience. We may not be able to identify at the time, or perhaps ever, the full or even partial extent of its role in God's plan for our lives, but the very belief that suffering is part of a divine plan, though incompletely understood, should be enough to make us question whether we as human beings ought to attempt to eliminate all suffering, a point Stanley Hauerwas has made in the context of the goal of Christian medicine. He writes:

> I want to at least raise the possibility that the most decisive challenge which medicine raises for Christian convictions and morality involves the attempt to make suffering pointless and thus subject to elimination. . . . I have always thought it odd that anyone should think it possible or even a good thing to eliminate all suffering. Suffering, I have been taught, is not something you eliminate but rather something with which you must learn to live.[1]

Additionally, we can learn much from the New Testament writers concerning God's perspective on human suffering, which would seem to support the contention that suffering is not meaningless and ought not necessarily be avoided or eradicated, at least not at all costs. According to Paul, our suffering is closely linked with that of Christ. By our own suffering, we share in some small part, or have "fellowship of sharing," in Christ's own passion and death (Phil. 3:10). Our shared suffering is intimately connected with, perhaps even causally related to, sharing his glory (Rom. 8:17). Further developing this notion of suffering's preceding glorification, Paul tells the Philippians that they should expect to suffer "on behalf of Christ" (Phil. 1:29) and should be prepared to "suffer the loss of all things" in order to "gain Christ" (Phil. 3:8). There appears, then, to be some mystical sense in which our temporal suffering enables us to have greater immediate union with Christ and ennobles us as we subsequently share in his eternal glory (2 Cor. 4:17).

This discovery of a sense of purpose confers on suffering meaning and value such that we should consider carefully whether or not the *summum bonum* of medicine, including genetic screening, is to eradicate all human suffering. However, God's Word does not only reveal to us the purposefulness of suffering but also encourages us in practical ways to persevere in the face of it. Peter promises us that while we will suffer for awhile, God will then "restore you and make you strong, firm and steadfast" (1 Peter 5:10), suggesting that God permits suffering to develop in his adopted children the same character as his firstborn Son possesses. Finally, when we cannot comprehend or accept God's purposes in allowing us to suffer, James encourages us to pray (James 5:13). Recognizing that it is human nature that causes us to seek to devalue and thus have reason to avoid and eliminate suffering, he exhorts us to speak to God and seek a divine, transcendent perspective that will enable us to make sense of our condition or the condition of a loved one.

I stated above that if we accept that the elimination of suffering is a good thing and that genetic screening allows us to eliminate or minimize suffering, then genetic screening must be morally acceptable, perhaps even morally required. Up to this point, I have argued that from a biblical perspective, there are no grounds for thinking suffering to be meaningless and, therefore, necessarily subject to elimination. Likewise, there appears to be good reason for accepting suffering as part of God's sovereign plan for both his firstborn and his adopted heirs. I have emphasized the positive, purposive aspects of human suffering chiefly to counter the commonly accepted notion that the human and, indeed, the Christian response to suffering should be immediate desire for its elimination.

This does not mean, however, that we ought to seek suffering out of some mistaken martyr complex or to allow others to suffer as we watch with detached and pious gaze. The compassion Christ showed for those who suffered physically, spiritually, and socially certainly precludes those of us who follow him from rejoicing in the suffering of others. Instead, we are called not so much to remove suffering from human life but rather to reconcile the sufferer to the sovereign God whose ultimate purpose is to restore and glorify her or him as he did his Son, Jesus. Should not suffering of any kind, whether from persecution or disease, remind each of us of our finite nature and, therefore, our need to become more dependent on God?

This leads us to consider the question of whether genetic screening truly promises the elimination of human suffering, and if so, through what means? In one sense, this is a moot point, for the argument I mounted above in defense of genetic screening relied on two premises, the first being the assumption that all suffering should be eliminated, which we have suggested is insupportable if we recognize God's sovereignty. The truth of the second premise, that genetic screening can eliminate human suffering, is, therefore, irrelevant to the validity of the argument. However, I believe it is worth exploring briefly as it reveals important presuppositions concerning human life and its value.

Certainly it is true that genetic screening is able to minimize, if not eradicate altogether, a great deal of human suffering if we are content to identify suffering with physical pain. If we were to screen every newborn for a host of genetic disorders, many of which are currently treatable or will be treatable in the near future, and some of which might be avoided by careful diet or other behavioral modifications, it is indisputable that the amount of *human suffering as defined as physical pain* would be greatly diminished. However, it is not so clear that neonatal screening would reduce human suffering more broadly defined, for instance by Hauerwas as "submitting or being forced to submit to and endure some particular set of circumstances."[2] Identifying an infant's predisposition to heart disease, for example, makes both infant and parents aware of just such a set of circumstances. Not only are those who are affected by this diagnosis forced to submit to and endure the knowledge that it is likely that the child will one day develop a fatal condition, but this awareness creates its own burdensome and accompanying circumstances—a restricted diet, carefully regimented exercise schedule, and regular doctor's visits. There is, of course, the possibility that such a circumspect lifestyle will enable the child to evade his genetic destiny in a manner of speaking, but it does not appear too unreasonable to ask whether we have enabled him to avoid or minimize suffering if we accept that suffering is more than just physical pain and is rather *any forced submission to one's circumstances*. It does not seem possible, then, to conclude that just because genetic screening of newborns (or, for that matter, adults) will enable us to minimize physical suffering in some cases that such a screening program allows us to minimize or eliminate suffering *in general*. Rather, the knowledge gained from screening may itself become a burden under which we suffer.

Thus far we have been thinking about genetic screening in the context of those *who are already born* and the effects such screening might have on them vis-à-vis suffering. However, many have contested that the real importance of genetic screening is its ability to identify genetic bases of disease and deformity *before birth*—the implication being that such conditions, if not correctable surgically or pharmaceutically before birth, might then be eliminated by the termination of the pregnancy. The assumption undergirding much of the scientific and medical establishments' views on prenatal screening, as Hauerwas has correctly identified, is that "when children will have only a life of suffering it is better that they die young."[3] The only way, then, for prenatal genetic screening to aid us in the elimination of suffering is to direct us to eliminate the sufferer. The implications of this statement for our understanding of the value of human life as well as for a eugenic reconstruction of society are beyond the scope of this chapter, but it is sufficient to say that these are matters of fundamental importance for our society that Christians ought to take the lead in addressing. It is also unwise to assume that the termination of a pregnancy that bears a genetically impaired child results in the suppression or elimination of suffering. Abortion often carries with it a lifetime of emotional scars.

## TECHNOLOGY AND TEMPTATION

Having evaluated and provided a proper perspective to the argument that genetic screening is morally acceptable because it aids the elimination of suffering, we should also briefly consider another argument that might be offered for the development and application of such technology. Technology, it is suggested, is in itself morally neutral; therefore, there is no reason why we should not pursue it as far as our minds are capable of taking it. Genetic screening is merely another tool at our disposal, another weapon in the doctor's armamentarium, another way of harnessing nature and putting science to work for us. Why should we not then take advantage of it? Are we not commanded in Genesis 1:22 to "fill the earth and subdue it?" We appear to be created by our Creator to create; we not only have minds capable of imagining possibilities but also hands with which to actualize the possible. As Christians, then, it would seem that our response to technology ought to be an enthusiastic unbridled affirmation of our God-given creativity.

While it is undoubtedly true that we have been endowed with creative gifts, it is important to remember that those gifts were given for a specific reason and are to be used only within certain parameters—those defined by our Creator. Our *raison d'être* is not to create but to glorify God (e.g., 1 Cor. 6:20; 1 Peter 4:11); that is, everything we do and, therefore, everything we create, should point to him to affirm his role as Lord of this earth. Furthermore, our creative gifts are to be used within the parameters of his redemptive plan as we join together with God in his restoration of a fallen world to its original pristine condition (2 Cor. 5:18–19). If technology assists us in breaking down divisions between people and God and between races and tribes, in protecting ourselves from once-peaceable animals who as a result of our fall became predators, and generally, in restoring a broken world to wholeness, then these are very good reasons for affirming technology.

However, if our creativity is used not to bring glory to the Creator nor to participate in his plan of restoration, then we must question its use. We must wonder whether the purveyors of technology, and particularly biotechnology, "are attempting to recreate nature in the image of efficiency" rather than restoring it to the image of God.[4] While this concern does not apply to genetic screening per se in that this technique only identifies genetic structure rather than directly altering it, it is relevant more indirectly as the ultimate purpose of screening is to create what is arguably a more efficient person, one not plagued by physical deformities or weaknesses.

Of course, we might argue that screening enables us to identify and treat conditions that exist only as a consequence of the Fall and, therefore, genetic screening fits into our restorative role. If this is our motivation, then we are on firmer theological ground. However, we ought to "think about technology with a view to how it affects the human condition in its totality, that is, in both its material and spiritual aspects."[5] Genetic screening and subsequent therapeutic interventions might enable us in some part to counteract only the physical consequences of the Fall, but they can certainly not restore the human spirit to unbroken and right relationship with the Creator. In fact, there is some danger that such technology might contribute to spiritual division as it shapes our thinking and realigns our priorities regarding the importance of physical health and our ability to control it. There is the temptation to think that as we become technologically more advanced, we and not God are in control of the natural world. There is the temptation to think that we can safely control and manage technology by using it only for restorative purposes and not for destructive ones, when arguably "we have never limited a technology to its beneficial uses."[6] And there is the temptation to devote inordinate amounts of attention to the restoration of physical wholeness such that we neglect spiritual unity. Steve Bruce observes that "our attention is further concentrated on the natural world by the success of technology in delivering the goods. Technically efficient machinery and procedures reduce uncertainty and our need for the supernatural."[7]

## CONCLUSION

While the progress of medicine has indeed been spectacular this century, both in terms of the acquisition of technological prowess and its subsequent usefulness in the alleviation of physical suffering, there are reasons why we ought to hesitate to embrace these developments wholeheartedly. I have just argued that technology that is not utilized for God's glory but rather for the elevation of humans to the status of creation's masters is an act of rebellion against the Creator. Further, even when our aim is to employ technology to assist the divine restorative project, there are inherent dangers we face— among them forgetting who is in charge of the project, wrongly believing ourselves able to limit technology to such good purposes, and neglecting the more fundamental role of reconciling people's minds and hearts to God in favor of restoring the health of the body.

Additionally, I have argued that the understanding of suffering as something that is pointless and ought necessarily to be eliminated finds no support in God's Word. Rather, in the life of Christ and the words of the apostles, we find evidence to the contrary—suffering is imbued with meaning because it is through suffering that we identify more closely with Christ and are, therefore, made capable of sharing in his glory. This is not to say that we should either seek our own suffering or shun others who suffer; rather, suffering must be met with Christlike compassion. There must be a balanced awareness of both the permissive purposes of God in allowing suffering and the mercy of God in bringing an end to it. In practice, it is difficult to know how to achieve this; my instinct is that we must compassionately seek to minimize the physical suffering of others but not at any cost and certainly not at the expense of eliminating the sufferer. The expanse of the genetic frontier, while visible today, is still ahead of us, but our motives for wanting to avail ourselves of its resources must be considered and understood now.

What then shall we conclude about genetic screening? There appear to be inherent dangers in accepting it unquestioningly, namely, (1) the pursuit of the elimination of suffering that concurrently renders meaningless God's sovereign purposes in allowing suffering and (2) a devotion to technology that persuades us that we and not God are the rulers of this world. I am not recommending that we reject genetic screening as inherently antithetical to God's plans and purposes, but, rather, I am proposing that we consider carefully not only the hows but also the whys of implementing this powerful tool in light of a scriptural understanding of God's sovereignty and human suffering and the very real temptation of rebellion that manifests itself whenever we become too enamored with our own knowledge and abilities. We cannot allow a potentially good and merciful technology to become a barrier between us and our need for God. No technology that God has allowed humanity to develop is intended to provoke a reliance on ourselves. Remember that "every good gift and every perfect gift is from above, and comes down from the Father of lights, with whom there is no variation or shadow of turning" (James 1:17 NKJV). Although medical advances have helped many live longer and more productively, we still succumb to injury and disease and, therefore, must initially rely on the eternal mercy of our compassionate God while we evaluate and use wisely the technologies he has allowed us to create.

## ENDNOTES

1. Stanley Hauerwas, *Suffering Presence: Theological Reflections on Medicine, the Mentally Handicapped, and the Church* (South Bend, Ind.: University of Notre Dame Press, 1986), 24.
2. Ibid., 28.
3. Ibid., 23.
4. Andrew Kimbrell, "Second Genesis: The Biotechnology Revolution," *The Intercollegiate Review* 28, no. 1 (fall 1992): 16–17.
5. Jeffrey O. Nelson, "Introduction to Technology and Ethics in a Brave New World Order: A Symposium," *The Intercollegiate Review*, 3–4.
6. Kimbrell, "Second Genesis," 14.
7. Steve Bruce, *Religion in the Modern World: From Cults to Cathedrals* (Oxford: Oxford University Press, 1996), 50.

# INDEX

Nazi 112, 118, 282
risks 163, 168
Expressed Sequence Tags (EST) 92

Familial Alzheimer's. *See* Alzheimer's
disease.
Familial benefit 177–80
Family
biblical view of 182–86
children's place in 170–86
discrimination against 36
faulty assumptions about 215–16
genetic history of 89–94, 117, 164–65,
183, 212, 248, 262, 288, 299, 305–6
in Bible 143, 145, 182–83
of dying child 196, 204–6
secular view of 180–82
Fascism 133
FDA 82
Fetal
anomaly 199
benefit 174
development 73–78, 209n
medicine 205
Fetoscopy 43
Fetus
genetic testing of 43, 62, 172–80
treatment options 35
manipulation of 73–74, 141
organ harvesting 228, 286–88
Folkism 134
Fragile X syndrome 30, 44, 184, 194
Frog research 76, 151, 262, 268, 270
Fukuyama, Francis 243–44
Fusion cell 146–47, 268, 270

Galton, Francis 31, 297
Gamete intrafallopian transfer. *See* GIFT.
Gammas 151
Gay rights. *See* Homosexuality.
Gender selection 140, 142, 146–47
Gene
as icon 242–43, 264
calf named 271
enhancements 303
mapping 132
molecular 243–46
patenting 89, 101n
splicing 140, 148–50
testing 27, 193
therapy 22, 26, 31, 41–43, 58, 65, 74,
117, 131–32, 163, 166–67, 191, 296,
299, 306
Genetic
abortion 34–37, 43–44, 172–79, 183–84,
190
counseling 24, 25, 44, 119, 189, 191,
193, 195n, 212–21

discrimination 61, 117–18, 127, 133–36,
191
engineering 29–32, 34–36, 38, 270–71,
275, 281, 296–303
essentialism 52–53, 55–67
ethics 45–47, 78, 80–84, 164–67, 173–80,
191–94, 240, 261, 263, 265, 267, 269,
271–73, 275, 278–92, 296–303
health factors 24–26, 61
inheritance 33, 86n, 248
justice 55–60, 160–62
patents 80, 89, 91–93, 95, 97, 99–100, 101n
prenatal screening 34–37, 43–44, 61–64,
165, 170–74, 183–86, 189, 212,
213–21, 266, 288–91, 304–13
privacy 36–38
property rights 80, 101n, 102n
repair 148
sequence 84n
technology types 142–52
technologies 142–52
testing before conception 25, 42–43, 56,
59, 131, 136, 164, 188, 189–94, 212,
278
therapy 40, 42, 64, 66, 74, 85n, 98, 117,
136, 142, 149, 160, 162, 188, 191,
193, 299, 302
Genetics,
medical 22, 23–27, 242–44
theology of 46–47
Genome Project 226
advances through 42, 47, 71, 117–18
genetics principles and 24, 27, 157, 299
potential misuse of 20, 28, 32, 34, 37, 38,
127, 173, 284
purpose of 19, 23–24, 30, 41, 84n, 306
scope of 22, 26, 29–30, 149
support for 90
Germ-line therapy 192–93
German eugenics 32, 112, 118, 134, 282, 297
GIFT 144, 158, 160, 170, 178, 284–85, 296,
298, 313
Glycogen storage disease 164
Gordon, Jean 106–9, 111, 120n
Graves, Bipp 114–16
Growth hormone therapy 64–65
Gurdon, J. B. 262
Gynecologists 218, 219
bias of 217–19
Gynecology 212, 214, 218

Haeckel, Ernst 134
Hall, Jerry 279–81, 289–90
Handicapped child. *See* Disabled.
Harvesting 41, 76, 228
Health-care cost 44, 56, 65, 218, 221. *See
also* Insurance coverage.
Hemophilia 164, 167, 184